Bovine Orthopedics

Editors

DAVID E. ANDERSON
ANDRÉ DESROCHERS

VETERINARY CLINICS OF NORTH AMERICA: FOOD ANIMAL PRACTICE

www.vetfood.theclinics.com

Consulting Editor
ROBERT A. SMITH

March 2014 • Volume 30 • Number 1

ELSEVIER

1600 John F. Kennedy Boulevard • Suite 1800 • Philadelphia, Pennsylvania, 19103-2899

http://www.vetfood.theclinics.com

VETERINARY CLINICS OF NORTH AMERICA: FOOD ANIMAL PRACTICE Volume 30, Number 1
March 2014 ISSN 0749-0720, ISBN-13: 978-0-323-28726-5

Editor: Patrick Manley
Developmental Editor: Yonah Korngold

Veterinary Clinics of North America: Food Animal Practice (ISSN 0749-0720) is published in March, July, and November by Elsevier Inc., 360 Park Avenue South, New York, NY 10010-1710. Subscription prices are $235.00 per year (domestic individuals), $326.00 per year (domestic institutions), $110.00 per year (domestic students/residents), $265.00 per year (Canadian individuals), $430.00 per year (Canadian institutions), $335.00 per year (international individuals), $430.00 per year (international institutions), and $165.00 per year (international and Canadian students/residents). To receive student/resident rate, orders must be accompanied by name of affiliated institution, date of term, and the signature of program/residency coordinator on institution letterhead. *Clinics* subscription prices. All prices are subject to change without notice. **POSTMASTER:** Send address changes to *Veterinary Clinics of North America: Food Animal Practice*, Elsevier Health Sciences Division, Subscription Customer Service, 3251 Riverport Lane, Maryland Heights, MO 63043. Customer Service (orders, claims, online, change of address): Elsevier Health Sciences Division, Subscription Customer Service, 3251 Riverport Lane, Maryland Heights, MO 63043. Tel: 1-800-654-2452 (U.S. and Canada); 314-447-8871 (ouside U.S. and Canada). Fax: 314-447-8029. E-mail: journalscustomerservice-usa@elsevier.com (for print support); journalsonlinesupport-usa@elsevier.com (for online support).

Reprints. For copies of 100 or more, of articles in this publication, please contact the Commercial Reprints Department, Elsevier Inc., 360 Park Avenue South, New York, NY 10010-1710. Tel.: 212-633-3874; Fax: 212-633-3820; E-mail: reprints@elsevier.com.

Veterinary Clinics of North America: Food Animal Practice is covered in *Current Contents/Agriculture, Biology and Environmental Sciences, MEDLINE/PubMed (Index Medicus),* and *Excerpta Medica.*

Printed and bound by CPI Group (UK) Ltd, Croydon, CR0 4YY

Contributors

CONSULTING EDITOR

ROBERT A. SMITH, DVM, MS
Diplomate, American Board of Veterinary Practitioners; Veterinary Research and Consulting Services, LLC, Greeley, Colorado

EDITORS

DAVID E. ANDERSON, DVM, MS
Diplomate, American College of Veterinary Surgeons; Professor and Head, Department of Large Animal Clinical Sciences, College of Veterinary Medicine, University of Tennessee, Knoxville, Tennessee

ANDRÉ DESROCHERS, DMV, MS
Diplomate, American College of Veterinary Surgeons; Diplomate, European College of Bovine Health Management; Professor of Farm Animal Surgery, Department of Clinical Sciences, Faculty of Veterinary Medicine, Université de Montréal, Saint-Hyacinthe, Quebec, Canada

AUTHORS

STEPHEN B. ADAMS, DVM, MS
Department of Veterinary Clinical Sciences, Purdue University School of Veterinary Medicine, West Lafayette, Indiana

DAVID E. ANDERSON, DVM, MS
Diplomate, American College of Veterinary Surgeons; Professor and Head, Department of Large Animal Clinical Sciences, College of Veterinary Medicine, University of Tennessee, Knoxville, Tennessee

AUBREY NICHOLAS BAIRD, DVM, MS
Department of Veterinary Clinical Sciences, Purdue University School of Veterinary Medicine, West Lafayette, Indiana

ANDRÉ DESROCHERS, DMV, MS
Diplomate, American College of Veterinary Surgeons; Diplomate, European College of Bovine Health Management; Professor of Farm Animal Surgery, Department of Clinical Sciences, Faculty of Veterinary Medicine, Université de Montréal, Saint-Hyacinthe, Quebec, Canada

GILLES FECTEAU, DMV
Diplomate, American College of Veterinary Internal Medicine; Department of Clinical Sciences, Faculty of Veterinary Medicine, Université de Montréal, Saint-Hyacinthe, Québec, Canada

DAVID FRANCOZ, DMV, DES, MSc
Diplomate, American College of Veterinary Internal Medicine; Faculty of Veterinary Medicine, Associate Professor, Department of Clinical Sciences, Université de Montréal, Saint-Hyacinthe, Quebec, Canada

URS GEISSBÜHLER, Dr med vet
Diplomate of the European College of Veterinary Diagnostic Imaging; Clinical Radiology, Department of Clinical Veterinary Medicine, Vetsuisse-Faculty, University of Bern, Berne, Switzerland

JOHANN KOFLER, Dr med vet
Diplomate of the European College of Bovine Health Management; Associate Professor, Department of Farm Animals and Veterinary Public Health, Clinic for Ruminants, University of Veterinary Medicine Vienna, Vienna, Austria

HÉLÈNE LARDÉ, Dr Med Vet, DES
Centre Hospitalier Universitaire Vétérinaire, Université de Montréal, Saint-Hyacinthe, Quebec, Canada

EMMA MARCHIONATTI, DMV
Department of Clinical Sciences, Faculty of Veterinary Medicine, Université de Montréal, Saint-Hyacinthe, Québec, Canada

PIERRE-YVES MULON, DMV, DES
Diplomate, American College of Veterinary Surgeons; Hôpital Vétérinaire Lachute, Lachute, Quebec, Canada

SYLVAIN NICHOLS, DMV, MS
Diplomate, American College of Veterinary Surgeons; Department of Clinical Sciences, Faculty of Veterinary Medicine, Université de Montréal, Saint-Hyacinthe, Quebec, Canada

ANDREW NIEHAUS, DVM, MS
Diplomate, American College of Veterinary Surgeons – Large Animal; Assistant Professor, Department of Veterinary Clinical Sciences, College of Veterinary Medicine, The Ohio State University, Columbus, Ohio

KARL NUSS, Dr Med Vet
Diplomate, European College of Veterinary Surgery; Section Head, Farm Animal Surgery, Department of Farm Animals, Vetsuisse-Faculty, University of Zurich, Zurich, Switzerland

REBECCA PENTECOST, DVM, MS
Department of Veterinary Clinical Sciences, College of Veterinary Medicine, The Ohio State University, Columbus, Ohio

GUY ST. JEAN, DMV, MS
Diplomate, American College of Veterinary Surgeons; Associate Dean for Academic Affairs and Professor of Surgery, Department of Veterinary Clinical Sciences, Ross University School of Veterinary Medicine, Basseterre, St. Kitts, West Indies

ADRIAN STEINER, Dr med vet, MS
Dr. habil., Diplomate, European College of Veterinary Surgeons; Diplomate, European College of Bovine Health Management; Professor and Head, Vetsuisse-Faculty, Farm Animal Clinic, Department of Clinical Veterinary Medicine, University of Bern, Bern, Switzerland

SUSAN R. VOGEL, DVM, MS
Senior Research Scientist, Elanco Animal Health, Greenfield, Indiana

Contents

The Walker splint has been specifically designed for treating tibial fractures and stifle injuries in cattle. It usually fits better in rear limbs of cattle than the TSCC and thus can provide more stability. Spica bandages combined with lateral splints placed over the dorsum of the affected limb and down the contralateral shoulder may be used for partial immobilization of humeral fractures in calves and small ruminants when surgical repair is not an option.

Evidence-based criteria that promise the best treatment outcome for bovine fracture patients have not been established. Internal fixation with plates and screws allows successful management of many long bone fractures in calves as well as in heavier cattle. Intramedullary pins may be better or equally suited for repair of humerus or femoral fractures in calves, respectively. In richly comminuted fractures in heavy cattle, methods of external fixation are still indicated. With newly introduced locking plates, treatment options for repair of long bone fractures in cattle have further improved, but high costs and a guarded prognosis limit their application.

External skeletal fixation (ESF) is a versatile method for rigid immobilization of long bone fractures in cattle. Traditional ESF devices may be used in young calves for clinical management of open fractures. Transfixation pinning and casting is an adaptation of ESF principles to improve versatility and clinical management of selected fractures.

Limb amputation is an alternative to euthanasia when catastrophic injury prevents successful restoration of the limb or when cost is an issue. Proximal limb disarticulation for amputation is preferred if a prosthesis is not considered. Distal amputations are needed to accommodate exoskeletal prosthesis. This article reviews the considerations and describes techniques for this surgery.

Contracted flexor tendon leading to flexural deformity is a common congenital defect in cattle. Arthrogryposis is a congenital syndrome of persistent joint contracture that occurs frequently in Europe as a consequence of Schmallenberg virus infection of the dam. Spastic paresis has a hereditary component, and affected cattle should not be used for breeding purposes. The most common tendon avulsion involves the deep digital flexor tendon. Tendon disruptions may be successfully managed by tenorrhaphy and external coaptation or by external coaptation alone. Medical management alone is unlikely to be effective for purulent tenosynovitis.

ligament injuries are among the most common traumatic injuries of the stifle joint. Although the prognosis is guarded, better success and less degenerative change are expected with early diagnosis and treatment. Meniscal injuries and upward fixation of the patella are less commonly diagnosed, but their clinical signs, treatment, and prognosis are discussed in this article.

VETERINARY CLINICS OF NORTH AMERICA: FOOD ANIMAL PRACTICE

THE CLINICS ARE NOW AVAILABLE ONLINE!
Access your subscription at:
www.theclinics.com

Preface

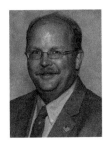 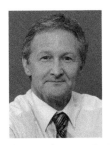

David E. Anderson, DVM, MS, DACVS
André Desrochers, DMV, MS, DACVS, DECBHM

Editors

The art and science of orthopedic surgery continue to grow with new principles, tools, and methods being developed. The cattle industry continues to expand markets and the value of genetically superior animals increases with these markets. As surgeons, the application of new techniques in bovine surgery presents unique challenges and exciting possibilities. The field surgeon is challenged with needing to practice economical, practical, and effective surgery. Surgeons in referral centers enjoy a greater variety of options because of the combination of facilities, personnel, and lessened pressure to contain costs of treatment. In this issue, we have attempted to bridge these gaps by developing information with which to perform decision analysis for orthopedic injuries, accurately determine treatment options, and understand prognosis with outcomes assessment. Our goal was to provide options and describe techniques applicable both to field treatment of orthopedic injuries in commercial cattle and for the advanced treatment of complex injuries in cattle. We hope that this edition of the *Veterinary Clinics of North America: Food Animal Practice* can serve as a resource to surgeons working in both environments. Also, we hope that this text may present new techniques and clarify options for clinicians struggling to decide how to treat cattle suffering from orthopedic disease.

David E. Anderson, DVM, MS, DACVS
Large Animal Clinical Sciences
College of Veterinary Medicine
University of Tennessee
2407 River Drive
Knoxville, TN 37996-4545, USA

Vet Clin Food Anim 30 (2014) xi–xii
http://dx.doi.org/10.1016/j.cvfa.2013.12.002
0749-0720/14/$ – see front matter

André Desrochers, DMV, MS, DACVS, DECBHM
Department of Clinical Sciences
Faculty of Veterinary Medicine
Université de Montréal
3200 Sicotte
St-Hyacinthe, Quebec, Canada, J2S 7C6

E-mail addresses:
dander48@utk.edu (D.E. Anderson)
andre.desrochers@umontreal.ca (A. Desrochers)

Decision Analysis for Fracture Management in Cattle

Guy St. Jean, DMV, MS[a],*, David E. Anderson, DVM, MS[b]

KEYWORDS

- Cattle • Fracture • Decision analysis • External coaptation • Internal fixation
- External fixator • Stall rest

KEY POINTS

- Bovine fractures are common and each bovine patient is unique, presents innumerable challenges, and requires careful judgment.
- In cattle the fracture repair usually should be of acceptable quality to not cause a decrease in milk or meat production or interfere with natural breeding.
- The decision to treat a fracture in cattle is made by evaluating the cost and success rates of the treatment, the value of the animal, and the location and type of fracture.
- Temporary stabilization of limb fractures often is the one difference between success and failure.
- External coaptation often is appropriate and an economic treatment to repair a fractured bone in cattle.
- Open fractures in cattle have guarded prognosis. The success rate often depends on the degree of contamination and the economic limitation of the owner.

Appendicular fractures (bones of the front limbs or hind limbs) are common in cattle, are commonly found in calves, and often occur following trauma during handling or a dystocia.[1] Fractures involving the axial skeleton (skull, spine, pelvis) are less common and less commonly treated. The most common bones involved in fractures of cattle are the metacarpus and metatarsus, followed by the tibia, radius and ulna, humerus, and femur.[1–5] Fractures of the axial skeleton and phalanges are rare, but the most common axial skeleton fractures are the sacrum, pelvis, and mandible.[1]

Each bovine patient with a fracture is unique and presents various challenges requiring careful judgment. Decision analysis is always part of clinical cases in any species, but economic factors are a particularly significant influence on decision analysis for cattle under consideration for treatment because of the requirement for

---

[a] Department of Veterinary Clinical Sciences, Ross University School of Veterinary Medicine, PO Box 334, Basseterre, St. Kitts, West Indies; [b] Department of Large Animal Clinical Sciences, College of Veterinary Medicine, University of Tennessee, Knoxville, TN 37996, USA
* Corresponding author.
E-mail address: GSt.Jean@rossvet.edu.kn

Vet Clin Food Anim 30 (2014) 1–10
http://dx.doi.org/10.1016/j.cvfa.2013.11.011   **vetfood.theclinics.com**

economic returns in nearly every case. Every animal with a fracture is different. Every owner, farm manager, and rancher brings a different set of circumstances and expectations. With the exception of rodeo livestock, cattle most often do not need to perform at the same athletic capacity as horses. In cattle, return to productivity after fracture repair should be of acceptable quality so as not to negatively impact growth for meat production, cause a decrease in milk production, or interfere with reproductive efficiency, including embryo or semen production and natural service breeding. Each veterinarian brings a different point of view to the decision analysis process, but there are common features to all cases that must be considered: owner expectations, perceived value of animal, prognosis for treatment, and likely outcome after successful treatment.

Most cattle are favorable patients for treatment of fractures because they have a calm demeanor, are capable of spending most of the time lying down during convalescence, have tremendous potential for bone healing because of vascular density and enhanced cambial layer to the periosteum, infrequently suffer permanent contralateral limb breakdown or stress laminitis in the unaffected limbs, and usually do not resist having orthopedic devices (eg, splints, casts, external skeletal fixators) on their limbs.[4,5]

ECONOMICS

In cattle, the decision to treat a fracture is made by evaluating the severity of the injury (eg, open vs closed fracture, neurovascular trauma), cost of treatment, expected success rate of treatment, perceived or potential economic and genetic value of the animal, and the location and type of fracture (eg, articular vs nonarticular, amenable to cast vs bone plate vs external skeletal fixation [ESF]). The presence of sepsis, nerve damage, and vascular trauma negatively impacts prognosis and significantly increases cost of treatment. Closed fractures are expected to heal in most cases, whereas open fractures are more likely to suffer complications such as sequestration of bone, delayed union, or nonunion. The temperament and behavior of the animal can improve or worsen prognosis. Cattle with aggressive behavior are more likely to maintain the ability to stand, walk, and care for themselves. However, these patients are more difficult and dangerous to treat and therefore may receive lesser quality care. Proximal limbs injuries, such as humeral or femoral fractures, have greater soft tissue support and collateral blood supply, but are more difficult to stabilize than more distal fractures. External coaptation devices are more easily adjusted to forelimb injuries than hind limb injuries. Fracture treatment in younger patients with lighter body weights is more easily healed because of their remarkable healing rate and greater stability of fixation devices than adult cattle. Although expensive, orthopedic implants designed for use in small animal and human surgery are often of adequate mechanical strength for use in young calves and have been used successfully in the management of various fractures in cattle. After the multitude of factors that affect prognosis has been considered, the veterinarian can offer options for the client to choose from. The veterinarian's responsibility is to ensure that the owner can make an informed decision about the cost of treatment as it relates to the ultimate outcome of the case.

In general, cattle producers will elect the least expensive treatment for any given fracture that still offers a reasonable success rate. Often, owners are willing to elect costly treatments, even when the prognosis is poor, when cattle are perceived to have high economic or genetic potential. Occasionally, these options are chosen because the animal has attained a "pet" status on the farm. In many cases, bulls carry the greatest perceived value, but cows that can be used for embryo transfer may be similarly viewed. Recently, cloning technology has tremendously enhanced the genetic merit of calves, which, in turn, has mandated veterinary orthopedic care that may not have been afforded in the past. Societal influences may also change the view of veterinary care for cattle and some veterinarians may be asked to treat orthopedic injuries regardless of their market value. In the authors' experience, it is not unusual for discretionary dollars to be allocated to the fracture repair of cattle that would have previously been slaughtered or euthanized. Also, cattle owners often will treat cattle that sustain injuries as a result of human error because of a sense of guilt or responsibility to make amends for their mistakes. In these cases veterinary surgeons may be asked to repair a fractured bone at an expense that far exceeds the value of the animal.

Ultimately, the veterinarian is charged with informing the client of the options, costs, and likely outcomes so that the client may choose the option that most closely matches their own risk-benefit analysis. Veterinary professionals often use "percentage" when conducting the decision analysis for fracture patients.[1–8] These percentages are based on personal and anecdotal experiences and literature.[1–8] Unfortunately, the evidence-based medicine for fracture treatment in cattle is lacking in regard to specific fractures and specific repair techniques because of the relatively small sample populations in various studies. Also, literature is expected to be biased toward successful outcomes and likely overestimates prognosis in many cases.

DIAGNOSTICS

Decision analysis in the management of individual patients initially must be based on a complete history and physical examination. Treatment options and prognosis are affected by concurrent injuries, disease status, or nutritional status of the patient. The identification of multiple injuries is not unusual in adult cattle. Adult cattle are expected to be able to rise, stand, and walk on 3 legs when the fourth limb is compromised. When cattle are examined for fracture in one limb (eg, tibial) but are unable to rise, stand, or walk, additional injuries should be suspected (eg, contralateral limb injury, pelvic injury, spine injury) and the prognosis should be adjusted. Evaluation of the fractured limb and surrounding soft tissues around the fracture requires diligence by the clinician. Open wounds, vascular compromise, and nerve injury increase the likelihood of complications. Assessment of the systemic health of the animal is especially critical in calves, and passive transfer of antibodies and immunity should be determined (eg, measurement of total protein, immunoglobulin G, and white blood cell count). Diagnosis of many fractures, especially those affecting the distal limbs, presents little diagnostic challenge and radiographic imaging often is not done. Radiographic assessment is done routinely in upper limbs injuries. However, the clinician must be cautious in that, although radiographs are helpful for planning treatment, these images relay little insight about other injuries, systemic health, or neurologic status of the animal.

Owners and farm managers that are fully informed and prepared for possible complications from the outset are better prepared to accept complications if they occur and can more easily make decisions regarding the course of action should they occur. Although adult cattle are less prone to systemic illness secondary to fracture, calves are vulnerable to pneumonia, enteritis, and septicemia.[7] These problems can be concurrent or unrelated to the fracture. These secondary problems require complete assessment and pre-emptive management. Fractures in neonates often preclude the ingestion of sufficient colostrum during the first 12 hours of life. The resulting failure of passive transfer may jeopardize the recovery to the calf and lead to their demise despite successful repair of the fracture.[7]

EMERGENCY TREATMENT

Treatment of the patient and injured limb including temporary stabilization of the fractured limb often makes the difference between success and failure. Temporary stabilization of limb fractures should be attempted before moving the animal or if possible before attempting to get the animal to stand. Immediate medical therapy may be required to treat shock or to stabilize the patient when hypovolemia or toxemia is present. In calves septicemia or lack of sufficient colostrum intake is a concern that should be addressed if present.

Fractures distal to the level of the mid radius or mid tibia may be temporarily stabilized with full-limb splints or casts. In the authors' experience, field stabilization of fractures proximal to this level should not be attempted in adults because these efforts often result in the creation of a fulcrum effect at or near the fracture site, exacerbating soft tissue trauma and increasing the risk of neurovascular damage or creation of an open wound. Adult cattle with proximal limb fracture should be carefully loaded into a trailer and allowed to lie down before beginning transport if the repair is not performed on the farm. The use of loading ramps may be required to ensure that the patient does not fall during loading.

Distal limb injuries are readily immobilized by the application of a rigid splint or a cast. Although these forms of external coaptation may be applied as a temporary means of immobilization of the limb, these appliances must be sufficiently strong to withstand the forces applied during rising, standing, and walking. Rigid splints are constructed by application of a Robert Jones bandage and including 2 splints placed 90° apart (eg, caudal and lateral aspect of the limb). Splint material can be made using 2 thick wooden boards or 2 halves of a large, thick polyvinyl chloride pipe placed on the caudal and lateral aspect of the limb to create a stable external coaptation. The splints are placed with 90° of separation so that bending forces can be effectively resisted in both the cranial-to-caudal and the lateral-to-medial planes. A padded bandage is placed on the limb; the splints are positioned, and elastic tape is applied firmly. Adequate padding around the limb before application of the splints helps to ensure that the elastic tape will not cause injury from excessive constriction of the limb. Excessive padding or inadequate tension will result in displacement of the splint and may exacerbate the injury. The integrity of the splint should be checked frequently. For fractures distal to the carpus or hock, the splints should be placed from the ground (even with the sole) proximally to the level of the elbow/proximal radius or stifle/proximal tibia, respectively. For fractures proximal to the carpus or hock and distal to the mid radius or mid tibia, the lateral splint should extend to the level of the proximal scapula or pelvis.

Alternatively, a cast may be used to provide external coaptation for temporary stabilization of the fracture. Casts should be constructed from fiberglass casting tape and be sufficiently thick so as to prevent failure. Cast fractures and failures most commonly occur at joints, especially when the angle changes markedly (eg, hock), and at the proximal and distal ends of the cast. The authors recommend encasing the entire foot within the cast to ensure maximum diversion of forces associated with weight and ground reaction force into the cast material.

In calves, proximal limb injuries may be temporarily protected using slings. A modified Velpeau sling can be applied to the forelimb for emergency immobilization of fractures of the radius, humerus, and scapula. These slings are constructed by application of an encircling bandage to the distal limb (metacarpus), then flexing the limb against the body, followed by an encircling bandage around the thorax. The splint can be further enhanced by including a "figure-of-8" wrap between the forelimbs and around the base of the neck. A modified Ehmer sling can be used to temporarily immobilize fractures of the tibia and femur. The modified Ehmer is constructed by applying an encircling bandage to the distal limb (metatarsus), then flexing the limb against the body, followed by an encircling bandage around the pelvis and abdomen. This sling may be further enhanced by wrapping a "figure-of-8" bandage between the rear limbs.

PRINCIPLES OF FRACTURE MANAGEMENT

When a bovine patient is presented with a fracture of the appendicular skeleton, the following questions must be answered. Is treatment required?[4] Can the fracture be acceptably reduced closed or is internal reduction required?[4] Can the fracture be adequately immobilized using external coaptation alone or is ESF or internal fixation, with or without external coaptation, required? What are the cost and benefits of treating this animal? A variety of methods for immobilization or stabilization of fractures in cattle is available for use. The selection of the method used may be based on the injury whereby best method may be chosen or may be based on economic constraints in which the minimum acceptable coaptation method is used (**Table 1**). The prognosis for fracture healing is affected by the location and severity of the injury, age of the patient, and integrity of the tissues (**Fig. 1**).

External coaptation in the form of rigid splints or cast immobilization often is an appropriate and economical way to stabilize fractures in cattle. Rigid splints are appropriate and effective for Salter-Harris type 1 and 2 fractures of the distal metacarpus or metatarsus only. When these physeal fractures are anatomically reduced, the interdigitation that is established within the physis allows full weight-bearing without displacement. These injuries heal rapidly and rigid splinting can achieve effective immobilization in lightweight calves. Fiberglass casts are far more effective at resisting bending forces and maintaining immobilization of the fracture site than splints. Thus, most fractures that are amenable to external coaptation should be treated using casts. Casts should be applied such that the articulation proximal and distal to the fracture is immobilized. The purpose of immobilizing a joint above and below the fracture is to minimize displacement of the proximal and distal fracture segment that would occur during joint movement and to maximize the likelihood of neutralizing weight-bearing force as the limb is loaded during standing and walking. The only fractures for which this rule may be violated are Salter-Harris type 1 or 2 fracture of the distal Metacarpus (MC) and Metatarsus (MT) physis when casts are stopped immediately distal to the carpus or tarsus and Salter-Harris type 1 or 2 fracture of the distal radius and tibia when casts are stopped immediately distal to the elbow or stifle. The materials for fabricating casts and splints are readily available and most cattle become accustomed to locomotion within a few days. When a patient fails to acclimate to the external coaptation device, the cast or splint should be re-evaluated and altered to improve patient care and outcome. External coaptation with casts alone cannot adequately immobilize fractures proximal to the distal radial physis or the distal tibial physis because there is not sufficient length of limb to capture forces and maintain fracture immobilization. Also, soft tissue injuries and open fractures may not be managed optimally by use of casts, splints, or splint-cast combinations. Complications of splinting and casting can include muscle-tendon contracture in the injured limb, muscle-tendon laxity in the contralateral limb, decreased range of motion of joints, degeneration of articular cartilage, skin sores or ulcers, damage to the

Table 1
Minimal acceptable techniques for stabilization of fractures based on location of the fracture

Long Bone	Fracture Site	Minimum Coaptation Method for Stabilization	Rigid Coaptation
Phalanges	P1, P2, P3	Walking block applied to companion digit	Half-limb cast ± lag screw fixation
Metacarpus/ Metatarsus III/IV	Distal physis	Half-limb cast or rigid splint	Half-limb cast
	Mid diaphysis: proximal MC/MT III/IV	Full-limb cast or rigid splint	Full limb cast ± pin-cast or DCP plate
Radius	Distal physis Salter-Harris type 1 fracture	Full-limb cast or Thomas splint	Pin-cast
	Distal metaphysis to proximal radius	Thomas splint or Hanging limb pin-cast	DCP plate or pin-cast
Humerus	Humerus	Young calves: Spica splint Cattle >6 mo old: stall confinement or open reduction with internal fixation	DCP plate or intramedullary interlocking nail or dynamic compression plating
Scapula	Scapula	Young calves: Spica splint Cattle >6 mo old: stall confinement or open reduction with internal fixation	DCP plate
Tibia	Distal physis, Salter-Harris type 1	Full-limb cast or Thomas splint	Hanging limb pin-cast
	Distal metaphysis: proximal tibia	Thomas splint or hanging limb pin-cast	DCP or pin-cast
Femur	Femur	Open reduction with internal fixation	Intramedullary interlocking nail or

soft tissue or vasculature because of the cast being too tight or constriction within the cast caused by swelling, instability within the appliance resulting in creation of an open wound that may communicate with the fracture, malalignment of the fracture, malunion, delayed union, or nonunion of the fracture, and prolonged convalescence. These complications can be diminished by careful attention to detail during application of the splint or cast and frequent careful re-evaluation of the patient. Although costly, failure of the patient to use the limb or a sudden change in the patient's ability to use the limb are indications for removal of the appliance and reassessment of the limb.

Cattle are amenable to application of some "high-order" or complex splints for immobilization of certain fractures. The most common complex splint used is the Thomas splint, but Spica splints are used occasionally as well. The use of a Thomas splint or a Thomas splint and cast combination is most often used for fractures of the radius and tibia.[2,3] Spica splints can be used effectively in young cattle for immobilization of humerus fractures. Seemingly simple to use, these complex splints must

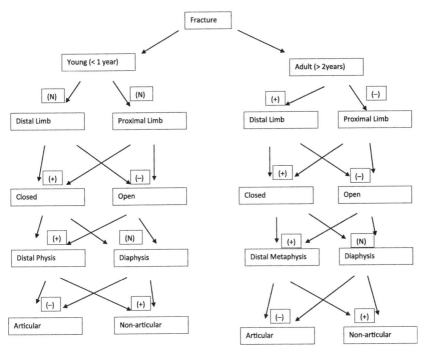

Fig. 1. Factors affecting prognosis for fracture healing in cattle. (N), no or minimal effect; (+), beneficial effect; (−), negative effect.

be meticulously applied to achieve success. High-order splints applied too long for the limb in an attempt to apply tension to the fractured limb often result in prolonged recumbency, and inability to stand, and excessive muscle contraction on the injured limb and "breakdown" of the contralateral limb. High-order splints that are applied too short in an attempt to ease patient mobility result in fracture displacement, open fractures, and nonunion or delayed union of the fracture. Cattle having a Thomas splint-cast or Spica splint-cast must be assisted to stand multiple times daily until they are capable and willing to rise under their own power and move about the stall. These patients must also be checked several times daily to ensure that they have not lain down on the splint such that they become cast and unable to rise. Patients that become unable to rise or attain sterna recumbency are at risk for bloat and death.

ESF refers to the stabilization of a fracture using transfixation pins and any external frame connecting the pins and spanning the region of instability. Examples of external frames used to connect transfixing pins include side bars, circular fixators, acrylic cement, and fiberglass casting tape. In cattle, transfixation pinning and casting of fractures often are often a more successful means to return the animal to weight-bearing rapidly after surgery. In young calves and depending on fracture configuration, these ESF appliances may be applied to the fractured bone without spanning adjacent joints such that joint mobility is preserved and more normal growth with fewer complications is encountered.[9] ESF techniques involve limited surgical invasiveness with reduced cost than open reduction and internal fixation techniques, such as intramedullary pinning, bone plating Dynamic Compression Plates (DCP), or intramedullary interlocking nail fixation. In most cases, ESF is simple and can be done in field settings. ESF is the preferred method for management of open fracture because the ability to maintain fracture immobilization is achieved while accommodating management of soft tissue wounds on the limb. Furthermore, ESF techniques permit easy implant removal after clinical union of the fracture and results in relatively few complications from the implants.[9] ESF easily can be used for fractures of the MC, MT, radius, or tibia. Although more difficult, ESF can be used for selected fractures of the humerus and femur as well. Disadvantages of ESF are suboptimal fracture reduction, absence of interfragmentary compression, lesser biomechanical stability than internal fixation with bone plates, increased postoperative management than rigid splints or casts, pain associated with motion of the pins at the bone interface, and bending or breakage of the implants. Economic constraints dictate that ESF most often is used in valuable cattle such as purebred cattle, show cattle, or in cattle perceived to have great value.[9]

Open fractures in cattle have a more guarded prognosis.[1,2] The success rate for treatment of open fractures depends on the severity of soft tissue damage, bones affected, duration of the injury, degree of contamination of the wound, and the economic limitation of the owner. The principles of treatment of open fractures are to thoroughly clean and debride the wound, copiously lavage the wound, and provide medical care such as antibiotics, frequent wound care, pain management, and local therapy for sepsis. Prolonged antibiotic treatment is indicated and selection for use in cattle must be made with consideration for extralabel use and potential antibiotic residues. Based on experience, the authors routinely initiate antibiotic therapy with procaine penicillin or sodium ceftiofur. Local treatment and copious lavage are performed frequently depending on the degree of contamination and the severity of infection. In one study, successful treatment of open fractures of the MC/MT in adult cattle was associated with careful cleaning and debridement of the open wound and fracture performed with the patient under general anesthesia (Tulleners). Open fractures often develop sequestration of large segments of cortical bone during healing (Valentino). Bone sequestra can adversely affect fracture treatment, but most often these sequestra can be removed without preventing bone healing. If sequestra are present, sequestrectomy should be performed to allow fracture healing to proceed. The fracture site is extensively debrided until healthy bone is exposed.

Osteomyelitis of the fractured bone can be challenging to treat successfully. Techniques used to treat bone infection include intravenous or intraosseous regional limb perfusion, implantation of antibiotic impregnated beads, and cancellous bone grafts. Regional intravenous perfusion of antibiotics distal to a tourniquet proximal to the infected bone is recommended to achieve high concentrations of antibiotics at the level of the bone. Most often, antibiotic-impregnated beads are handmade using polymethylmethacrylate cement at the time of use. Orthopedic-grade polymethylmethacrylate bone cement is prepared and powdered antibiotics are mixed into the cement before it hardens. Also before hardening, the beads are made small enough to be placed into multiple soft tissue sites surrounding the fracture. Therapeutic concentrations of antibiotics are expected to be achieved locally for up to 2 weeks after implantation. Cancellous bone grafting is also performed to facilitate bone healing. A fresh autologous cancellous bone graft is harvested from the sternum, iliac crest, proximal tibia, or proximal humerus and implanted into the fracture site. Cancellous bone grafts stimulate neovascularization and osteogenesis, which indirectly enhance clearance of infection. Open fractures are expected to have a prolonged healing time and may require 12 weeks or more for clinical bone union versus 4 to 8 weeks for closed fractures.[10]

Femoral and humeral fractures usually will require some form of internal fixation. In young cattle having fracture with minimal displacement, the bone may heal with stall confinement alone (Nichols and another recent paper). In most cases, femoral fractures sustain considerable fragment displacement and overriding.[7] Although successful treatment of femoral fractures using stall rest has been reported,[7] open reduction and internal fixation are advised to optimize humane patient care and improve functional outcome.[6,7] Although humerus fractures are less likely to become significantly displaced, the prognosis for healing after surgical versus conservative management is similar. Surgical treatment of humeral and femoral fracture varies depending on the age of the animal, configuration of the fracture, and the surgeon's experience. Open reduction and internal fixations are usually attempted in young, lightweight cattle. Surgery for mid diaphyseal fracture of the femur has a significantly better surgical outcome than distal diaphyseal fractures.[7] Stabilization of the femur and humerus can be achieved by intramedullary stack pinning, intramedullary pinning and cerclage wire, intramedullary pinning and type I ESF, intramedullary interlocking nail fixation, rush pin fixation, or specialized bone plates and screws. Dynamic compression plates, cobrahead plates, angled blade plates, and condylar bone plates have had limited success in repairing femoral and humeral fractures in cattle. Failure of these devices has been attributed to the limited holding power of young calf bone for orthopedic screws. Recently, locking screw plates have been developed to improve holding power of screws in weak bone and may offer significant advantages for the repair of upper limb fractures in valuable cattle. Fracture of the femoral head or capital physeal fractures occur in young calves after forced extractions during dystocia associated with "hip lock" and in cattle less than 24 months old associated with peer trauma in group housing. Literature reports include stabilization using multiple Steinmann pins or lag screw fixation using 6.5-mm cancellous end-threaded screws or 7.0-mm cannulated screws (ref StJean and Ewoldt and Edwards). In young bulls in a semen collection facility, 70% of the bulls with slipped capital physis treated with 7.0-mm cannulated screws had successful outcomes and were serviceable for semen collection.[8]

In some patients, successful treatment of the fracture is not possible. These unmanageable fractures occur as a result of the severity of the fracture, compromise to soft tissues, loss of neurovascular integrity, or overwhelming infection. In these cases, limb amputation or euthanasia of the patient must be considered. Surgeons have performed limb amputations in cattle for purposes of preservation of genetics or because the animal has sentimental value for the client. Limb amputation can be done initially or following unsuccessful fracture repair procedures. In highly valuable cattle or "pets," limb prosthesis can be offered to the client. This option must be discussed before amputation so that the amputation can be done in such a manner that the prosthesis can be fitted to the limb. The best long-term results are achieved when a prosthetic team consists of a professional orthotic and prosthetic specialist, ensuring customization of the prosthetic to maximize patient comfort and limb utilization.

In conclusion, decision analysis for fracture management depends on the animal, injury, owner, and veterinarian. The goals of the client for that individual animal, the economic constraints impacting treatment, and the enthusiasm of the veterinarian to pursue treatment options will remain a driving force in the future of bovine orthopedics.

REFERENCES

1. Tulleners EP. Management of bovine orthopedic problems, part 1: fractures. The Comp Cont Educ Pract 1986;8:69–79.

Diagnostic Imaging in Bovine Orthopedics

Johann Kofler, Dr med vet[a],*, Urs Geissbühler, Dr med vet[b],
Adrian Steiner, Dr med vet, MS[c]

KEYWORDS

- Radiology • Ultrasonography • Computed tomography
- Magnetic resonance imaging • Musculoskeletal disorders • Cattle

KEY POINTS

- Ultrasonography is an imaging modality that can be applied anywhere in bovine practice and allows rapid, noninvasive differentiation of soft-tissue structures of the bovine musculoskeletal system.
- Ultrasound units with 5.0- to 7.5-MHz linear transducers, commonly used in large animal reproduction, are well suited for rapid and straightforward differentiation of soft-tissue swelling in the limbs. In addition, ultrasonography can be very helpful for detection of foreign bodies in the limbs or trunk that cannot be diagnosed radiographically.[39]
- Ultrasonography provides accurate information about the location, size, and the nature of the content of lesions or fluid-filled cavities and the surrounding tissues, making puncture precise and safer.
- The physiologic amount of synovial fluid of normal synovial cavities in cattle cannot be imaged by ultrasonography; visualization of effusion is easy and usually indicates an inflammatory process.
- Ultrasonography can detect early stages of inflammation of synovial cavities based on an increased amount of effusion and distension of the synovial pouch.
- However, radiography remains still the method of choice for evaluation of bone lesions, such as fractures, luxation, and osteomyelitis.
- An early diagnosis, accurate anatomic differentiation of the soft-tissue structures involved, characterization of the lesions, and a thorough preoperative inspection of incriminated regions are of enormous benefit in determining an accurate prognosis and for planning surgery and treatment.

[a] Department of Farm Animals and Veterinary Public Health, Clinic for Ruminants, University of Veterinary Medicine Vienna, Veterinärplatz 1, A-1210 Vienna, Austria; [b] Department of Clinical Veterinary Medicine, Vetsuisse-Faculty, University of Bern, Länggassstrasse 124, CH-3001 Berne, Switzerland; [c] Clinical Radiology, Department of Clinical Veterinary Medicine, Farm Animal Clinic, Vetsuisse-Faculty, University of Bern, Länggassstrasse 124, CH-3001 Berne, Switzerland
* Corresponding author.
E-mail address: Johann.Kofler@vetmeduni.ac.at

Vet Clin Food Anim 30 (2014) 11–53
http://dx.doi.org/10.1016/j.cvfa.2013.11.003
0749-0720/14/$ – see front matter © 2014 Elsevier Inc. All rights reserved.
vetfood.theclinics.com

INTRODUCTION

A careful clinical and orthopedic examination is always the first step in making a diagnosis of bovine limb disorders before diagnostic imaging techniques are applied.[1–5] A radiographic unit is not standard equipment for bovine practitioners in hospital or field situations.[6,7] However, ultrasound machines with 7.5-MHz (multifrequency) linear transducers have been used in bovine reproduction for many years, and are eminently suitable for evaluation of orthopedic disorders.[8,9]

The goal of this article is to encourage veterinarians to use radiology and ultrasonography for the evaluation of bovine orthopedic disorders. These diagnostic imaging techniques improve the likelihood of a definitive diagnosis in every bovine patient, but especially in highly valuable cattle, whose owners demand increasingly more diagnostic and surgical interventions that require high-level specialized techniques.[10]

RADIOGRAPHY IN BOVINE ORTHOPEDICS

During the last years and decades radiography has established itself as a standard diagnostic procedure in veterinary medicine. Nevertheless, up to now it has not become a routine procedure in bovine practice, particularly because of its cost. This situation is also reflected in the scientific literature. Until now, only few books and articles have been published about diagnostic radiography in cattle. To date only 2 cattle radiography reference works have appeared: the textbook *Bovine Radiology* by Uri Bargai from 1989,[11] and the other recently published DVD "Bovine Radiology: Digital Diagnostic Atlas" from the Vetsuisse-Faculty of the University of Berne, Switzerland.[7] One finds otherwise several articles and publications which deal with orthopedic topics in cattle radiography.[6,12–23]

Radiography Equipment and Imaging Systems

In practice, portable machines with a performance of 3.5 to 4 kW are used to produce radiologic images of cattle. These devices are very practical for taking radiographic images in the area of the distal limbs and the skull of adult cattle, as well as for imaging calves. However, when one wishes to examine the proximal limb skeleton, the limits of this equipment's performance is reached very soon, owing to the very thick layers of tissue to be penetrated by the x-rays. Only with very powerful, mainly stationary radiologic equipment, such as one finds in large clinics, is it possible to produce reasonable images of these body parts. The imaging systems used in farm animal radiography are not different from those in equine radiography. In addition to conventional film-screen combinations, digital imaging systems (computed radiography or direct radiography) are being used increasingly more frequently.

Radiation Protection

There are 3 main principal recommendations made by the International Commission on Radiological Protection (ICRP) to minimize the radiation exposure of persons involved in radiographic studies,[24] namely:

- Justification
- Optimization
- Dose limitation

Justification implies that any radiologic examination must yield a benefit sufficient to justify the risks of the radiation exposure. Radiography should only be performed if, according to the case history and clinical examination, radiographic alterations can be expected and if the radiologic diagnosis will have consequences for the further treatment of the animal.

Optimization is also known as the principle of ALARA (As Low As Reasonably Achievable), which means that all reasonable measures should be taken to keep radiation doses at the lowest level possible.

The concept of dose limitation addresses the maximum permissible dose that an individual may receive annually or accumulate over a working lifetime. These doses should be within the limits established by international organizations such as the ICRP and national bodies. These limits are intended to reduce the probability of conjecture and to prevent deleterious deterministic radiation effects.

While radiographing cattle, particularly adult animals, one is almost always reliant on assistants who stay in the radiography room during the recording. One person usually has to hold the animal still while another holds the imaging plate. The only alternative is to examine under general anesthesia, which in adult ruminants should be avoided whenever possible because of the risks of anesthesia complications (ruminal bloat; regurgitation and aspiration of the rumen contents).

Radiation-protective apparel must be worn by all personnel involved and in the vicinity of the animal examined. The minimal outfit consists of a lead apron and, if the cassette is hand held, lead gloves. A thyroid shield is strongly recommended. Always be aware that protective clothing provides protection only against scattered radiation; it does not shield from the primary radiation beam! Protective clothing must be stored and maintained according to manufacturer's recommendations. It should be inspected annually for shielding protection or when damage is suspected. Another measure to reduce the radiation dosage is to use devices such as cassette holders with long extension poles, which enable staff to place themselves at the greatest possible distance from the source of radiation. The optimal selection of the parameters minimizes the radiation dose for a radiograph as well as the risk of unnecessary repetition of images. The most important points in this context[24]:

- Careful choice of film-screen combination (conventional radiography)
- Radiographic examination technique: radiation doses and patient's positioning
- Adequate film development technique or algorithms

Planning a Radiographic Study

The planning of a radiographic study is an important part of radiation protection in bovine radiography that may help to avoid unnecessary repetition of radiographs. The most important points to be considered are:

- In field situations, an adequate location has to be chosen for the radiologic examination (plane floor, dark room, concrete building).
- To avoid artifacts, dirt should be brushed out of the animal's fur before radiographs are taken.
- Nervous or frightened animals should be sedated to reduce the risk of movement blur and to reduce the number of auxiliary persons present in the radiography room.
- Positioning of the animal and the x-ray machine should be done very carefully to avoid unnecessary repetition of radiographs.
- Optimal exposure settings should be applied to obtain radiographs of good quality and to avoid repetition of the images.

Special Radiography in Cattle

Feet

Feet are one of the most frequently radiographed body parts in cattle. Very often the cause of lameness is located in this area. The most common indications are the suspicion of a pedal bone fracture or a deep septic process involving the pedal bone, the distal sesamoid bone, and/or the distal interphalangeal joint.

As a standard procedure, a dorsal 65° proximal-palmaro-/plantarodistal and a lateral 30° dorsal-mediodistal oblique radiographic image will be taken (**Figs. 1** and **2**). For these 2 radiographic views the imaging plate has to be protected by an overlaid fiber-glass tunnel. These 2 projections allow the pedal bone and distal sesamoid bone, as well as the distal interphalangeal joint, to be displayed and evaluated in 2 different planes. A further possibility of obtaining an image of the distal phalanx and the neighboring joints without superimpositions is the lateromedial or mediolateral projection with a film placed in the interdigital space. The most convenient way to achieve this is to put the cow into a trimming chute and hoist up the limb to be examined. In such a case, a screenless radiographic film can be positioned in the interdigital space without any difficulty and the image taken.

In the healthy limb, the individual bones are clearly differentiated, the bone structure homogeneous, and the joint contours smooth and clearly defined. In the pedal bone, the vessel canals are clearly visible and well delineated. When suspecting deep septic processes in the region of the feet, the main interest lies in whether and to what extent the bones and the distal interphalangeal joint are affected. Osteitis of the pedal bone shows up as unclearly defined, irregular, and heterogeneous radiolucency of the bone (**Fig. 3**). Periosteal new bone formations are often observed at the edges of the defect, depending of the age of the lesion. Radiographic images of a sepsis of the distal interphalangeal joint will show a diffuse soft-tissue swelling proximal to the coronary band and enlargement of the joint space as a first sign. The joint space may eventually narrow down because the joint cartilage is destroyed in chronic cases, but this depends

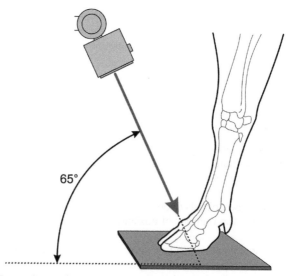

Fig. 1. Dorsal 65° proximo-palmarodistal oblique view of the third phalanx; the cow stands weight bearing on the cassette.

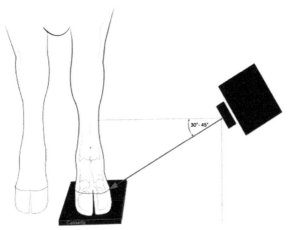

Fig. 2. Lateral 30° proximal-mediodistal oblique view for evaluation of the lateral third phalanx; the cow stands weight bearing on the cassette.

on the infectious agent involved and its bacterial production. The joint contours become irregular, and when the disease is chronic the infection often spreads to the subchondral bone plates of the second and third phalanx as well as the distal sesamoid bone.[14,20,21,25] The septic arthritis gradually develops into an osteitis (pedal bone) and/or osteomyelitis (second phalanx) (**Fig. 4**). Fractures of the pedal bone are usually clearly visible by the characteristic depiction of 1 or more radiolucent lines (fracture lines), which may be more or less clearly defined. The horn capsule mostly does not permit a dislocation of the fragments (**Fig. 5**). Evidence of an open fracture includes gas inclusions and defects of the horn capsule.

Long bones
Suspected fractures and sequester formation in the area of the long bones are the most common indications for a radiologic examination in adult cows. Growth disorders and infectious processes in the area of the growth plate are frequent indications for a radiologic examination of young animals.

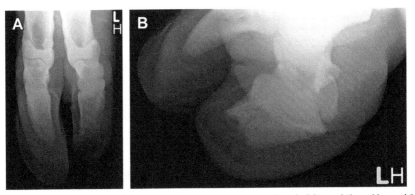

Fig. 3. Cow, Angus, 3 years old; dorsal 65° proximo-plantarodistal oblique (*A*) and lateral 30° proximal-mediodistal oblique view of the third phalanx (*B*); bone defect and osteitis of the lateral distal phalanx and horn defect of the lateral claw of the left hindlimb.

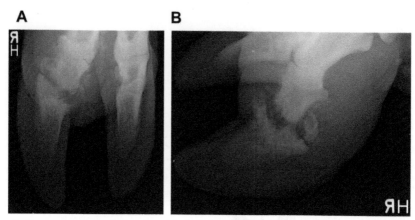

Fig. 4. Cow, mixed breed, 3 years old; dorsal 65° proximo-plantarodistal oblique (*A*) and lateral 30° proximal-mediodistal oblique view of the third phalanx (*B*); erosive arthritis of the lateral distal interphalangeal joint of the right hindlimb with concurrent osteomyelitis of the lateral navicular bone.

As standard projections, dorsopalmar/dorsoplantar (craniocaudal) and lateromedial/mediolateral radiographs are taken. If necessary, these can be supplemented by various oblique projections (usually dorsolateral-palmaro-/-plantaromedial and/or palmaro-/plantarolateral-dorsomedial oblique). All these radiographs are normally taken on the standing animal. The exceptions are radiographs of the humerus and femur. In cooperative cattle, the humerus can be depicted in the standing animal, but uncooperative patients must be positioned in lateral recumbency under deep sedation for radiographic examination. When depicting the femur, the animal must always be laid down. A mediolateral radiograph will usually be taken (**Fig. 6**).

In the healthy animal, only the cortical (compacta) and cancellous (spongiosa) bone are recognizable on the radiographic images of the long bones. The compacta shows up as a homogeneous, mineral opaque outer layer of the bone. The outer surface is

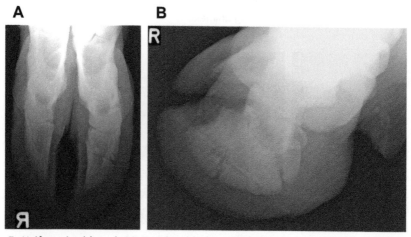

Fig. 5. Heifer, mixed breed, 20 months old; dorsal 65° proximo-palmarodistal oblique (*A*) and medial 30° proximal-laterodistal oblique view of the third phalanx (*B*); subacute transverse fracture of the medial distal phalanx of the right forelimb.

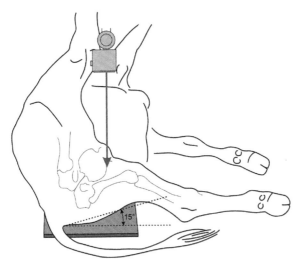

Fig. 6. Mediolateral projection (faux profile) of the femur. Under general anesthesia, the animal is positioned first in dorsal recumbency. The cassette is set on the floor and the affected limb is laid down on it, keeping the upper leg abducted. The affected limb has an angle of 10° to 15° to the floor.

sharply defined while endosteally, one observes a more fluent transition. Mainly in older animals, new bone formations may sometimes be visible at the insertions of tendons and ligaments. The clinical significance of such enthesophytes must be evaluated with care because they are not necessarily associated with clinical symptoms. The spongiosa shows up as the summation of many bone trabeculae; the bone marrow lying in between has a soft-tissue density. The opacity of the spongiosa varies according to the location within the long bone; according to Wolff's Law, more trabeculae are produced at sites of high strain than at sites of less strain. Overall, in healthy cattle the spongiosa shows up as regularly structured with fluent transitions. The transition to the central bone marrow cavity is also smooth. The surrounding soft tissues appear homogeneous in normal cattle.

Fractures are characterized by interruptions in the continuity of bony structures, and fracture lines are visible as radiolucent lines. Normally a soft-tissue swelling is also visible. Gas inclusions point to an injury of the soft-tissue coat, and are therefore very important in guiding toward an adequate therapy (**Fig. 7**). The individual fracture fragments can be dislocated at various degrees. To determine the direction and the degree of rotation, dislocation, and/or angulation of fracture fragments, it is important to take at least 2 radiographic images perpendicular to each other. Radiographic images must be repeated to control the progress of healing in a stabilized fracture. At the beginning of the fracture-healing process, the fracture line/crack widens as a result of low perfusion of bony tissue being depleted by macrophages, and only later narrows again. Compared with other species, such as horses, cattle react with a considerable amount of mineralized callus formation even with internal fixation (**Fig. 8**).[26] The first signs of mineralized callus are radiologically visible at 7 to 10 days after the trauma, which is a very short time span in comparison with equines.

Another long-bone abnormality often diagnosed in adult cattle is the formation of a bone sequestrum, generally caused by a severe blunt impact on the periosteum and bone.[17] In the acute stage, sequestra are not recognizable on radiographic images. At

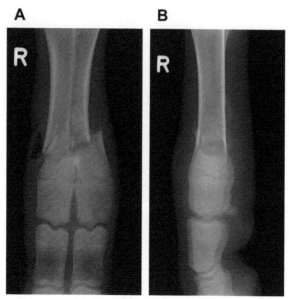

Fig. 7. Dorsopalmar (*A*) and lateromedial (*B*) projections of metacarpus III/IV; Simmental calf, 11 days old; subacute comminuted fracture of the left metacarpal metaphysis with slight dislocation of the distal main fragment and gas pockets within the soft tissues.

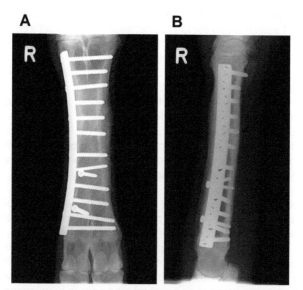

Fig. 8. Dorsopalmar (*A*) and lateromedial (*B*) projections of metacarpus III/IV; Red Holstein heifer, 18 months old; 3 months after internal fracture fixation; moderate amount of partially inhomogeneous (especially at the level of the screw tips), irregular, and sharply defined new bone formation dorsally, medially, and palmarly at the metacarpus III/IV.

first, mostly discrete radiolucent lines and incomplete structural interruptions are visible, which affect the periosteal aspect of the cortex. Multiple radiographic images can be necessary to find such discrete lines. Later on, the typical radiographic signs of a sequestrum formation become evident. At least 1 nondislocated bone fragment becomes progressively demarcated (sequestrum), surrounded by a radiolucent area (cloaca). Massive periosteal reactions (involucrum) form around the sequestrum. After about 7 to 10 days, these new bone formations are mineralized and become radiographically visible. The soft tissue is considerably thickened in the area of the lesion (**Fig. 9**). Afterward a radiolucent band can be identified in some cases from the radiolucent area to the bone surface (sinus tract).

Infections of the growth plates are often seen in young animals.[6,23] In healthy young animals, the physis shows up as an overlapping, soft-tissue opaque, well-defined curved line (cartilage). The physis narrows with aging until only a thin line of increased radiopacity, the so-called physeal scar, remains. In the case of sepsis the following lesions can be observed: broadened physis, vaguely delineated and irregular lysis, sclerotic zones, and soft-tissue swelling (**Figs. 10** and **24A**). Irregular, opaque new bone formations may appear at the edges of the growth plate.

Joints

To depict joints, 2 projections perpendicular to each other are usually performed. With complex joints such as carpus or tarsus, additional oblique radiographs must also be made so that all joint edges and contours may be reliably evaluated. In adult cattle, all joints distal to elbow and stifle can be radiographed in the standing position. It is possible to depict the hip, stifle, shoulder, and elbow joints in the standing animal,

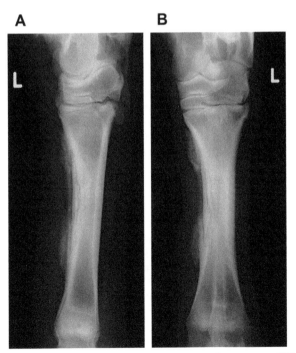

Fig. 9. Dorsoplantar (*A*) and lateromedial (*B*) projections of metatarsus III/IV; Red Holstein calf, 3.5 months old; bone fragment demarcation with significant callus formation of the left metatarsus III/IV.

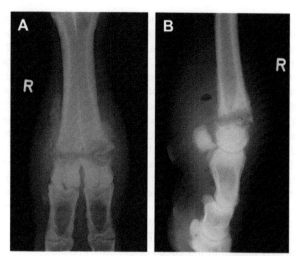

Fig. 10. Dorsopalmar (*A*) and lateromedial (*B*) projections of metacarpus III/IV; Red Holstein heifer, 2 years old; aggressive bone lesion at the level of the right distal metacarpal growth plate with emphysematous soft-tissue swelling and abscess formation; Salter-Harris type I fracture of the right distal metacarpus III/IV.

but the quality is poor, lacking in contrast when compared with radiographic images taken with the animal lying down. Joints of calves, in contrast to adult cattle, are better radiographed with the calf sedated and recumbent, which is done mainly to optimize radiation protection. With the calf sedated, it can be positioned in such a way that radiographs of high quality are the result; moreover, no assistants need be present in the radiography room during the examination.

In healthy cattle, the following joint structures are radiographically visible, and should be routinely evaluated: the position of the bones constituting the joint, the width of the joint space, the appearance of the joint contours, the width of the subchondral bone plates, the joint edges, and the periarticular soft tissues.

Increased soft-tissue opacity in the area of a joint may be due to a space-occupying process in the joint capsule and/or in the joint cavity and/or in the periarticular soft tissue (**Fig. 11**).[19,20,22] Intra-articular soft-tissue swelling is mainly caused by a joint effusion. Important information concerning the integrity of the ligaments is provided by evaluating the position and angle of the joint-forming bones (**Fig. 12**). Deviations from the axis indicate ligament ruptures. Such instabilities may be more reliably diagnosed by means of stress radiographs or when the limb is weight bearing. The radiologically visible joint space comprises all tissues present between the opposing subchondral bone plates including the joint cartilage, the synovial fluid, and possibly intracapsular ligaments or menisci. If the joint space appears to be narrowed, this indicates the destruction of the joint cartilage, for example in a case of advanced osteoarthritis (**Fig. 13**). Widening of the joint space, on the other hand, is a sign of joint effusion (**Fig. 14**). When the limb is not weight bearing, widening of the joint space may not represent a pathologic process. The age of the animal must also be taken into account; calves have a thicker joint cartilage than adults, which makes the joint space appear radiographically wider. It is therefore often advisable to produce a comparative radiographic image of the contralateral limb in growing animals, so that diagnostic uncertainties may be eliminated. Next to be evaluated are the joint contours, which appear sharply defined and smooth in the healthy animal. An irregular surface of the

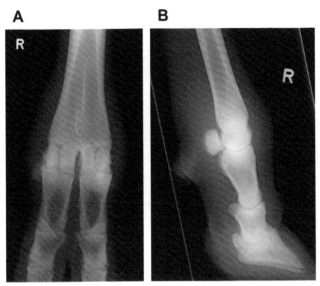

Fig. 11. Dorsopalmar (*A*) and lateromedial (*B*) projections of the metacarpophalangeal joint; Red Holstein cow, 3 years old; pronounced soft-tissue swelling in the area of the right metacarpophalangeal joint.

subchondral bone plate can be termed an erosive arthropathy, the cause of which in cattle is almost always a septic articular process. Attention must also be paid to the joint edges. If these appear irregular because of new bone formation (osteophytes), this indicates a chronic joint instability; osteophytes are interpreted as signs of osteo-arthritis (see **Fig. 13**).

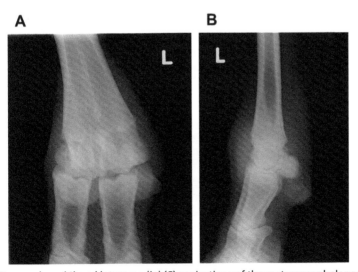

Fig. 12. Dorsopalmar (*A*) and lateromedial (*B*) projections of the metacarpophalangeal joint; Holstein-Friesian heifer, 2 years old; medial subluxation and osteoarthritis of the left meta-carpophalangeal joint; moderate osteoarthritis of the left metacarpophalangeal joint.

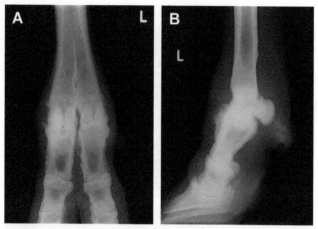

Fig. 13. Dorsopalmar (*A*) and lateromedial (*B*) projections of the metacarpophalangeal joint; Holstein-Friesian cow, 6 years old; moderate axial and abaxial osteoarthritis of the left metacarpophalangeal joint and severe ossifying periostitis of the proximal phalanges and the distal part of metacarpus III/IV.

Finally, the subchondral bone plates are evaluated. Thickening or sclerosis is a sign of increased stress, which typically shows up when joint cartilage is lost. There may be a generalized or localized reduction in the opacity of the subchondral bone plate. Localized increased radiopacity of the subchondral bone plate (lytic zones) mostly

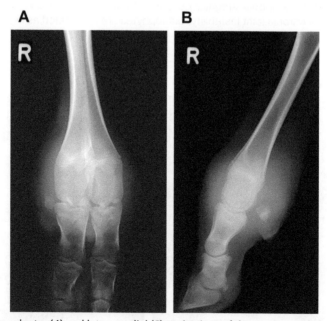

Fig. 14. Dorsoplantar (*A*) and lateromedial (*B*) projections of the metatarsophalangeal joint; Red Holstein calf, female, 5 weeks old; distinct effusion of the right metatarsophalangeal joint; slight erosion of the lateral subchondral bone plate and the axial medial proximal sesamoid bone.

appears with septic articular processes or degenerative joint disease. A generalized reduction in the opacity or width of the subchondral bone plates can be seen in cases of long-lasting reduction of weight bearing occurring following severe lameness or after administration of a walking cast (inactivity hypotrophy).

DIAGNOSTIC ULTRASONOGRAPHY IN BOVINE ORTHOPEDICS

In recent years, ultrasonography has been introduced as a routinely applied diagnostic imaging method for bovine limb disorders in many veterinary teaching hospitals globally.[8,9,27–40] Making a clinical diagnosis in limbs with diffuse soft-tissue swelling and in cattle with disorders of the proximal limb is often challenging. It is frequently impossible to identify with certainty the incriminated anatomic structures where 2 or more adjacent synovial cavities (joints, tendon sheaths, bursae) or adjoining muscles are involved.[8,30,41–45] Ultrasonography is superior to radiography for the diagnosis of conditions affecting the soft tissues.[2,46,47] It is ideal for evaluation of musculoskeletal disorders such as arthritis, tenosynovitis, bursitis, and tendon and muscle lesions, because they are frequently associated with extensive soft-tissue swelling and inflammatory exudation (**Figs. 15–44**).[8,19,27,30,31,35–37,41–45,48–53]

Preparation of the Patient

Ultrasonography of the bovine limbs, except the digits, is best achieved with the patient standing. For evaluation of the digits, particularly the metacarpo-/metatarsophalangeal and interphalangeal joints, the animal can be confined in a chute with the affected limb raised and secured, or placed in lateral recumbency on a hoof-trimming table.[8,9] If sedation is required, xylazine (0.05–0.1 mg/kg) or detomidine (10 μg/kg) may be administered intravenously.[54] Calves can be examined standing or restrained in lateral recumbency.[8,9] The region of interest is clipped, washed, and cleaned with alcohol, and coupling gel is applied.

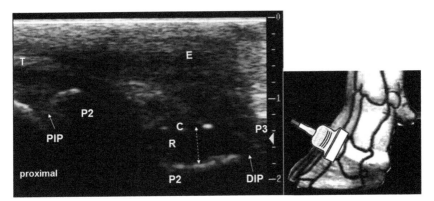

Fig. 15. Each schematic drawing in all the sonograms shows the corresponding position of the transducer in the standing animal to achieve the depicted sonogram. Longitudinal sonogram (7.5-MHz linear transducer) of the dorsal aspect of the right digital region showing a serous arthritis of the distal interphalangeal (DIP) joint in a 2.5-year-old Holstein-Friesian cow. C, capsule and dorsal border of the distended joint pouch (R), which contains an anechoic effusion (*dashed line between arrows*); DIP, distal interphalangeal joint space between the extensor process of phalanx 3 (P3) and the articular surface of phalanx 2 (P2); E, subcutaneous edema; PIP, proximal interphalangeal joint; T, extensor tendon.

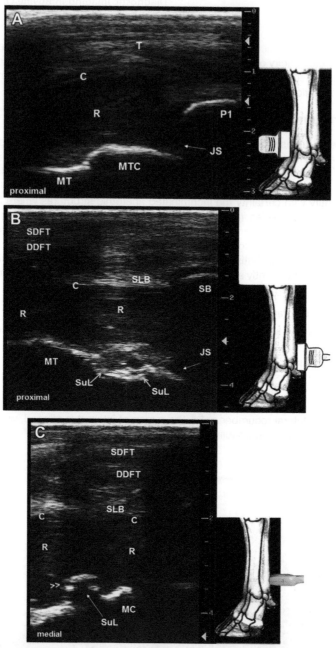

Fig. 16. (*A*) Longitudinal sonogram (7.5-MHz linear transducer) of the dorsal aspect of the metatarsophalangeal joint of the left, lateral digit with a fibrinopurulent arthritis in a 3.5-month-old Simmental bull calf. C, joint capsule; JS, joint space; MT, metatarsus; MTC, convex condyle of the metatarsus; P1, phalanx 1 with normal smooth bone contour; R, severely distended dorsal recess containing hypoechoic effusion; T, extensor tendon. (*B, C*) Longitudinal (*B*) and transverse (*C*) sonograms (7.5-MHz linear transducer) of the plantar aspect of the metatarsophalangeal joint of *A*. C, joint capsule; DDFT, deep digital flexor tendon; JS, joint space; MT, metatarsus; R, severely distended plantar recess of the fetlock joint containing a heterogeneous hypoechoic effusion (*arrowheads*); SB, proximal sesamoidal bone; SDFT, superficial digital flexor tendon; SLB, suspensory ligament branch; SuL, subchondral bone lesion due to osteolysis.

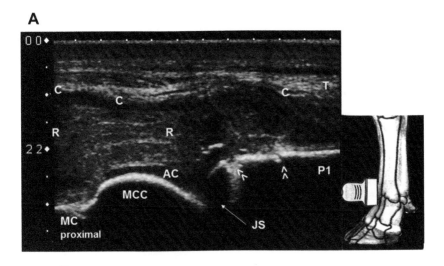

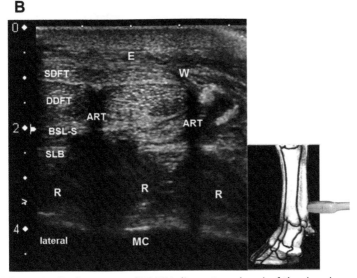

Fig. 17. (*A*) Longitudinal sonogram (7.5-MHz linear transducer) of the dorsal aspect of the metacarpophalangeal joint of the right, lateral digit with a septic fibrinous arthritis and bone sequestration in a 6.5-month-old Simmental bull caused by trauma. AC, anechoic articular cartilage; C, joint capsule; JS, joint space; MC, metacarpus; MCC, convex condyle of the metacarpus; P1, phalanx 1 with irregular contour of the bone due to osteolysis of a sequestrated small bone area (*arrowheads*) at the proximal aspect; R, severely distended dorsal recess of the fetlock joint containing heterogeneous hypoechoic effusion without flow phenomena; T, extensor tendon. (*B*) Transverse sonogram (7.5-MHz linear transducer) of the palmar aspect of the right metacarpal region of the calf in *A*, showing the severely distended palmar pouch of the fetlock joint with normal appearance of the digital flexor tendons and the flexor tendon sheaths (DFTS). ART, edge-shadowing artifact; BSL-S, branch of the suspensory ligament to the SDFT; C, palmar joint capsule of the fetlock joint; DDFT, deep digital flexor tendon; E, subcutaneous edema; MC, plantar surface of the metacarpus; SDFT, superficial digital flexor tendon; SLB, branches of the suspensory ligament; R, severely distended palmar recess of the fetlock joint containing mainly hypoechoic effusion; W, wall of the DFTS.

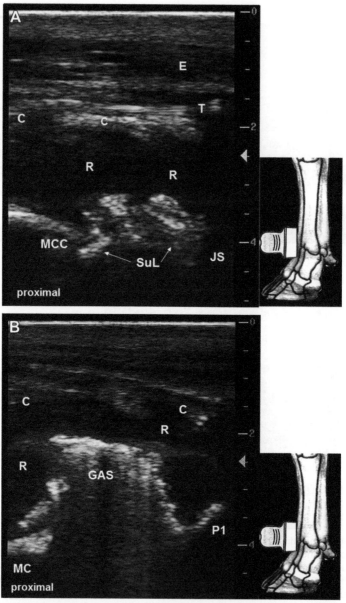

Fig. 18. (*A*, *B*) Longitudinal sonograms (7.5-MHz linear transducer) of the dorsal aspect of the metacarpophalangeal joint of the right, lateral digit with a purulent arthritis and osteomyelitis in a 2.8-year-old Simmental cow caused by trauma. C, joint capsule; E, subcutaneous edema; JS, joint space; MCC, convex condyle of the medial metacarpus; P1, proximal phalanx; R, severely distended dorsal recess containing a heterogeneous hypoechoic effusion without flow phenomena; SuL, subchondral bone lesion of the condyle with osteolysis and bone fragments; T, extensor tendon. Sonogram *B* shows the medial dorsal pouch with a large gas accumulation (GAS) represented by the hyperechoic band creating artifacts distally.

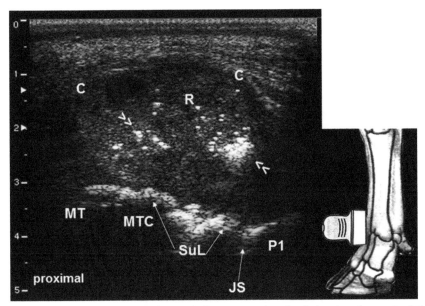

Fig. 19. Longitudinal sonogram (7.5-MHz linear transducer) of the dorsal aspect of the metatarsophalangeal joint of the left, medial digit with a purulent arthritis and osteomyelitis in a 4.8-year-old Simmental cow caused by a laceration wound. C, joint capsule; JS, joint space; MTC, condyle of the medial metatarsus; P1, proximal phalanx; R, severely distended dorsal recess containing a heterogeneous hypoechoic effusion with flow phenomena and many small hyperechoic reflexes (*arrowheads*); SuL, subchondral bone lesion of the condyle with severe osteolysis. The normal convex contour (see **Fig. 17A**) is destroyed.

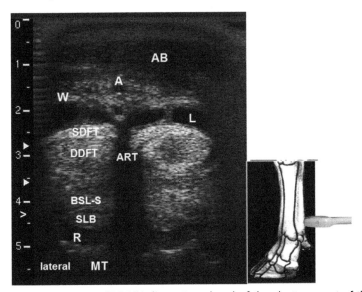

Fig. 20. Transverse sonogram (7.5-MHz linear transducer) of the plantar aspect of the distal left metatarsus showing the lateral and medial digital flexor tendon sheath (DFTS), the digital flexor tendons, and the plantar pouch of the fetlock joint in a 4.5-year-old Red Friesian cow with septic serous tenosynovitis of the DFTS. A, common digital plantar artery III; AB, subcutaneous abscess; ART, edge-shadowing artifact; BSL-S, branch of the suspensory ligament to the superficial flexor tendon; DDFT, deep digital flexor tendon; L, lumen of the DFTS with anechoic effusion; MT, plantar surface of the metatarsus; R, normal plantar pouch of the fetlock joint; SDFT, superficial digital flexor tendon; SLB, abaxial branch of the suspensory ligament; W, DFTS wall.

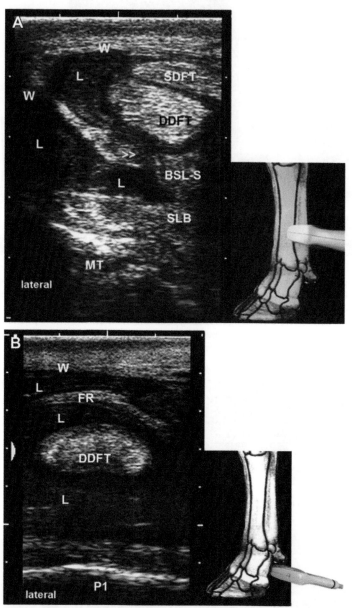

Fig. 21. (*A, B*) Transverse sonograms (7.5-MHz linear transducer) of the lateral DFTS of the left hindlimb with a septic, fibrinous tenosynovitis in a 3.5-year-old Simmental cow. (*A*) Plantar aspect of the distal metatarsal region. BSL-S, branch of the suspensory ligament to the SDFT; DDFT, deep digital flexor tendon; L, distended lumen of DFTS compartments with hypoechoic effusion without flow phenomena; MT, plantar surface of the metatarsus; SLB, axial branch of the suspensory ligament; SDFT, superficial digital flexor tendon; W, DFTS wall. (*B*) Distal compartment of the DFTS in the lateral pastern region with the severely distended lumen (L); the DDFT; the DFTS wall (W); the flexor retinaculum (FR); and the plantar contour of the proximal phalanx (P1).

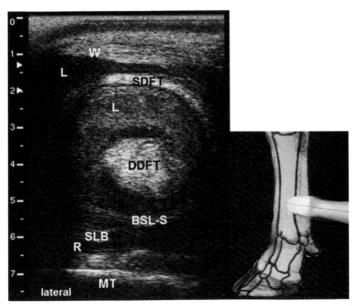

Fig. 22. Transverse sonogram (7.5-MHz linear transducer) of the plantar aspect of the distal right metatarsal region in a 6-year-old Simmental cow with purulent tenosynovitis of the lateral DFTS. BSL-S, branch of the suspensory ligament to the SDFT; DDFT, deep digital flexor tendon; L, highly distended outer and inner compartments of DFTS with hypoechoic effusion; MT, plantar metatarsal surface; SDFT, superficial digital flexor tendon; SLB, abaxial branch of the suspensory ligament; R, normal plantar fetlock joint pouch; W, DFTS wall.

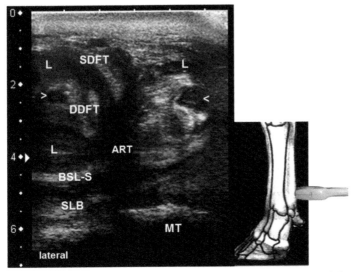

Fig. 23. Transverse sonogram (7.5 MHz linear transducer) of the distal plantar left metatarsal region in a 4.5-year-old Simmental cow with a fibrinopurulent tenosynovitis of the lateral and medial digital flexor tendon sheath (DFTS) and a purulent inflammation and necrosis of parts of the deep digital flexor tendon fibers (DDFT). ART, edge-shadowing artifact; BSL-S, branch of the suspensory ligament to the SDFT; L, highly distended outer and inner compartments of DFTS with hypoechoic effusion; MT, metatarsal surface; SDFT, superficial digital flexor tendon; SLB, abaxial branch of the suspensory ligament. Area between arrowheads indicates core lesions in the medial and lateral DDFT due to purulent inflammation of tendon fibers.

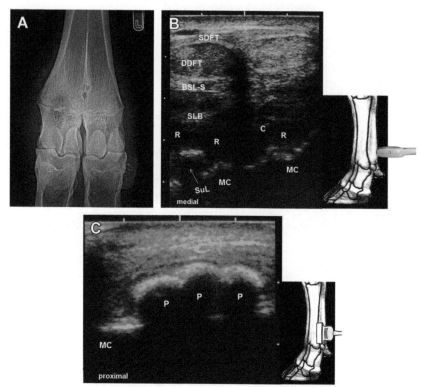

Fig. 24. (*A*) Dorsoplantar radiograph of the distal left metacarpal region and the metacarpophalangeal joint of a 12-month-old Holstein-Friesian heifer showing a radiolucent, well-demarcated osteomyelitic lesion involving parts of the medial metaphysis, physis, and epiphysis, periosteal bone proliferation at the medial bone surface, and soft-tissue swelling, caused by a hematogenous infection. The fetlock joint space appears normal. (*B*) Transverse sonogram (7.5-MHz linear transducer) of the plantar aspect of the metacarpophalangeal joint of the heifer in *A* showing a serofibrinous arthritis of the fetlock joint, which could not be assessed by radiography. BSL-S, branch of the suspensory ligament to the SDFT; C, joint capsule; DDFT, deep digital flexor tendon; MC, metacarpus; R, distended plantar recess containing an anechoic effusion; SDFT, superficial digital flexor tendon; SLB, suspensory ligament branch; SuL, subchondral bone lesion due to periosteal bone proliferation. (*C*) Longitudinal sonogram (7.5-MHz linear transducer) of the medial aspect of the distal metacarpal bone of the heifer in *A* showing the normal smooth contour of the bone proximally (MC) and an altered bone surface with periosteal proliferations (P), consistent with the radiographically assessed periosteal bone proliferations in *A*.

Method of Ultrasonographic Examination

A 7.5-MHz (5–8 MHz with a multifrequency probe) linear transducer is recommended for examination of superficial structures that are less than approximately 6 cm from the skin surface. This frequency can also be used to examine all the joint regions of calves that are only a few weeks old.[8,9,41,49,55,56] For evaluation of thick muscle bellies of the trunk, hip, thigh, and shoulder region in adult cattle and severe swelling anywhere on the limb, the use of a 5.0- or 3.5-MHz convex transducer is advised.[8,31,35–38,41,45,57,58]

The examiner starts by obtaining a general overview of the region of interest for orientation purposes by locating and imaging anatomic landmarks, such as bone

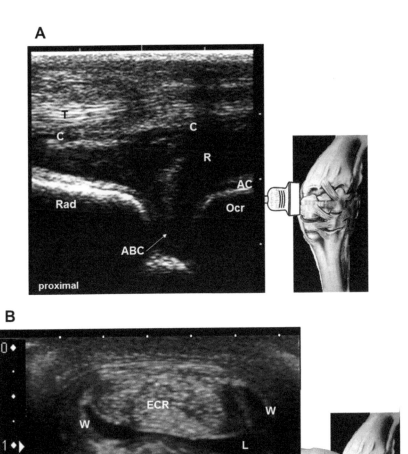

Fig. 25. (A) Longitudinal sonogram (7.5-MHz linear transducer) of the dorsal left carpal region in a 5-week-old Limousin bull calf with fibrinopurulent arthritis of the left antebrachiocarpal (ABC) joint. ABC, joint space of ABC joint; AC, anechoic articular cartilage; C, joint capsule; Ocr, radial carpal bone; R, clearly distended joint recess with a heterogeneous anechoic and hypoechoic appearance; Rad, surface of radius; T, extensor carpi radialis tendon. (B) Transverse sonogram (7.5-MHz linear transducer) of the left cranial distal antebrachial region of the calf in A showing the extensor carpi radialis tendon (ECR) and its tendon sheath with a septic serous inflammation. Rad, surface of radius; W, wall of the tendon sheath clearly differentiated because of the distended lumen (L) with anechoic effusion.

surfaces, cartilaginous growth plates of long bones, joint spaces, tendons, ligaments, or large blood vessels. These features are easy to identify because of their location, shape, or surface characteristics.[8,9,46] Once the anatomic landmarks in the area of interest have been identified, the search for pathologic changes begins.[8,9,31,47]

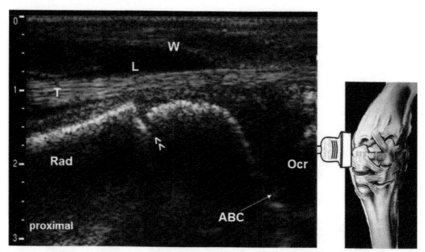

Fig. 26. Longitudinal sonogram (7.5-MHz linear transducer) of the dorsal aspect of the left carpus of a 10-week-old Simmental bull calf showing a fibrinopurulent arthritis of the ante-brachiocarpal (ABC) joint. ABC, joint space of ABC joint; C, joint capsule; Ocr, radial carpal bone; R, distended joint recesses with heterogeneous hypoechoic effusion without acoustic enhancement and without flow phenomena; Rad, surface of radius; T, extensor carpi radialis tendon with a slight, mainly anechoic effusion of the tendon sheath; W, wall of the tendon sheath. Double arrowhead indicates cartilaginous growth plate of the distal radius.

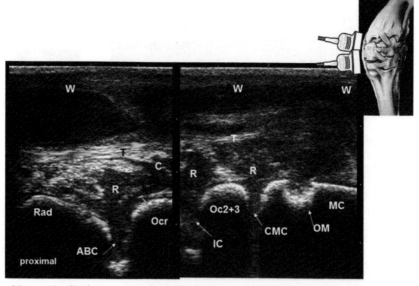

Fig. 27. Longitudinal sonograms (7.5-MHz linear transducer) of the dorsal aspect of the left carpus of a 2-week-old Simmental calf with fibrinopurulent arthritis of the antebrachiocarpal (ABC), intercarpal (IC), and carpometacarpal (CMC) joints and with osteomyelitis of the prox-imal metacarpus. ABC, IC, CMC, joint spaces of ABC, IC, and CMC joints; C, joint capsule; MC, metacarpal surface with normal hyperechoic smooth contour; Ocr, radial carpal bone; Oc2+3, second and third carpal bone; OM, osteomyelitic bone lesion; R, distended joint recesses with heterogeneous hypoechoic effusion without acoustic enhancement and without flow phenomena; Rad, surface of radius; T, extensor carpi radialis tendon with mainly anechoic effusion in the tendon sheath; W, wall of the highly distended tendon sheath.

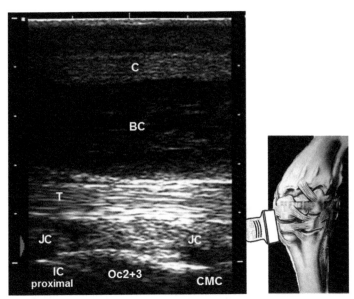

Fig. 28. Longitudinal sonogram (7.5-MHz linear transducer) of the dorsal aspect of the right carpal region showing normal intercarpal (IC) and carpometacarpal (CMC) joints and a purulent carpal hygroma (bursitis) in a 2.5-year-old Simmental cow. BC, severely distended bursa cavity with mainly anechoic effusion; C, capsule of the bursa; C, joint capsule in direct contact with the articular surface; Oc2+3, second and third carpal bones; T, extensor carpi radialis tendon.

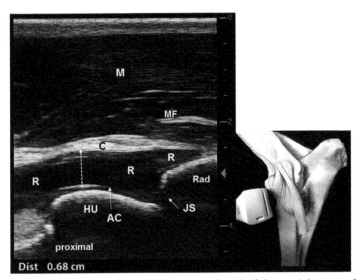

Fig. 29. Longitudinal sonogram (7.5-MHz linear transducer) of the cranial aspect of the right elbow joint of a 6-week-old Holstein-Friesian calf with a septic serous arthritis. AC, articular cartilage; C, joint capsule; Dist, width of the distended pouch (6.8 mm); HU, convex surface of the humeral condyle; JS, joint space of the elbow joint; M, extensor carpi radialis muscle; MF, muscle fascia; R, clearly distended cranial recess with anechoic effusion (*dashed arrow*); Rad, surface of radius.

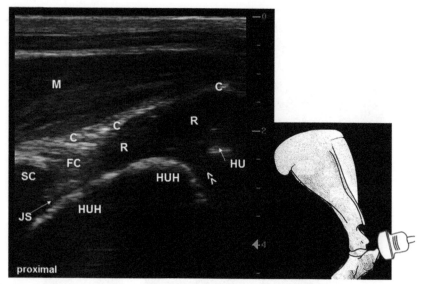

Fig. 30. Longitudinal sonogram (3.5-MHz convex transducer) of the craniolateral aspect of the left scapulohumeral joint of a 4-month-old Brown-Swiss calf with a septic, serous arthritis. C, joint capsule; FC, hypoechoic cartilage covering the distal rim of scapula; HU, hyperechoic surface of the humerus distal of the growth plate; HUH, hyperechoic convex surface of humeral head; JS, joint space of the scapulohumeral joint; M, supraspinatus muscle; R, the recess, which is slightly distended in the distal aspect with an anechoic effusion; SC, hyperechoic surface of the distal scapula. Double arrowhead indicates cartilaginous (anechoic) growth plate of the humeral head, making the contour of the humeral head appear interrupted.

The region of interest must be examined systematically: always examined longitudinally, transversely, and sometimes obliquely, proximal to distal, cranial to caudal, and medial to lateral. The entire length of ligaments, tendons, and tendon sheaths is examined, and all joint pouches (dorsal/cranial, palmar/plantar/caudal, lateral, medial) are inspected. Just as the clinical examination follows a standardized protocol, so too should the ultrasonographic examination, ensuring that all anatomic structures in the region of interest are carefully inspected.[8,9,46,47]

The following criteria must be evaluated:

The exact anatomic location of the structure/lesion
Echogenicity, echo pattern, size of the structure/lesion
Type of border of the lesion/cavity and of the soft-tissue swelling
The presence or absence of flow phenomena
The presence of artifacts such as acoustic enhancement or acoustic shadowing (see **Figs. 15–44**).[8,9,31]

Flow phenomena can be elicited by balloting or compressing a fluid-filled cavity with the transducer or manually, and by passive flexion or extension of the joint.[8,9,31,43,44,46,55,56] The presence of flow phenomena indicates liquid content, which may be serous, serofibrinous, purulent, or hemorrhagic.[30,31,41,43,44,48,49] Absence of flow phenomena indicates a semisolid to solid content, such as fibrinous clotted exudate or clotted blood.[30,31,41,43,44,49,50]

The size of distended synovial cavities, abscesses, hematomas, and other fluid accumulations as well as the distance between the skin surface and lesion can be

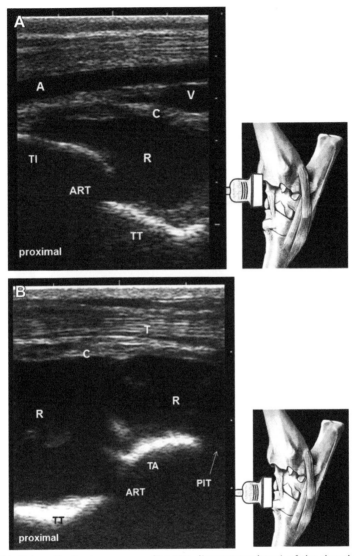

Fig. 31. (A, B) Longitudinal sonograms (7.5-MHz linear transducer) of the dorsal aspect of the left tarsocrural joint showing the dorsal joint pouch with septic serofibrinous arthritis (polyarthritis) in a 3-year-old Simmental cow. A, dorsal pedal artery; ART, artifact caused by the perpendicular course of the bone surface impeding ultrasound-wave reflection; C, joint capsule; PIT, joint space of the proximal intertarsal joint; R, distended joint recess with a mainly anechoic effusion and acoustic enhancement indicated by the broad hyper-echoic band of reflection on the lateral ridge of the talus and trochlea tali (TT); T, extensor tendon; TI, tibia; V, vein.

accurately measured using the electronic cursors (see **Figs. 15** and **29**). Comparison with the contralateral normal limb is recommended in cases of doubt.[8,9] Joints should be examined in the normal and flexed positions (see **Fig. 38**) to allow inspection of as much articular surface as possible and to detect possible subchondral lesions.[8,9,31,41,49]

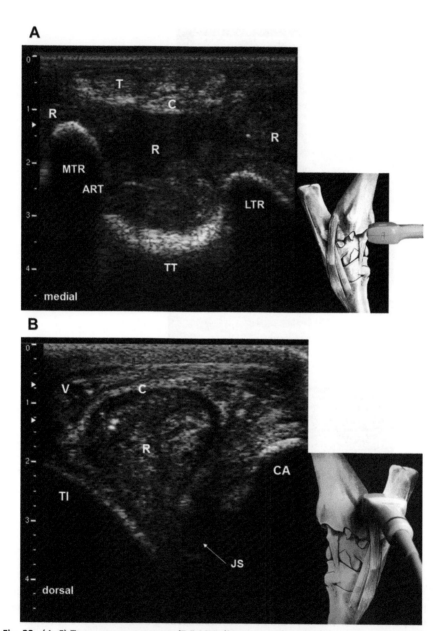

Fig. 32. (*A, B*) Transverse sonograms (7.5-MHz linear transducer) of the dorsal (*A*) and laterocaudal joint pouches (*B*) of the right tarsocrural joint in a 6-week-old Simmental bull calf with a fibrinopurulent arthritis. ART, artifact caused by the perpendicular position of the bone surface of MTK/LTK and TT impeding ultrasound-wave reflection; C, joint capsule; JS, joint space; LTR, lateral ridge of the talus; MTR, medial ridge of the talus; R, dorsal/laterocaudal pouch with heterogeneous effusion without flow phenomena; T, extensor tendon; TI and CA, hyperechoic surfaces of tibia and calcaneus; TT, trochlea tali; V, vein.

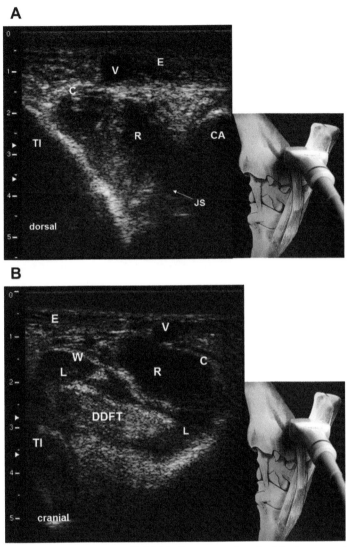

Fig. 33. (*A, B*) Transverse sonograms (7.5-MHz linear transducer) of the laterocaudal (*A*) and mediocaudal (*B*) aspects of the left tarsocrural joint of a 6.5-year-old Simmental cow showing a serofibrinous arthritis of the tarsocrural joint and a concurrent serofibrinous tenosynovitis of the directly adjoining tarsal flexor tendon sheath (TFTS). C, joint capsule; E, subcutaneous edema; R, severely distended joint recess in the triangle between the hyperechoic tibial surface (TI) cranially and the hyperechoic calcaneal surface (CA) caudally, the effusion showing a heterogeneous appearance with anechoic and hypoechoic zones; DDFT, digital flexor tendon and flexor hallucis longus tendon; JS, joint space; L, distended lumen of TFTS; V, lateral/medial saphenous vein; W, wall of TFTS.

Many large vessels (medial and lateral saphenous artery and vein, median artery and vein) and smaller distal vessels can be inspected ultrasonographically (see **Figs. 20**, **31**A, **32**B, **33**A, B).[53,59–61] Each vessel is evaluated along its course (see **Fig. 31**A), noting pulsation of arteries, compressibility of veins, and the presence of

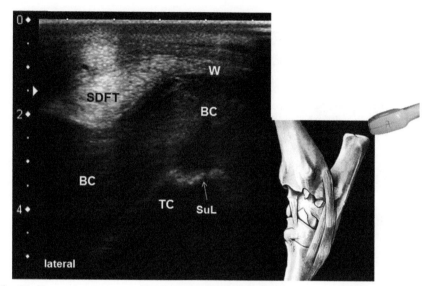

Fig. 34. Transverse sonogram (7.5-MHz linear transducer) of the caudal aspect of the left tarsus showing a purulent inflammation of the bursa subtendinea calcanei and a small osteolytic area of the tuber calcis in a 5-year-old Simmental cow. BC, distended bursa cavity with a heterogeneous hypoechoic effusion; SDFT, superficial digital flexor tendon; SuL, lysis of the fibrocartilage of the tuber calcis and subchondral osteolysis; TC, tuber calcis; W, wall of the bursa.

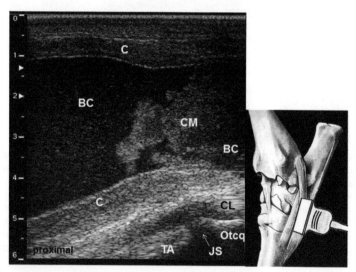

Fig. 35. Longitudinal sonogram (7.5-MHz linear transducer) of the lateral aspect of the right tarsus showing a purulent bursitis (bursitis tarsalis lateralis) in a 3.5-year-old Simmental cow. BC, highly distended bursa cavity with a heterogeneous mainly anechoic effusion with many minute echoic reflexes in the proximal part, and a more hypoechoic effusion with clotted masses (CM) distally; C, thick capsule of bursa; CL, lateral collateral ligament; JS, normal joint space between the talus (TA) and the centroquartal tarsal bone (Otcp).

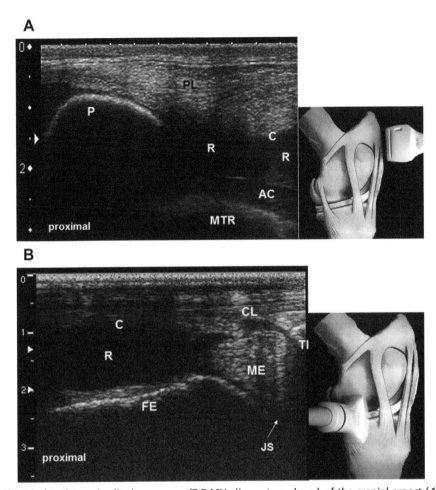

Fig. 36. (A, B) Longitudinal sonogram (7.5-MHz linear transducer) of the cranial aspect (A) of the left femoropatellar joint (A) and the medial aspect of the left femorotibial joint (B) showing serous inflammation of both joint recesses in a 10-week-old Simmental bull calf (same as in **Fig. 26**). AC, articular cartilage; C, joint capsule; CL, medial collateral ligament; JS, joint space; ME, medial meniscus; MTR, hyperechoic surface of the medial trochlear ridge of the femur (FE); P, surface of the basis of patella; PL, intermediate patellar ligament; R, markedly distended recess of the femoropatellar/medial femorotibial joint with anechoic effusion; TI, tibial surface.

intraluminal thrombi, which are associated with loss of compressibility and increased intraluminal echogenicity.[8,53,59–61] For the evaluation of blood flow, color Doppler can be applied.[47]

Ultrasonographic standard examination planes in bovine limbs
The region of interest and all anatomic structures within should always be viewed longitudinally and transversely in their entirety. However, for practical purposes there are certain ultrasonographic planes that facilitate orientation, making identification and evaluation of the region of interest easier for the operator.[8,9,28,29,55–58]

For all the joint regions (joint-associated structures such as joint capsule, joint-forming bone surfaces, joint pouches, collateral ligaments) of the bovine limbs, the

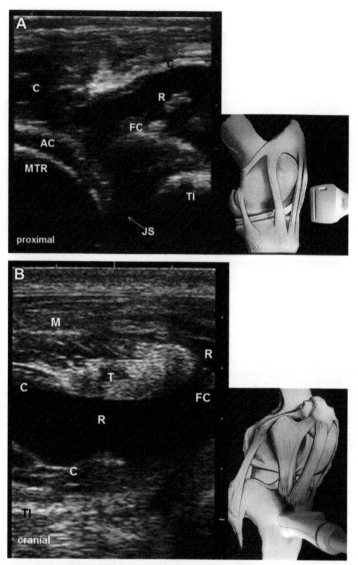

Fig. 37. (*A, B*) Longitudinal sonogram (7.5-MHz linear transducer) of the craniolateral aspect of the right femoropatellar joint (*A*) and transverse sonogram of the distal pouch of the lateral femorotibial joint (*B*) showing a serofibrinous arthritis in a 4-month-old Simmental calf. AC, articular cartilage; C, joint capsule; JS, joint space; M, long digital extensor muscle; MTR-FE, hyperechoic surface of the medial trochlear ridge of the femur; R, markedly distended recess with anechoic effusion and some hypoechoic fibrin clots (FC); T, tendon of peroneus muscle; TI, tibial surface.

standard examination plane of choice is the longitudinal for the dorsal (cranial), lateral, palmar/plantar (caudal), and medial aspects, depending on the anatomy (see **Figs. 15, 16**A, B, **17**A, **18**A, **19, 25**A, **26, 27, 29, 30, 31**A, **36**A, B, **37**A).[8,9,28,35,43,44,55,56,58,62] Cartilaginous growth plates at the distal and/or proximal ends of the long bones in calves are also imaged longitudinally (see **Figs. 26** and **40**).[8,9,49]

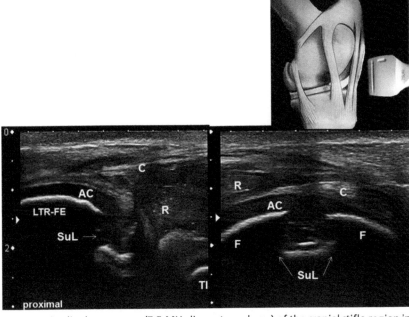

Fig. 38. Longitudinal sonograms (7.5-MHz linear transducer) of the cranial stifle region in an 8-day-old Scottish Highland bull calf with a fibrinopurulent arthritis of the left femoropatellar joint and osteomyelitis. AC, articular cartilage; C, joint capsule; LTR-FE, hyperechoic surface of the lateral trochlear ridge of femur; R, recess with heterogeneous mainly echoic effusion difficult to differentiate from the surrounding tissue; SuL, subchondral osteolysis of the lateral femoral condyle with interruption of the normal hyperechoic bone surface and convex contour of the condyle caused by bone infection; TI, proximal surface of tibia. The right sonogram shows the same bone lesion in the flexed stifle joint allowing a much better imaging of the condyle; F, lateral trochlear ridge of the femur.

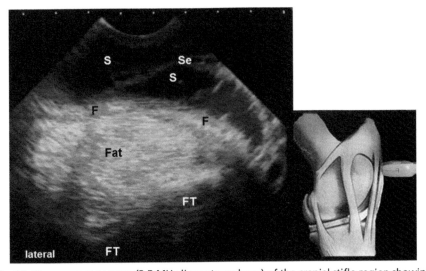

Fig. 39. Transverse sonogram (3.5-MHz linear transducer) of the cranial stifle region showing a subcutaneous seroma located cranially of the femoropatellar joint in a 5-year-old cow. F, stifle fascia; Fat, fatty tissue; FT, typical sinusoidal contour of femoral trochlea (the normal femoropatellar joint recess cannot be visualized); S, seroma with mainly anechoic fluid; Se, thin septa of connective tissue.

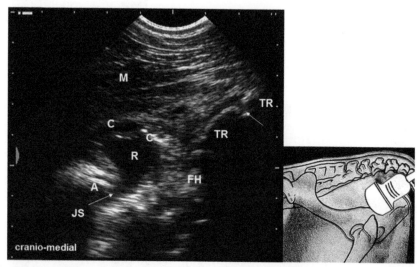

Fig. 40. Longitudinal-oblique sonogram (3.5-MHz linear transducer) showing a purulent arthritis of the right coxofemoral joint and osteolysis of the femoral head in a 6-month-old Brown-Swiss calf. Arrow on right indicates apophyseal growth plate A, surface of acetabulum; C, coxofemoral joint capsule; JS, joint space between the acetabulum and femoral head (FH), which shows a completely irregular raw surface indicating osteolysis; M, gluteal muscles; R, distended joint recess with anechoic effusion; TR, trochanter major.

Transverse planes are the standard examination planes of choice for the suspensory ligament, the digital, carpal, and tarsal tendons, and their tendon sheaths, and for muscles, because they allow a better overview (see **Figs. 17**B, **20, 21**A, B, **22, 23, 24**B, **25**B, **33**B, **37**B).[8,9,28,33,39,43,44,48,63–65]

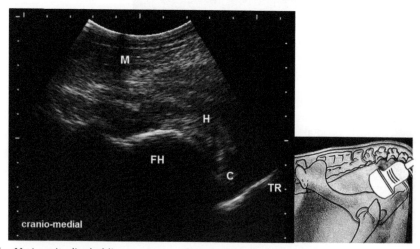

Fig. 41. Longitudinal-oblique sonogram (3.5-MHz linear transducer) showing a coxofemoral luxation in a 6-month-old Simmental calf. The surface of the acetabulum cannot be imaged. C, lacerated joint capsule; FH, dislocated femoral head, more than 3 cm distant from the normal position; H, coagulated blood indicating a hematoma; M, gluteus medius muscle; TR, surface of trochanter major.

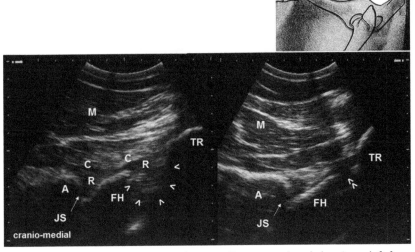

Fig. 42. Longitudinal-oblique sonogram (3.5-MHz linear transducer) showing a left femoral capital physeal fracture in an 8-week-old Holstein-Friesian calf. Pattern of arrowheads point to fracture cleft indicated by the wide distance between the femoral head and the contour of the trochanter major (TR). A, surface of acetabulum; C, coxofemoral joint capsule; JS, joint space between the acetabulum and femoral head (FH); M, gluteus medius muscle; R, slightly distended joint recess with hypoechoic effusion. By careful manipulation (flexion and extension) of the left hindlimb during sonography, an abnormal movement could be assessed in the fracture zone. The sonogram on the right shows the normal appearance of the right coxofemoral joint in the same calf. Double arrowhead indicates normal epiphyseal growth plate.

The oblique longitudinal plane along the femoral neck axis is suited best for the inspection of the coxofemoral joint. The transducer is placed on the trochanter major and moved craniomedially toward the cranial end of the sacrum.[8,9,57] This action allows one to image the surface of trochanter major, femoral neck and head, joint space, acetabulum, and the joint capsule (see **Figs. 40–42**). In adult cattle, a 3.5-MHz convex transducer is required to image the coxofemoral joint, which usually lies 12 to 18 cm distant from the skin surface.[38,57]

Transrectal ultrasonography (4–8-MHz linear rectal probe) allows evaluation of the entire bony pelvic girdle, the ventral aspect of the caudal lumbar vertebrae and sacrum, the iliosacral joints, and the abdominal aorta and its proximal branches.[57]

Ultrasonographic Appearance of Musculoskeletal Disorders

Table 1 lists the normal ultrasonographic appearance of the structures of the musculoskeletal system. Normal synovial cavities in cattle are difficult or impossible to visualize via ultrasonography because of the very small physiologic amount of synovial fluid.[8,9,28,55,56,58] Inflammatory (septic) processes and traumatic soft-tissue injuries are especially suitable to be diagnosed with the aid of ultrasonography because of fluid accumulation in the affected tissues.[30,37,41–44,48–53,63,65,66] As the pathologic

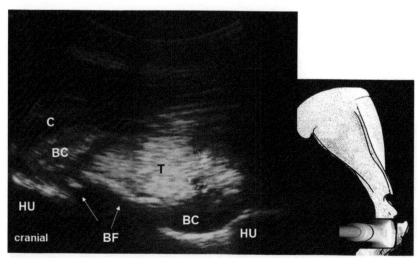

Fig. 43. Transverse sonogram (3.5-MHz convex transducer) of the lateral aspect of the left scapulohumeral joint region of a 4-year-old Charolais bull with a traumatic bursitis of the tendon of infraspinatus muscle with a concurrent avulsion fracture of a part of the insertion site of the tendon. BC, the bursa cavity is clearly distended and shows a heterogeneous hypoechoic effusion caused by clotted blood; BF, a large and a small avulsed bone fragment at the insertion site of the tendon branch; C, capsule of bursa; HU, surface of humerus; M, deltoid muscle; T, superficial branch of tendon of infraspinatus muscle.

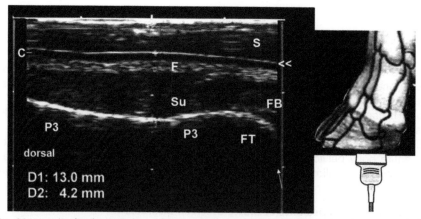

Fig. 44. Longitudinal sonogram of the middle and plantar weight-bearing area of the medial claw of a right hindlimb showing the 4.2-mm thick sole horn layer (S), a thin echogenic line indicating the sole horn/corium border (*arrowheads*), the very thin, anechoic corium layer (C), the less echogenic, reticular patterned outer layer of the subcutis (fascia: F), and the main anechoic part of the subcutis (Su) with hypoechoic columns. FB, fat pad; P3, clearly outlined, hyperechoic solar surface of the distal phalanx (P3) reaching to the flexor tubercle (FT).

Table 1 Normal ultrasonographic appearance of important structures of the musculoskeletal system	
Skin	Thin Echoic Line
Connective tissue	Echogenicity varies from hypoechoic to echoic, depending on the density of the tissue
Fat tissue	Echogenicity varies from nearly anechoic to hypoechoic
Muscle	Less hypoechoic with characteristic echoic to hyperechoic striations caused by the muscle septa in longitudinal planes; and small irregular, pinpoint, echoic to hyperechoic reflections of the septa in transverse planes
Tendon, ligament	Homogeneous echoic structure of varying size with a distinct, linear, and parallel arrangement of the fiber bundles
Bone surface	Smooth hyperechoic reflective band with total acoustic shadowing distally
Growth plate in calves	Cartilaginous growth plates of long bones and the apophyseal growth plates of the olecranon, the greater tubercle of the humerus, calcaneus, tibial tuberosity, and trochanter major appear as short anechoic interruptions of the hyperechoic bone surface in the longitudinal plane
Articular cartilage	Thin anechoic seam over the subchondral hyperechoic bone of the joint
Joint space	Narrow interruption of the hyperechoic bone surfaces with funnel-shaped inward-curved contours of the joint-forming bones
Joint recess (pouch)	Normally, the joint cavity cannot be imaged; sometimes only very small anechoic zones at the level of the joint space can be identified
Joint capsule	Thin echoic structure lying close to the articular surface in healthy joints
Meniscus	Homogeneous echoic triangular-shaped structure
Vessels	Anechoic tubular or band-shaped structures enveloped by thin echoic lines (wall; seen especially in arteries); arteries show pulsations, veins can be compressed completely

Data from Refs.[8,9,19,28,29,31–33,55–59]

changes are ultrasonographically very similar in all inflamed synovial cavities, they are discussed here as one.

Arthritis, tenosynovitis, and bursitis

Septic disorders of synovial cavities occur frequently in cattle.[1,2,30,35–37,41–45,51,54,67–69] Traumatic arthritis is often associated with tearing or rupture of collateral (cruciate) ligaments, the joint capsule, and luxation or subluxation.[2,8,38,69,70] Synovial effusion can be detected reliably using ultrasonography even in the early stages.[8,9,19,29–32,35–37,39,41–45,48,49,51,52,63,66] The diseased synovial cavity (joint recess, tendon sheath, bursa) appears mildly to severely dilated with a thin echoic capsule, which is distinctly displaced from the articular surface (see **Figs. 15–23, 24**B, **25–38, 40, 43**). The echogenicity of the effusion ranges from anechoic to echoic depending on its nature (serous, serofibrinous, fibrinous, purulent).[8] Anechoic or hypoechoic content allows good differentiation of the synovial cavity from surrounding tissues, which are generally echoic (see **Figs. 15–18, 20, 21**B, **24**B, **25**A, B, **26, 28–31**A, B, **35, 36**A, B, **40**), whereas echoic content does not (see **Figs. 19, 38, 43**).[30,31,36,41,43,44,49] Liquid content can be identified based on flow phenomena, which are characterized by small and large hypoechoic to echoic particles or clots that are seen floating in the anechoic fluid (see **Figs. 16**A, B, **19, 21**A, B, **25**A, **28, 31**B, **33**A, **35, 37**A). In long-standing cases of sepsis, the precipitated gelatinous masses of fibrin impair or prevent aspiration of fluid, and these semisolid masses appear hypoechoic to echoic and show no flow phenomena (see **Figs. 17**A, **32**A, B, **38**).[19,30,31,35–37,41,43,44,46,48,49,51,54,63] Based on history, physical examination, and the cause of the disorder, the experienced clinician has a relatively good idea of the consistency and nature of the synovial fluid. A definitive answer is provided by centesis.[4,5,8]

Fresh blood in the joint cavity caused by trauma (hemarthrosis) appears homogeneously anechoic, similar to hematomas that are only a few hours old.[50,71] Later on in the disease process, the ultrasonographic appearance becomes similar to that of coagulated blood, characterized by heterogeneous hypoechoic masses (see **Fig. 43**) with well-demarcated anechoic areas.[41,50,71] An accurate ultrasonographic diagnosis of traumatic arthritis or bursitis can be made when lesions of the joint capsule, tendon (see **Figs. 41** and **43**), bone, the collateral and cruciate ligaments or the menisci can be identified[8,9,70,72]; centesis might reveal a hemorrhagic sample.[4,5]

In cattle with swollen joints, the differential diagnosis includes concurrent tenosynovitis, hematoma, seroma, periarticular abscess, or edema. In cases of periarticular disorders without any involvement of the articular structures, the joint pouch appears normal and the fluid accumulation is located completely extra-articularly (eg, tenosynovitis, bursitis, or subcutaneous seroma) (see **Figs. 21**A, **22, 28, 35, 39**).[8,9]

The most commonly affected tendon sheath in cattle is the digital flexor tendon sheath of the hindlimbs (see **Figs. 20–23**).[30,33,39,48,63,65,68,69,73,74] Septic disorders of other tendon sheaths are uncommon, but occasionally occur in the sheaths of the tendons of the extensor carpi radialis muscle and the common and lateral digital extensor muscles, the carpal flexor muscles, and the tendons of the flexor hallucis longus and tibialis caudalis muscles in the tarsus (see **Figs. 25**B, **26, 33**B).[43,44,48,52,68,69,73,74] Aseptic tenosynovitis of the tendon of the extensor carpi radialis muscle has also been described.[43,48,75]

The most commonly incriminated bursae are the bursa subcutanea and subtendinea calcanei (see **Fig. 34**), the bursa tarsalis lateralis (see **Fig. 35**), and the bursa praecarpalis (carpal hygroma) (see **Fig. 28**).[35,43,44,48,68,70] The bursa intertubercularis, the bursa of the tendon of the infraspinatus (see **Fig. 43**), and the biceps femoris muscle[36,37] are rarely affected. The involved bursae can be identified using anatomic landmarks such as tendons that run below or above them, and the characteristic bone contours.[8,9,36,37]

Tendinitis and desmitis

The main indications for ultrasonography are swellings along the course of tendons or ligaments with a history of trauma, wounds with possible damage to tendons and/or ligaments, and suspected tenosynovitis.[8,9,36,37] The diagnosis of aseptic tendinitis or desmitis with partial fiber rupture and/or avulsion fracture of their insertion site (see **Fig. 43**) has been documented in cattle.[73,74] The sonographic appearance can be expected to be similar to that in horses.[76,77] The sonographic appearance of diseased flexor tendons is well documented in cattle,[28,30,33] including infection of the digital flexor tendon sheaths with purulent necrosis of the tendon, and tendons with circular defects caused by a penetrating foreign body.[8,9] These defects were characterized by a circumscribed, diffuse decrease or complete loss of echogenicity, loss of the parallel fiber arrangement, or the presence of anechoic focal lesions extending over a considerable length, caused by purulent infection (see **Fig. 23**).[8,9,30,63]

Muscle disorders

One of the main indications for ultrasonography is swelling involving muscles, decubital ulcers of the skin over muscle bellies, and septic tendinitis and tenosynovitis at the transition from muscle to the tendon of origin.[8,9] Depending on the causative event (eg, trauma, chronic ischemia and hypoxia owing to continuous pressure, severe udder edema, iatrogenic origin), muscle trauma may result in the formation of hematomas, muscle tears, compartment syndrome, muscle necrosis, or abscess.[68,76–79] Various ultrasonographic patterns have been described, including anechoic fluid accumulations of various sizes in fresh muscle hematomas, irregularly shaped lesions with scattered low-level echoes (muscle tears), ill-defined echoic areas with loss of normal muscle striations and overall increase in muscle echogenicity (muscle compartment syndrome, muscle necrosis), and highly reflective zones with acoustic shadowing and loss of normal muscle architecture.[76,78–81] Chronic muscle injuries develop fibrosis and scarring characterized by heterogeneous areas of increased echoes.[76,79]

Bone lesions

Radiography is the method of choice for the evaluation of bone lesions, such as fractures, luxation, and osteomyelitis (see **Fig. 24**A).[6,7,11] Some bones are difficult to assess with radiography, such as the scapula, ribs, and pelvis, as well as the bones of distal limbs. These bones can be examined ultrasonographically if a radiographic unit is not available.[8,9] The pelvis may be examined transcutaneously and transrectally.[8,9,57] Ultrasound waves are reflected by the bone surface and are completely absorbed, so that only the bone surface can be evaluated.[47,66] The normal bone contour appears as a smooth hyperechoic reflective band (see **Figs. 16**A, **25**A, B, **26**, **29**, **36**A, B).[31,41,55,56,66,82] Fractures are characterized by an abnormal interruption or a step in the smooth contour of the bone (see **Figs. 42** and **43**). Careful manipulation of the affected limb may exacerbate this gap during ultrasonography. In other cases, a bone structure might be found in an abnormal area or position, as in the case of coxofemoral luxation whereby the femoral head is displaced into the gluteal muscles (see **Fig. 41**).[38] Small bone fragments in the soft tissues produce hyperechoic reflections with distal acoustic shadowing (see **Fig. 43**).[70,82,83] Concurrent fracture-associated hematomas appear as anechoic to hypoechoic areas of varying size around the fracture site (see **Figs. 41** and **42**).[77,82,83]

Early ultrasonographic signs of osteitis and osteomyelitis, before they can be detected radiographically, include thickening and displacement of the echoic periosteum from the bone by anechoic exudate, and swelling of the surrounding soft tissue.[77,79,84] Bone lysis and periosteal reaction appear later as irregular roughening and interruption of the normal contour of the bone surface (see **Figs. 17**A, **18**A, **24**B, C, **27**, **34**, **38**).[8,9,31,49]

A new and interesting application of ultrasonography is the evaluation of the thickness of the claw sole horn and the underlying soft-tissue layer, and the assessment of changes of the distal pedal bone surface, in dairy cattle in the context of laminitis (see **Fig. 44**).[34,40,85,86]

Abscess and hematoma

Because of their morphology, abscesses generally have a heterogeneous appearance.[8,9,43,44,50,79] Abscesses are characterized by a predominantly anechoic content, which is well demarcated from the surrounding tissues and may contain unevenly distributed, small, floating hypoechoic reflections (see **Fig. 20**). Furthermore, many minute echoic to hyperechoic reflections (gas bubbles) or large dorsal gas pockets can be seen, and flow phenomena can also be elicited.[8,9,50] Therefore, abscesses are echogenically similar to a purulent arthritis (see **Figs. 18**B and **19**).

Fresh hematomas have an anechoic appearance, flow phenomena, and some acoustic enhancement. With progressive coagulation, heterogeneous areas are noted with alternating anechoic (fluid), hypoechoic, and echoic (organized) zones.[8,9,50,71] Ultrasonography facilitates differentiation of abscesses, hematomas, and seromas (see **Fig. 39**), especially when they are located near joints, tendon sheaths, bones, and vessels. Subsequent needle aspiration should confirm the diagnosis.[8,47]

Ultrasound-Assisted Needle Aspiration or Biopsy

If the unit is available, ultrasonographic inspection of the structure of interest should always be carried out before centesis.[8,9] The position and size of the distended cavity and the location of liquid effusion within, as well as its distance and direction from a set point on the skin surface, can be determined accurately using the electronic cursors. After assessing the direction and depth of the structure to be punctured by ultrasound guidance,[8,9,31] the needle may be inserted with or without (free hand) ultrasound guidance.[8,9,47,84,87,88] The same technique can also be used for puncture or biopsy collection of veins suspected of containing septic thrombi or any abnormal masses.[8,9]

Summary

Ultrasonography is an imaging modality that can be applied anywhere in bovine practice and allows rapid noninvasive differentiation of soft-tissue structures of the bovine musculoskeletal system.[8,9] Ultrasound units with linear transducers of 5.0 to 7.5 MHz, commonly used in large animal reproduction, are well suited for rapid and straightforward differentiation of soft-tissue swelling in the limbs.[8,9,31,35,36,43,44,52–54] In addition, ultrasonography can be very helpful in detecting foreign bodies in the limbs or trunk that cannot be diagnosed radiographically.[39]

Ultrasonography provides accurate information about the location and size of lesions or fluid-filled cavities, the surrounding tissues, and the nature of the content, making puncture more precise and safer.[8,9,47] The physiologic amount of synovial fluid of normal synovial cavities in cattle cannot be imaged by ultrasonography; visualization of effusion is easy and usually indicates an inflammatory process (see **Table 1**).[8,9] Therefore, ultrasonography can detect early stages of inflammation of synovial cavities (see **Fig. 24**), based on an increased amount of effusion and distension of the synovial pouch.

An early diagnosis, accurate anatomic differentiation of the soft-tissue structures involved, characterization of the lesions, and a thorough preoperative inspection of incriminated regions are of enormous benefit in determining an accurate prognosis as well as planning surgery and treatment.[8,9]

COMPUTED TOMOGRAPHY AND MAGNETIC RESONANCE IMAGING IN BOVINE ORTHOPEDICS

The use of computed tomography (CT) and magnetic resonance imaging (MRI) in bovine orthopedics is limited to well-equipped veterinary clinics, mainly because of the high costs of the units and the need for general anesthesia.[89–91] Nevertheless, these imaging techniques can be an option in highly valuable cattle[10] for achieving a comprehensive diagnosis needed for preoperative planning of a surgical intervention.[90,91] The technical preconditions for CT and MRI in bovines were described by Ehlert and colleagues[90] and Nuss and colleagues.[91] Indications for the use of CT and MRI in bovine limbs/digits that have been reported include anatomic studies,[85,89,90,92–95] and only rarely clinical applications such as evaluation of the tympanic bulla in calves with otitis media.[96–98]

REFERENCES

1. Bailey JV. Bovine arthritides: classification, diagnosis, prognosis, treatment. Vet Clin North Am Food Anim Pract 1985;1(1):39–51.
2. Weaver AD. Joint conditions. In: Greenough PR, Weaver AD, editors. Lameness in cattle. 3rd edition. Philadelphia: WB Saunders; 1997. p. 162–70.
3. Stanek C. Examination of the locomotor system. In: Greenough PR, Weaver AD, editors. Lameness in cattle. 3rd edition. Philadelphia: WB Saunders; 1997. p. 14–23.
4. Dirksen G. Bewegungsapparat. In: Dirksen G, Gründer HD, Stöber M, editors. Die klinische Untersuchung des Rindes. 3rd edition. Berlin: Parey; 1990. p. 549–91.
5. Rohde C, Anderson DE, Desrochers A, et al. Synovial fluid analysis in cattle: a review of 130 cases. Vet Surg 2000;29(4):341–6.
6. Farrow CS. The radiologic investigation of bovine lameness associated with infection. Vet Clin North Am Food Anim Pract 1985;1(1):67–81.
7. Steiner A, Geissbühler U, Stoffel MH, et al. Bovine radiology—digital diagnostic atlas. In: Steiner A, Geissbühler U, Stoffel MH, et al, editors. 1st edition. Bern (Switzerland): University of Berne; 2010.
8. Kofler J. Ultrasonography as a diagnostic aid in bovine musculoskeletal disorders. Vet Clin North Am Food Anim Pract 2009;25(3):687–731.
9. Kofler J. Ultrasonographic examination of the musculoskeletal system in cattle. Tierarztl Prax Ausg G Grosstiere Nutztiere 2011;39(5):299–313 [in German].
10. Steiner A. Current concepts and future developments in surgery, anaesthesia and pain management. In: Proceedings/keynote lectures of the 27th World Buiatrics Congress. Lisbon (Portugal): admédic; ISSN 0873/6758; 2012. p. 137–8.
11. Bargai U, Pharr JW, Morgan JP. Bovine radiology. 1st edition. Iowa State University Press; 1989.
12. Bargai U, Shamir I, Lublin A, et al. Winter outbreaks of laminitis in dairy calves: aetiology and laboratory, radiological and pathological findings. Vet Rec 1992; 131(18):411–4.
13. Dietz O, Prietz G, Haette R. Serial radiological examinations of the phalanges of A.I. bulls for judgement limb soundness. Wien Tierarztl Monatsschr 1971;58(4): 163–7 [in German].
14. Farrow CS. Digital infections in cattle. Their radiologic spectrum. Vet Clin North Am Food Anim Pract 1985;1(1):53–65.
15. Farrow CS. Calving chain fractures. Radiographic assessment of healing. Vet Clin North Am Food Anim Pract 1999;15(2):221–30.
16. Gantke S, Nuss K, Kostlin R. Radiologic findings in bovine laminitis. Tierarztl Prax Ausg G Grosstiere Nutztiere 1998;26(5):239–46 [in German].
17. Hirsbrunner G, Steiner A, Martig J. Diaphyseal sequestration of the hollow bones in cattle. Tierarztl Prax 1995;23(3):251–8 [in German].
18. Irwin MR, Poulos PW Jr, Smith BP, et al. Radiology and histopathology of lameness in young cattle with secondary copper deficiency. J Comp Pathol 1974; 84(4):611–21.
19. Kofler J. Septic arthritis of the proximal interphalangeal (pastern) joint in cattle - clinical, radiological and sonographic findings and treatment. Berl Munch Tierarztl Wochenschr 1995;108(8):281–9 [in German].

20. Stanek C, Kofler J. On the classification of radiological changes in septic arthritis of the distal interphalangeal joint in cattle: comparison of two scoring systems. Wien Tierarztl Monatsschr 1995;82:390–6.
21. Nigam JM, Singh AP. Radiographic interpretation: radiography of bovine foot disorders. Mod Vet Pract 1980;61(7):621–4.
22. Verschooten F, DeMoor A. Infectious arthritis in cattle: a radiographic study. Vet Radiol Ultrasound 1974;15(1):60–9.
23. Verschooten F, Vermeiren D, Devriese L. Bone infection in the bovine appendicular skeleton: a clinical, radiographic, and experimental study. Vet Radiol Ultrasound 2000;41(3):250–60.
24. ICRP. The 2007 Recommendations of the International Commission on Radiological Protection. ICRP Publication 103. Ann ICRP 2007;37:2–4.
25. Starke A, Heppelmann M, Beyerbach M, et al. Septic arthritis of the distal interphalangeal joint in cattle: comparison of digital amputation and joint resection by solar approach. Vet Surg 2007;36(4):350–9.
26. Gamper S, Steiner A, Nuss K, et al. Clinical evaluation of the CRIF 4.5/5.5 system for long-bone fracture repair in cattle. Vet Surg 2006;35(4):361–8.
27. Munroe GA, Cauvin ER. The use of arthroscopy in the treatment of septic arthritis in two highland calves. Br Vet J 1994;150(5):439–49.
28. Kofler J, Edinger H. Diagnostic ultrasound imaging of the soft tissues in distal bovine limb. Vet Radiol Ultrasound 1995;36(3):246–52.
29. Flury S. Ultrasonographic imaging of the tarsus in cattle [thesis]. Bern (Switzerland): Veterinary Medicine; 1996.
30. Kofler J. Ultrasonographic imaging of pathology of digital flexor tendon sheath in cattle. Vet Rec 1996;139(2):36–41.
31. Kofler J. Ultraschalluntersuchung am Bewegungsapparat. In: Braun U, editor. Atlas und Lehrbuch der Ultraschalldiagnostik beim Rind. Berlin: Parey Buchverlag; 1997. p. 253–68.
32. Schock B, Nuss K, Koestlin R. Ultrasonographic examination of the stifle in the calf. In: Proceedings of the 10th International Symposium on Lameness in Ruminants. Lucerne (Switzerland): 1998. p. 311–3.
33. Tryon KA, Clark CR. Ultrasonographic examination of the distal limb of cattle. Vet Clin North Am Food Anim Pract 1999;15(2):275–300.
34. Van Amstel SR, Palin FL, Rohrbach BW, et al. Ultrasound measurement of sole horn thickness in trimmed claws of dairy cows. J Am Vet Med Assoc 2003; 223(4):492–4.
35. Seyrek-Intas D, Celimli N, Gorgul OS, et al. Comparison of clinical, ultrasonographic, and postoperative macroscopic findings in cows with bursitis. Vet Radiol Ultrasound 2005;46(2):143–5.
36. Nuss K, Ringer S, Meyer SW, et al. Lameness caused by infection of the subtendinous bursa of the infraspinatus muscle in three cows. Vet Rec 2007;160(6): 198–200.
37. Nuss K, Räber M, Sydler T, et al. Bursitis mit schwerwiegenden Sehnen- und Muskelnekrosen an der Außenseite der Kniegelenke beim Rind. [Bursitis with severe tendon and muscle necrosis on the lateral stifle area in cattle]. Schweiz Arch Tierheilkd 2011;153:520–5 [in German].
38. Starke A, Herzog K, Sohrt J, et al. Diagnostic procedures and surgical treatment of craniodorsal coxofemoral luxation in calves. Vet Surg 2007;36(2):99–106.
39. Mulon PY, Achard D, Babkine M. Ultrasonographic diagnosis of porcupine quill foreign bodies in the plantar flexor tendon sheath region in a heifer. Can Vet J 2010;51(8):888–90.

40. Laven LJ, Laven RA, Parkinson TJ, et al. An evaluation of the changes in distance from the external sole surface to the distal phalanx in heifers in their first lactation. Vet J 2012;193(3):639–43.

41. Kofler J. Arthrosonography: the use of diagnostic ultrasound in septic and traumatic arthritis in cattle - a retrospective study of 25 patients. Br Vet J 1996;152(6):683–98.

42. Nuss K. Septic arthritis of the shoulder and hip joint in cattle: diagnosis and therapy. Schweiz Arch Tierheilkd 2003;145(10):455–63 [in German].

43. Kofler J, Martinek B. Ultrasonographic imaging of disorders of the carpal region in 42 cattle—arthritis, tenosynovitis, precarpal hygroma, periarticular abscess. Tierarztl Prax 2004;32(2):61–72 [in German].

44. Kofler J, Altenbrunner-Martinek B. Ultrasonographic findings of disorders of the tarsal region in 97 cattle—arthritis, bursitis, tenosynovitis, periarticular abscess and vein thrombosis. Berl Munch Tierarztl Wochenschr 2008;121(3–4):145–58 [in German].

45. Starke A, Heppelmann M, Meyer H, et al. Diagnosis and therapy of septic arthritis in cattle. Cattle Pract 2008;16(1):36–43.

46. Kofler J, Hittmair K. Diagnostic ultrasonography in animals—continuation of the clinical examination? Vet J 2006;171(3):393–5.

47. King AM. Development, advances and applications of diagnostic ultrasound in animals. Vet J 2006;171(3):408–20.

48. Kofler J. Application of ultrasonic examination in the diagnosis of bovine locomotory system disorders. Schweiz Arch Tierheilkd 1995;137(8):369–80 [in German].

49. Kofler J. Ultrasonography in haematogeneous septic arthritis, polyarthritis and osteomyelitis in calves. Wien Tierarztl Monatsschr 1997;84(5):129–39 [in German].

50. Kofler J, Buchner A. Ultrasonic differential diagnostic examination of abscesses, haematomas and seromas in cattle. Wien Tierarztl Monatsschr 1995;82(5):159–68 [in German].

51. Roth M, Nuss K. Der klinische Fall: septische Arthritis beider Tarsokruralgelenke metastatischen Ursprungs bei einem Kalb. Tierarztl Prax 1999;21(5):287, 379–81.

52. Nuss K, Maierl J. Tenosynovitis of the deep flexor tendon sheath (M. flexor digitalis lateralis et M. tibialis caudalis) at the bovine tarsus (16 cases). Tierarztl Prax 2000;28(6):299–306.

53. Kofler J, Martinek B, Kuebber-Heiss A, et al. Generalised distal limb vessel thrombosis in two cows with digital and inner organ infections. Vet J 2004;167(1):107–10.

54. Heppelmann M, Rehage J, Kofler J, et al. Ultrasonographic diagnosis of the septic arthritis of the distal interphalangeal joint in cattle. Vet J 2009;179(3):407–16.

55. Kofler J. Ultrasonographic examination of the stifle region in cattle—normal appearance. Vet J 1999;158(1):21–32.

56. Kofler J. Ultrasonographic examination of the carpal region in cattle—normal appearance. Vet J 2000;159(1):85–96.

57. Grubelnik M, Kofler J, Martinek B, et al. Ultrasonographic examination of the hip joint and the pelvic region in cattle. Berl Munch Tierarztl Wochenschr 2002;115(5–6):209–20 [in German].

58. Altenbrunner-Martinek B, Grubelnik M, Kofler J. Ultrasonographic examination of important aspects of the bovine shoulder—physiological findings. Vet J 2007;173(2):317–24.

59. Kofler J. Description and determination of the diameter of arteries and veins in the hindlimb of cattle using B-mode ultrasonography. J Vet Med A 1995;42(4):253–66 [in German].

60. Kofler J, Buchner A, Sendlhofer A. Application of real-time ultrasonography for the detection of tarsal vein thrombosis in cattle. Vet Rec 1996;138(2):34–8.
61. Kofler J, Kuebber-Heiss A. Long-term ultrasonographic and venographic study of the development of tarsal vein thrombosis in a cow. Vet Rec 1997;140(26): 676–8.
62. Saule C, Nuss K, Köstlin RG, et al. Ultrasonographic anatomy of the bovine carpal joint. Tierarztl Prax 2005;33(6):364–72 [in German].
63. Kofler J. Sonography as a new diagnostic tool for septic tenosynovitis of the digital flexor tendon sheath in cattle—therapy and long term follow-up. Dtsch Tierarztl Wochenschr 1994;101(6):215–22 [in German].
64. Martinek B, Zoltan B, Floeck M, et al. Chondrosarcoma in a Simmental cow—clinical, ultrasonographic, radiographic and pathological findings. Vet J 2006;172(1):181–4.
65. Bertagnoli A, Räber M, Morandi N, et al. Tenovaginoscopic approach to the common digital flexor tendon sheath of adult cattle: technique, normal findings and preliminary results in four clinical cases. Vet J 2012;191(1):121–7.
66. Chhem RK, Kaplan PA, Dussault RG. Ultrasonography of the musculoskeletal system. Radiol Clin North Am 1994;32(2):275–89.
67. Trent AM, Plumb D. Treatment of infectious arthritis and osteomyelitis. Vet Clin North Am Food Anim Pract 1991;7(3):747–78.
68. Dirksen G. Krankheiten der Bewegungsorgane. In: Dirksen G, Gründer HD, Stöber M, editors. Innere Medizin und Chirurgie des Rindes. 4th edition. Berlin: Parey; 2002. p. 764–975.
69. Stanek C. Tendons and tendon sheaths. In: Greenough PR, Weaver AD, editors. Lameness in cattle. 3rd edition. Philadelphia: WB Saunders; 1997. p. 188–94.
70. Martinek B, Huber J, Kofler J, et al. Bilateral avulsion fracture (apophyseolysis) of the calcaneal tuber in a heifer. Berl Munch Tierarztl Wochenschr 2003; 116(7–8):328–32 [in German].
71. Aufschnaiter M. Sonography of coagulating blood: experimental and clinical findings. Ultraschall Med 1983;4(2):110–3 [in German].
72. Dik KJ. Ultrasonography of the equine stifle. Equine Vet Educ 1995;7(3):154–60.
73. Anderson DE, St-Jean G, Morin DE, et al. Traumatic flexor tendon injuries in 27 cattle. Vet Surg 1996;25(4):320–6.
74. Anderson DE, Desrochers A, St Jean G. Management of tendon disorders in cattle. Vet Clin North Am Food Anim Pract 2008;24(3):551–66.
75. Klee W, Hänichen T. Epidemiologische, klinische und pathologisch-anatomische Untersuchungen über die Entzündung der Karpalgelenkstrecker beim Rind. [Epidemiologic, clinical and pathologo-anatomic studies of the inflammation of the carpal joint extensors in cattle]. Schweiz Arch Tierheilkd 1989;131(3):151–7.
76. Genovese RL, Rantanen NW. The superficial digital flexor tendon & The deep digital flexor tendon, carpal sheath, and accessory ligament of the deep digital flexor tendon (check ligament). In: Nyland TG, Mattoon JS, editors. Veterinary diagnostic ultrasound. Philadelphia: WB Saunders; 1998. p. 289–445.
77. Reef VB. Equine diagnostic ultrasound. Philadelphia: WB Saunders; 1998. p. 39–186.
78. Fornage BD, Touche DH, Segal P, et al. Ultrasonography in the evaluation of muscular trauma. J Ultrasound Med 1983;2(12):549–54.
79. Léveillé R, Biller DS. Muscle evaluation, foreign bodies and miscellaneous swellings. In: Nyland TG, Mattoon JS, editors. Veterinary diagnostic ultrasound. Philadelphia: WB Saunders; 1998. p. 515–21.
80. Reimers K, Reimers CD, Wagner S, et al. Skeletal muscle sonography: a correlative study of echogenicity and morphology. J Ultrasound Med 1993;12(2):73–7.

81. Smith RK, Dyson SJ, Head MJ, et al. Ultrasonography of the equine triceps muscle before and after general anaesthesia and in post anaesthetic myopathy. Equine Vet J 1996;28(4):311–9.

82. Shepherd MC, Pilsworth RC. The use of ultrasound in the diagnosis of pelvic fractures. Equine Vet Educ 1994;6(4):223–7.

83. Reisinger R, Altenbrunner-Martinek B, Kofler J. Sternal recumbency after traumatic injury of the caudal thoracic spine with fracture of the dorsal spinous processes of the thoracic vertebrae 11 to 13 in a heifer. Wien Tierarztl Monatsschr 2008;95(3–4):72–9 [in German].

84. Howard CB, Einhorn M, Dagan R, et al. Ultrasound in diagnosis and management of acute haematogenous osteomyelitis in children. J Bone Joint Surg Br 1993;75(1):79–82.

85. Kofler J, Kuebber P, Henninger W. Ultrasonographic imaging and thickness measurement of the sole horn and the underlying soft tissue layer in bovine claws. Vet J 1999;157(3):322–31.

86. Laven LJ, Margerison JK, Laven RA. Validation of a portable ultrasound machine for estimating sole thickness in dairy cattle in New Zealand. N Z Vet J 2012;60(2):123–8.

87. Tucker R. Ultrasound-guided biopsy. In: Nyland TG, Mattoon JS, editors. Veterinary diagnostic ultrasound. Philadelphia: WB Saunders; 1998. p. 649–53.

88. David F, Rougier M, Morisset S. Ultrasound-guided coxofemoral arthrocentesis in horses. Equine Vet J 2007;39(1):79–83.

89. Schwarze I. Computed tomography of the bovine tarsus [thesis]. Vet Med 1998. Faculty of Veterinary Medicine Munich, LMU University Munich, Germany. [in German].

90. Ehlert A, Ferguson J, Gerlach K. Magnetic resonance imaging and cross-sectional anatomy of the normal bovine tarsus. Anat Histol Embryol 2011; 40(3):234–40.

91. Nuss K, Schnetzler C, Hagen R, et al. Clinical application of computed tomography in cattle. Tierarztl Prax Ausg G Grosstiere Nutztiere 2011;39(5):317–24 [in German].

92. Raij AR, Sardari K, Mohammadi H. Normal cross-sectional anatomy of the bovine digit: comparison of computed tomography and limb anatomy. Anat Histol Embryol 2008;37(3):188–91.

93. Raji AR, Sardari K, Mirmahmoob P. Magnetic resonance imaging of the normal bovine digit. Vet Res Commun 2009;33(6):515–20.

94. El-Shafey A, Sayed-Ahmed A. Computed tomography and cross sectional anatomy of the metacarpus and digits of the one humped camel and Egyptian water buffalo. Int J Morphol 2012;30(2):473–82.

95. Tsuka T, Ooshita K, Sugiyama A, et al. Quantitative evaluation of bone development of the distal phalanx of the cow hind limb using computed tomography. J Dairy Sci 2012;95(1):127–38.

96. Bernier Gosselin V, Francoz D, Babkine M, et al. A retrospective study of 29 cases of otitis media/interna in dairy calves. Can Vet J 2012;53(9):957–62.

97. Wenzinger B, Hagen R, Schmid T, et al. Coxofemoral joint radiography in standing cattle. Vet Radiol Ultrasound 2012;53(4):424–9.

98. Siegrist A, Geissbühler U. Radiographic examination of cattle. Tierarztl Prax Ausg G Grosstiere Nutztiere 2011;39(5):331–40 [in German].

Indications and Limitations of Splints and Casts

Pierre-Yves Mulon, DMV, DES[a],*, André Desrochers, DMV, MS[b]

KEYWORDS

- Cattle • Fracture • Cast • Orthopedic • Lameness

KEY POINTS

- Simple casts are indicated for close transverse or short oblique fractures and carries an excellent prognosis.
- The foot should always be included with full or short limb casts.
- A transfixation pinning and casting technique avoids collapse of the comminuted fracture or severe overriding of long oblique fractures during weight-bearing.
- The cast should be changed every 3 to 4 weeks in newborn calves to avoid complications regarding their fast growing rate.

 Videos of full limb casting on a young calf and a young heifer with a full limb cast with a quasi-normal gait accompany this article at http://www.vetfood.theclinics.com/

Long bone fractures are relatively common in cattle whether they result from a self-inflicted trauma or from external factors (herd mate or farm machinery).[1] Various advanced orthopedic techniques have been described to stabilize and treat fractures in cattle with success. Unfortunately the use of most of those techniques remains unrealistic in a field setting, rendering the realization of splints and casts still accurate for the treatment of long bone fracture in cattle. However despite that use of cast is reported in cattle for more than a century,[2] some guidelines need to be followed to assure the best results to the investment made by the owner. This article refers to the use of all external coaptations and their specific indications as well as their limitations.

USE OF CASTS IN CATTLE

The goal of casting is to provide early weight-bearing and achieve adequate bone healing rapidly. Most patients are young with a strong periosteal healing potential.

[a] Hôpital Vétérinaire Lachute, 431 Prinicipale, Lachute, Quebec J8H 1Y4, Canada;
[b] Department of Clinical Sciences, Faculty of Veterinary Medicine, Université de Montréal, 3200 Sicotte, St-Hyacinthe, Quebec J2S 7C6, Canada
* Corresponding author.
E-mail address: pymulon@gmail.com

Vet Clin Food Anim 30 (2014) 55–76
http://dx.doi.org/10.1016/j.cvfa.2013.11.007   **vetfood.theclinics.com**
0749-0720/14/$ – see front matter © 2014 Elsevier Inc. All rights reserved.

Therefore, cattle are great orthopedic patients regarding fracture repair.[1] Compared with other species, they tolerate limb immobilization very well because of their calm nature, making the use of casts common in field conditions as well as in referral centers.

The principle of the application of a cast to treat a fractured limb is to immobilize the joints distally and proximally to the fractured bone so that once reduced and imbedded in the cast the bone fragments stay aligned for a sufficient period of time to allow secondary bone healing. Based on the anatomy of cattle, the most proximal joints that can be immobilized in a cast are the carpus in forelimbs and the tarsus in hindlimbs. Therefore fractures of the metacarpus and metatarsus III–IV are best suited to be treated with simple external coaptation.

Plaster of Paris and synthetic casting tapes have been commonly used in cattle. Plaster cast is cheap and easy to conform to the limb, but it is not waterproof and it is weaker and heavier than synthetic casts. Moreover, it takes 24 hours to cure and to gain its final strength-retarding weight-bearing.[3] It is still in used in neonates but it should never be used in an older, heavy animal. Nowadays synthetic casting is routinely used in farm animals. The conformability has been greatly improved over the years by using fiberglass or polyester fiber with polyurethane resin. Although more expansive, fiberglass casting is used more often because of its rapid curing, light weight, permeability, and radiolucent property. An in vitro study tested a synthetic cast cylinder under compression and torsion.[3] After 10, 30, 60, and 120 minutes of curing, the cast cylinder was at 30%, 62%, 70%, and 100% of its strength, respectively. Considering the time it takes to conform the casting tape and getting the animal standing, the cast can support the weight of the animals after 30 minutes. Fiberglass casting tapes keep 70% to 90% of their strength after being immersed in water and dried out. Even with this loss of strength, a wet fiberglass cast is 33% stronger than a dry plaster cast.[4]

Casting tapes come in different widths (2, 3, 4, and 5 inches) to fit different patient sizes. The appropriate width that will allow perfect conformability without any fold should be used. Usually smaller tapes are used first to better conform the limb, followed by wider tape. It was shown in an in vitro cast cylinder model that 5-inch casts were stronger.[5] The tape is spiraled around the limb with a 50% overlap from bottom to top.

SELECTION OF THE PATIENTS

The fractured animal should be carefully examined before attempting to put a cast on the leg. Characterization of the fracture with 2 orthogonal radiographic views (dorso-palmar/plantar and lateromedial) should be performed. Casts are especially indicated for simple transverse or short oblique diaphyseal fractures (**Fig. 1**) and metaphyseal fractures (Salter-Harris type 1 and 2) (**Fig. 2**). The use of a simple cast in the case of compound diaphyseal fractures and long oblique fracture is debatable as reinforcement with a walking bar or use of the transphyseal pinning and casting technique may be more appropriate if external coaptation has been chosen for treatment to external skeletal fixators; the use of open reduction and internal fixation will provide a better stability to the fracture.[6]

Examination of skin integrity is extremely important because casts are indicated for a closed fracture. The distal limb is not well protected by soft tissue, increasing the risk of open fracture, and contamination is highly probable in farm injuries. Any skin injury around the fracture line should be carefully examined. If doubtful, the hair should be clipped, and the wound cleaned and probed to evaluate its depth.

Alteration of the vasculature in the case of chain-induced fracture in newborn calves during forced extraction may occur without a clear break of the skin barrier (**Fig. 3**).

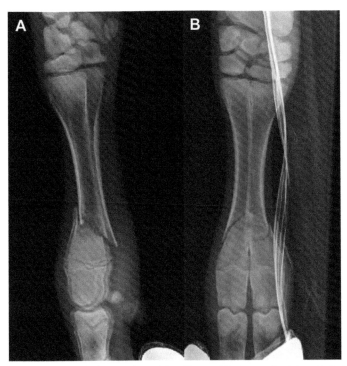

Fig. 1. Lateromedial (*A*) and dorsopalmar (*B*) radiographic views of calving chain fracture of the metacarpus III–IV in a 1-day-old Holstein heifer. It is a closed complete short oblique fracture of the distal metaphysis with a small dorsal displacement overriding the dorsal cortex of the proximal bone segment on the lateral-medial view.

The distal portion of the limb below the chain mark is usually swollen and might be cold to the touch if there is already thrombosis of the digital arteries.[7] Scintigraphy and arteriography can be used to objectively evaluate distal vasculature; however, it requires special equipment and is not easy to perform (**Fig. 4**). Moreover, treatment is extremely limited as far as specific treatment to vascular damage or thrombosis. It should be mentioned to the owner because it may lead to a necrosis of the distal aspect of the leg over time, which usually is unnoticed until cast removal.

GENERAL CAST TECHNIQUE

The material needed to create a cast is very simple: surgical stockinet, protecting felt pieces, and multiple rolls of fiberglass cast material. The animal should be placed in lateral recumbency with the affected leg uppermost. Heavy sedation or short-term intravenous general anesthesia is mandatory to reduce the fracture by traction and prevent inadvertent movements during the application of the cast and its hardening time. Two holes are drilled through the claw wall from the white line either at the toe or through the abaxial walls of each digit. A strong wire is passed through those holes and a rope is passed through the loop (**Fig. 5**). Moderate traction can then be applied while reducing the fracture of casting the limb. If more powerful traction is necessary, a rope is circled around the pastern or the fetlock, depending where is the fracture (**Fig. 6**).

Fracture reduction in a large animal is a combination of traction and fracture manipulation. Soft tissue swelling and muscle contraction initiate overriding of the bone

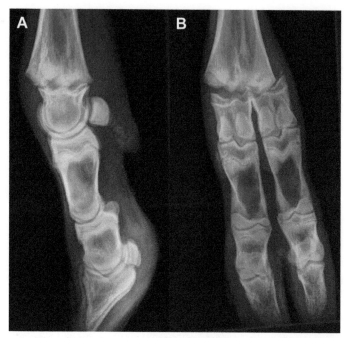

Fig. 2. Lateromedial (*A*) and dorsopalmar (*B*) radiographic views of a close complete distal physeal fracture of the metacarpus III–IV Salter-Harris type 2 on a 14-month-old Holstein heifer.

fragments to naturally stabilize the fracture. The goal of the reduction is to align the cortices and correct the rotation, as inadequate traction direction or strength can be detrimental. Physeal, overriding transverse, or short oblique fractures are reduced with the same technique. After correction of rotational alignment and with the limb under moderate traction, the fracture site is bent, until cortices of the compression side (concave side) are touching. Then the fractured bone is straightened and mild traction is kept to maintain the reduction. Reduction is assessed by palpation or with radiographs.

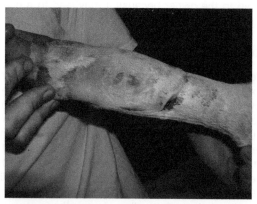

Fig. 3. Calving chain marks on the skin proximal to the swollen fetlock in a 1-day-old Holstein heifer. Those compression marks are sufficient to jeopardize the underlying vasculature of the distal extremity of the limb.

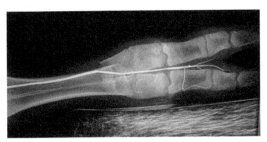

Fig. 4. A newborn calf with an obstetric fracture of the distal diaphysis of the metacarpi. An angiogram was performed to evaluate the distal limb perfusion. The contrast material is observed all the way down the digit, indicating that arterial perfusion is normal.

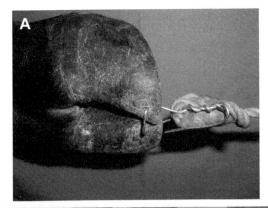

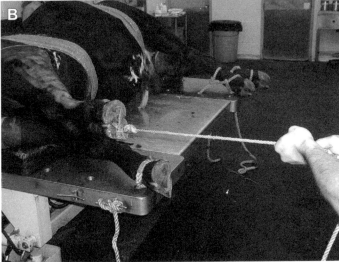

Fig. 5. (*A*) A heavy wire was passed through drill holes to allow traction (*B*) before reduction of the fracture.

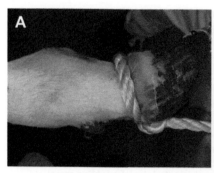
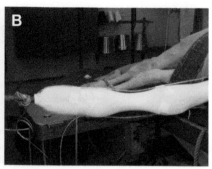

Fig. 6. (*A*) A Holstein heifer was presented with a distal physeal fracture of the metacarpus. A rope was used to reduce the fracture because more force was necessary and the wire though the claw could have failed under tension. (*B*) After reduction, the rope is removed and the reduction is stabilized by moderate traction on a claw wire loop.

Some basic principles must be strictly respected while immobilizing a fracture with a cast in large animals. The foot is always included in the cast. The proximal portion of the cast ends at the proximal aspect of a bone. The limb should be in a neutral position, respecting the normal biomechanic when the animal stands. Abnormal limb angulation will create undesired increased pressure under the cast and potential painful skin lesions.

Once the fracture is adequately reduced, a gentle tension is maintained on the leg by an assistant (Video 1). Pieces of felt of variable sizes are then placed over bony prominences and kept in place with white tape, taking care not to override the tape's extremities (**Fig. 7**). The tape must be loose, otherwise skin necrosis may occur. A triangular piece is inserted between the claws and a small rectangular piece is maintained just below the dewclaws (**Fig. 8**A). On forelimbs, the accessory carpal bone prominence is also a specific area to protect with a large square felt piece eventually thinned at its center for a better fit (see **Fig. 8**B). On hindlimbs both tibial malleoli should be protected as the tip of the calcaneus bone. Finally, the proximal aspect of the limb is protected by a 7- to 10-cm-wide band of felt. A double layer of stockinet or orthopedic felt is fit around the leg from the foot to the proximal aspect of the limb (**Fig. 9**). Then fiberglass tape is applied on the leg, starting at the fracture site. Each roll should overlap the previous one by 50%, as described earlier. Application of the cast must be fast enough so that all layers of casting material polymerize together, creating

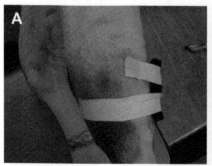
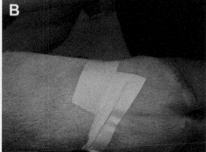

Fig. 7. (*A*) Tape of the accessory carpal bone padding as well as underneath the dewclaws (*B*) is not touching to avoid any stricture while drying or if the animal growth is rapid.

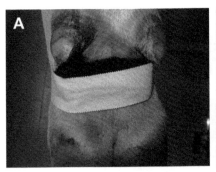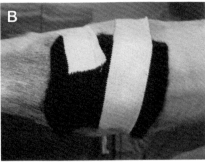

Fig. 8. (A) Padding just underneath the dewclaws to avoid skin ulceration from compression. (B) Padding over the accessory carpal bone.

a strong tubular structure. Otherwise the cast will laminate and will lose considerable strength. Tension applied to the first layer of casting material should be minimal to avoid folds in close contact with the limb. Tension is progressively increased to assure as much stability as possible to the fractured bone. The thickness of the fiberglass cast varies according to the weight of the animal. Animals weighting less than 150 kg should have between 6 and 8 layers; adult casts may have up to 16 layers of roll to assure sufficient strength.

Fiberglass casts are extremely strong in tension (convex side of the cast) and weaker in compression (concave side of the cast), rendering the risk of acute break of the cast at those specific locations. Practically, cast breakage will occur caudal to the carpus on flexion or cranial to tarsus (**Fig. 10**). Reinforcement of the concave side of the cast is important in adults to avoid such a complication. Reinforcement can be done by the

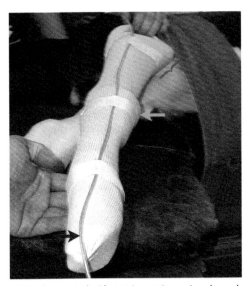

Fig. 9. The limb is ready to be casted. Obstetric cutting wires have been inserted in an IV extension set and placed on the lateral and medial sides of the leg (*blue arrow*). The piece of felt protecting the accessory carpal bone is in placed under the stockinet (*green arrow*). The red curly bracket is the location of the circular piece of felt that should protect the proximal aspect of the cast.

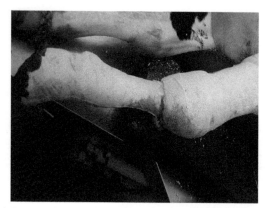

Fig. 10. An adult dairy cow that was immobilized with a cast for a comminuted diaphyseal metacarpal fracture. Catastrophic cast failure is just below the carpus, where flexion is important. The soft tissue was likely damaged because of the blood coming from the crack and surrounding cast.

inclusion of a metallic bar in the cast or more simply by the application of a thick band of fiberglass cast material.[5] Inclusion of the foot in the cast is mandatory in all cases. The cast surrounding the foot is also protected by some poly(methyl methacrylate) (Technovit), because the animal will put weight on the cast and wear off its bottom quickly if not protected. The authors have used pieces of innertubing to waterproof the bottom, decrease wear, and prevent slippage on a wet concrete floor.

FRACTURE REDUCTION EVALUATION

With the exception of physeal fractures that remain stable, fractures are unstable under the cast despite the close reduction that is performed before the application of the cast. Therefore the bone fragments may collapse and override during the first steps of the animal. It will result in an alteration of the reduction. Assessing the variation of the reduction 24 hours after the completion of the cast is not always possible, but could be of great value in case of major displacement to decide whether the cast should be changed (**Fig. 11**).

It is the authors' opinion that the cast should be changed or therapeutic plan modified with more advanced orthopedic techniques if displacement of the bone fragments is such that less than 50% of the fracture surface area is overlapped. A retrospective study on 58 animals with metacarpal or metatarsal fractures showed a significant correlation between the quality of fracture reduction and the long-term prognosis.[8,9]

Displacement of the bone fragments may lead to angular limb deformities. Wolff's law of bone healing results in a bone remodeling over time to adapt the strength of the bone cortices to the load under which they are placed. Minor angulation noticed immediately after weight-bearing on the cast may be corrected according to Wolff's law without necessitating modification of the cast and result in a complete functional bone segment when healed (**Fig. 12**). However, abnormal limb angulation can be a major flaw in show animals. Other fracture immobilization techniques might be considered to achieve a perfect alignment of bone fragments.[10,11]

AFTERCARE

After completion of the cast, the animal is left to recover without assistance. The animal should be kept in a small stall for a period of 8 weeks. Comfort should be

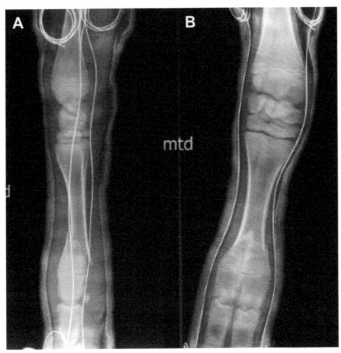

Fig. 11. Post-weight-bearing lateromedial (*A*) and dorsopalmar (*B*) control radiographic views of heifer from **Fig. 1** after reduction of the fracture and external coaptation with a full limb cast. Alignment of the cortices is adequate on both views. The overriding of the 2 bone segments is small and there is a light angle axial plane; those 2 minor imperfections in the reduction of the fracture will be corrected over time with compensatory growth and bone remodeling.

evaluated daily. Daily examination of the cast is also mandatory to evaluate the absence of cracks in the cast or wet spots, indicating exudate traveling from the inside to the outside. Animals usually put 100% of their weight on the fracture limb in the few days following application of the cast (Video 2). A sudden alteration of the use of the limb is an indication that the cast should be removed to assess the limb because it is likely a complication occurred.

Casts in adults may be kept for the entire time of bone healing if no complications occur. The authors prefer to change the cast after 4 weeks to assess the stability of the fracture and the stage of the callus and therefore better evaluate the duration of the remaining time needed for immobilization.

Casts in young calves should be changed every 3 to 4 weeks because of their fast growing rate. Attempting to extend the interval between cast changes may lead to severe limb compression and the development of cast injury.

COMPLICATIONS

Breakage of the cast is the most catastrophic complication and must be addressed immediately to prevent further soft tissue or bone damage. The area that concentrates the compression forces on the concave side of the leg is the weakest point of the cast (see **Fig. 10**). Removal of the cast is mandatory and urgent. The soft tissue injuries are treated if possible and a new cast should be applied on the fracture limb. Cast sores

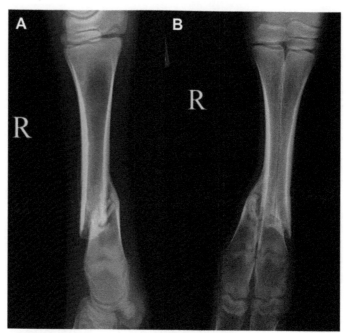

Fig. 12. Secondary bone healing process 8 weeks after fracture immobilization. The fracture healed despite a moderate palmar and lateral displacement as seen on the lateromedial (*A*) and dorsoplantar (*B*) radiographic views, respectively. Callus is minimal and calcified. Bone remodeling has started.

are uncommon in cattle compared with horses because of their thick skin. If padding over bone prominences is adequate and the cast tape well conforms during immobilization, cast sores are rarely seen.

Exudating cast sores may take a while to show up as cast color or odor changes. Serous fluids may accumulate in the stockinet before being visible on the outside of the cast. If the animal bears less weight on his leg because of a cast sore, it may be indicated to take 2 orthogonal radiographic views to outline the contrast between the skin and the cast material. On an unproblematic cast the stockinet layer appears as a very narrow radiolucent line between the skin and the cast material. This narrow radiolucent line will disappear as the stockinet will become soaked by exudate with a fluidlike opacity. It is always recommended to change the cast when an alteration of the weight-bearing occurs. The wound should be treated adequately with lavage and eventually with surgical debridement. Cast sores generally occur after more than 4 weeks (**Fig. 13**). Fracture stability is initiated at this time with a strong cartilaginous callus and foci of mineralization along the edges. A second cast can therefore be reapplied on the limb to allow immobilization for a longer time. In rare cases, the wound might be extensive and require daily care. The limb is therefore immobilized in a splint for the time necessary to control the infected of necrotic wound. The limb is immobilized in a cast immediately unless there is obvious signs of fracture healing.

Contralateral limb problems are rare. Dropped fetlock due to compensatory over-weight-bearing is sometimes encountered (**Fig. 14**). It does indicate that the healing process underneath is altered because the animal does not use its cast appropriately and cast revision should be performed. Contralateral fetlock should regain a more physiologic angle as the healing process is complete; however, some animals remain

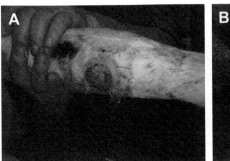
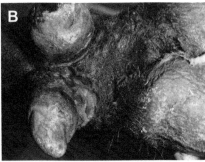

Fig. 13. (*A*) Cast sore on the accessory carpal bone discovered at cast change after 4 weeks of external coaptation with a full limb cast. (*B*) Ulceration underneath the dewclaw. The padding slipped underneath the cast.

with this default even several months after the final cast removal. The limb deformation is generally caused by soft tissue laxity rather than bone deformation.

Animals with a front limb immobilization become accustomed to it rapidly. Depending on the size of the animal and the weight of the cast, they can flex the elbow and the shoulder and have a decent gait. Other animals will either drag the cast or they will do a circumduction. While lying down, young animals can place the affected limb in all kinds of abnormal positions, especially if they are neonates. It is important to replace the limb in a normal position. With the immobilization of the hock, the reciprocal apparatus is maintained in a determined angle. Some cattle may lay down with their limb extended caudally, which may lead to a self-inflicted partial or complete rupture of the peroneus tertius muscle. This rupture is a minor complication and the animal will benefit from an extra 4 weeks of stall rest before returning to its normal environment. Angular limb deformities may occur if improper reduction stayed unnoticed under the cast, potentially leading to severe malunion.[10]

PROGNOSIS

Prognosis is excellent for a closed fracture of the metacarpus and metatarsus.[8,9,12,13] A success rate of 80% to 90% after cast immobilization has been reported (**Fig 15**).[12,13]

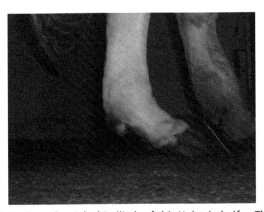

Fig. 14. Dropped fetlock on the right hindlimb of this Holstein heifer. The metatarsal fracture on the left hindlimb has been completely healed; a voluminous callus is present and external deformation of the distal aspect of the limb is noticeable.

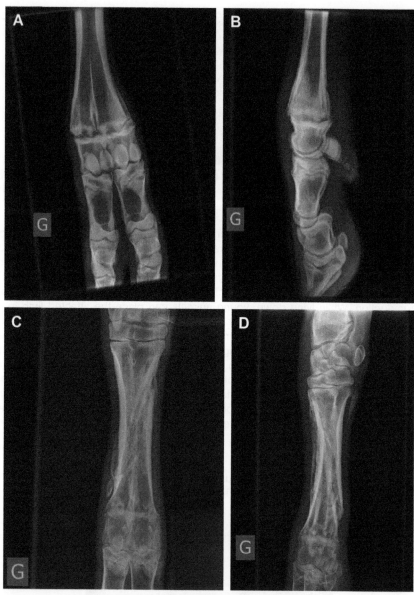

Fig. 15. A young female Holstein that was treated for a distal physeal fracture of the left metacarpi. Radiographic control after 4 weeks of immobilization at cast removal. On the dorsopalmar (*A*) and the lateromedial (*B*) views there is evidence of a small callus. An 18-month-old female Holstein with a long diaphyseal oblique fracture of the metacarpi. Radiographic control after 8 weeks of immobilization. On the dorsopalmar (*C*) and the lateromedial (*D*) views the callus is distributed along the diaphysis. The alignment is adequate considering the fracture configuration.

It has been the authors' observation that animals suffering from fractures located at the proximal third of the diaphysis, close to the carpus or tarsus, tend to be less comfortable in their cast initially and often require an extended period of immobilization compared with the distal metaphyseal or diaphyseal fractures (**Fig. 16**).

FULL LIMB CAST AND SHORT LIMB CAST

Full limb cast should always be favored in large animals for metacarpal and metatarsal fractures. It respects basic cast principles by annihilating the range of motion of the 2 adjacent joints (**Fig. 17**).

In cases of type 1 or type 2 Salter-Harris fractures of the metacarpus/tarsus III–IV, closed reduction by traction usually results in a complete anatomic alignment of the bone fragments as well as a strong stabilization of the fracture. This particular stabilization may allow the realization of a short limb cast, including the hoof to the proximal aspect of the metacarpus/tarsus III–IV. This stabilization will keep the carpus or tarsus free, limiting joint contracture that follows every long-term immobilization. A half limb cast may also be used after cast removal if callus formation is sufficient and fracture stabilization is strong enough to sustain a higher load (**Fig. 18**). There is also an economic reason in using a short limb cast because fewer rolls are being used. However, it should never outweigh the need of a full limb cast.

REINFORCED CAST—WALKING CAST

Walking bars have been associated with casts in an aim of shunting the loading forces on the fracture by transferring those forces from the distal aspect of the U bar to the transversal bars at the most proximal aspect of the U bar.[8] This type of reinforced cast may be used in cases of compound fracture of the metacarpus and metatarsus III–IV (**Fig. 19**). It is the authors' opinion that transfixation pinning and casting technique is

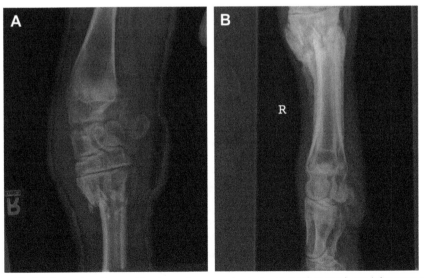

Fig. 16. (*A*) Lateral radiographic view of a comminuted proximal metaphyseal fracture of the metacarpi immobilized with a full limb cast. (*B*) The same animal radiographed 2 months after immobilization at cast removal. The callus is large and it is proximal to the carpometacarpal joint.

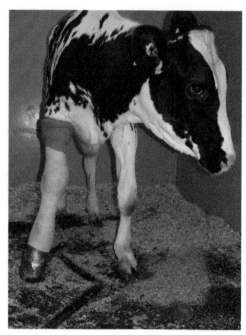

Fig. 17. A full limb cast on the right thoracic limb of a young Holstein heifer. Although she is bearing weight on the limb, the left front fetlock is slightly dropped and the carpus is flexed, indicating overload on this limb.

more appropriate for those cases. A cast with a U bar is heavier and longer, making the limb movement and gait very difficult for some animals. However, it is another means of strengthen the cast at a low cost.

TRANSFIXATION PINNING AND CASTING TECHNIQUE

The addition of 2 transcortical pins in the proximal adjacent bone to the fracture bone to the full limb cast is midway between simple external immobilization technique and external skeletal fixators. Indications for this specific orthopedic combination are a

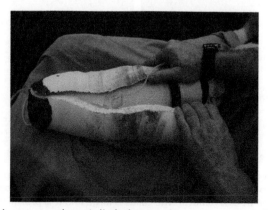

Fig. 18. A half limb cast on a thoracic limb that was just cut out open with obstetric wires.

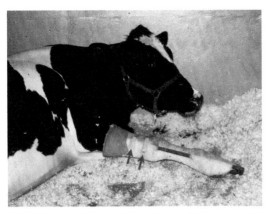

Fig. 19. Reinforced full limb cast with a walking bar applied on a yearling heifer to treat a comminuted metacarpal fracture. The metallic bar transfers the loading forces from the distal aspect of the bar to the transverse rods at the proximal aspect of the cast (*red arrows*).

highly comminuted closed fracture that will collapse with the use of a simple fiberglass cast and a long oblique or spiral fracture for which overriding of the bone segments when loaded will be important and at risk of perforating the skin (**Fig. 20**). The principle behind this orthopedic construct is to hang the distal portion of the limb by transferring the loading forces from the distal tip of the cast to the proximal transcortical pins.

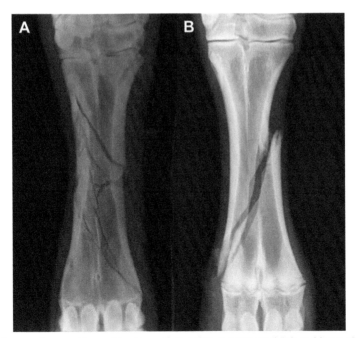

Fig. 20. Dorsopalmar radiographic views of complex comminuted (*A*) and long oblique (*B*) metacarpal fractures. Those fractures are at high risk of severe collapse (*A*) or significant overriding (*B*) during weight-bearing if treated with simple external coaptation. Transfixation pinning and casting are indicated for those fractures.

With the animal under general anesthesia with the fractured limb uppermost, the limb is surgically prepared for aseptic orthopedic surgery. Alternatively the use of a heavy sedation in combination with regional anesthesia such as brachial nerve block or epidural anesthesia may be sufficient to proceed to this technique.

The bone and distal physis are located with insertion of multiple hypodermic needles: the needle inserted in the physis will penetrate deeper in the tissue. Preoperative radiographs with needles preplaced will help the surgeon ascertain an accurate location of the pins (**Fig. 21**). Then 2 transcortical pins are inserted proximal to the physis with an angle of 30° between each other in the frontal plane. Diameter of the pins is critical because the hole will become stress concentrators, potentially leading to fatal fracture through the pin holes. The size should not exceed 20% of the diaphyseal diameter at the site of insertion. In calves 3/16-inch-diameter pins that are positively threaded at their center (thread larger than pin shaft) are used. In larger animals $^1/_4$-inch centrally threaded pins are used or none at all. During insertion of the pins, care should be taken to minimize heat production because it may induce circular bone necrosis with ultimately ring bone sequestration.

The pins insertion sites are covered with a square of nonadherent bandage maintained by a sterile Kling gauze and then the cast is created as described previously. It may be necessary to cut the pins approximately 2 inches from the skin to facilitate the wrapping of the fiberglass casting material around them. With the cast completed, the animal is allowed to recover in his stall and stall confinement is initiated as described for the regular cast (**Fig. 22**).

Removal of the cast at cast change may be a little bit more challenging because the cast should be cut with an oscillating saw around each pin. Depending on the stabilization of the fracture, the decision is made to remove the pins with the application

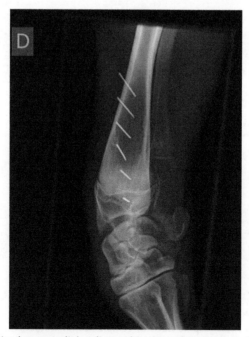

Fig. 21. Intraoperative lateromedial radiographic view of the radius of a yearling Holstein heifer before insertion of transcortical pins. Six 18-G needles have been inserted on the lateral aspect of the leg to serve as landmarks for appropriate location of the pins.

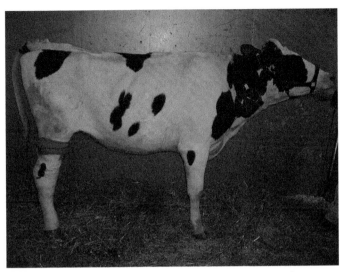

Fig. 22. A 16-month-old Holstein heifer suffering from a compound metatarsal fracture bearing full weight on the injured right hindlimb treated with transfixation pinning and casting technique.

a second full limb cast for an additional period of 4 weeks or possibly not remove the pins.

COMPLICATIONS

Complications related to the pins are mainly early pin loosening, pin bending, fracture through pin holes, infection, and development of ring sequestrum.[14]

Early pin loosening occurs mainly due to the extreme high strain at the bone-implant interface leading to a certain degree of bone necrosis. If one pin gets loose in the early weeks of immobilization, the animal should be reanesthetized, the cast removed, and the pin changed. Recently a pin-sleeve transfixation system was developed to reduce pin-bone interface strain and minimize early pin loosening.[15,16] Pin bending may occur if pin selection was inadequate or the animal is overly active. Some degree of bending is acceptable; however, it should be monitored closely as acute breakage of the pin would necessitate immediate cast change. The quality of fracture reduction (collapse of the compound fracture of overriding of the bone segments) should be assessed as the bend in the pin may have modified the internal architecture of the reduction from the immediate post-coaptation period.

Fracture through the pin hole is more of a risk to happen if the location of the pins is at the mid diaphysis. Insertion of pins into the metaphysis provides a more secure construct regarding decreasing the chance of secondary fracture. Those fractures are a major complication because they usually force the owner to make the decision of euthanasia.

Ring sequestrum is rare but will develop if improper technique during drilling is used (**Fig. 23**). Constant cooling of the drill bits, tapes, and pins during drilling with sterile saline allows control of the heat generated by the friction at the pin-bone interface.

Pin holes or pin tract infection may occur despite the best protection of the entry wound and sterile coverage of the pins exiting the cast. It may remain unnoticed until the cast change at 4 weeks. It should not be considered a sign of osteomyelitis

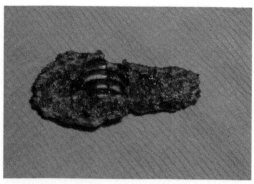

Fig. 23. Complication related to transfixation pinning and casting. Ring sequestrum removed from the parent bone weeks after removal of the centrally threaded positive-profile transfixation pins.

because there is rarely a communication between the tract and the medullary cavity. Removal of the pins, flushing of the tract, and systemic antimicrobial therapy usually are sufficient to control the infection.

PROGNOSIS

Prognosis of closed fracture treated by means of a transfixating pinning and casting technique is good. However, the morbidity is higher compared with a simple cast. The immobilization period is usually longer because the configuration of the fracture is more complex and healing is slower. The volume of the callus in those fractures is larger. This technique is really versatile and can be adapted to a great variety of cases; initially this technique was used to treat radial and tibial fractures.[14,17,18]

CASTING AN OPEN FRACTURE?

Open fractures occur on a regular basis in cattle. They have been categorized by Gustilo and Anderson as 3 different types (see table in article by Gustilo and Anderson in this issue).

Open fractures are best treated using an external fixator (see article by Gustillo and Anderson in this issue). However, it is difficult to manage without appropriate training and experience. The options left are casting, amputation, or euthanasia. Case selection is crucial and the authors think that treatment should only be attempted for type 1 open fractures (**Fig. 24**A).[19–21]

The wound should be cleaned of dirt and foreign material and then surgically prepared for surgical exploration, debridement, and lavage. Control of the infection is primordial in such cases. Local delivery of antibiotics may be provided by the use of antibiotic impregnated poly(methyl methacrylate) beads (see **Fig. 24**B; **Fig. 25**). However, the use of such a carrier of antibiotics is off-label. Therefore, the use of this administration route should respect the regulations for antimicrobial use of the state and country. The same limitation and consideration apply to the preventive or curative use of antibiotics for bone infection.

An open fracture may take longer to heal because of the infection. One or 2 more months of immobilization might be necessary to achieve bone healing compared with a closed fracture of the same bone and configuration. The authors favor an early cast change at 10 to 12 days after the trauma to assess the evolution of the wound,

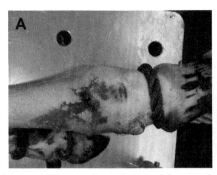
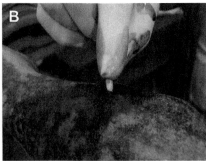

Fig. 24. A young Holstein heifer with a distal metacarpal open fracture type 1. (*A*) Wound is less than 1 cm in diameter and contamination is minimal. The wound was cleaned, debrided, and lavaged and antibiotics impregnated beads (*B*) were inserted through the incision around the fracture.

making a decision whether the infection is under control. At this point, antibiotic therapy can be adjusted based on clinical findings. If there are no clinical or radiographic signs of infection on the first cast change, the antibiotics can be terminated. Then, a second cast is applied for 4 more weeks and the cast is changed a second time. A third cast is applied to complete the remaining time necessary for the stabilization of the fracture. Eventually the cast could also be fenestrated in relation to the wound

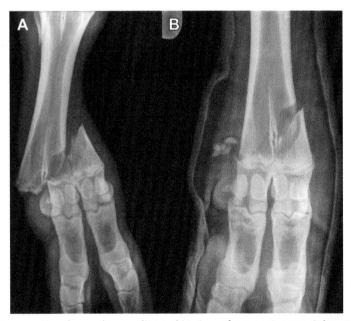

Fig. 25. Preoperative dorsopalmar radiographic view of a type 1 open, Salter-Harris type 2 fracture in a yearling heifer (*A*). Medial displacement is moderate. Postreduction and external coaptation with a full limb cast of the fracture (*B*). Reduction is optimal in the dorsopalmar projection. Five beads of antibiotic-impregnated poly(methyl methacrylate) beads have been inserted in the wound after cleaning and debridement. The wound was protected by a thick bandage as shown by the radiolucent section in regard to the poly(methyl methacrylate) beads.

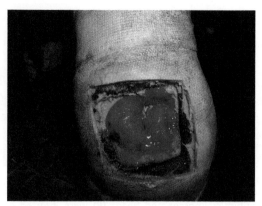

Fig. 26. Treatment of open fracture with a fenestrated cast. The square section of the cast can be removed daily to provide appropriate care to the wound. Constant pressure from the edges of the window stimulates granulation.

to provide daily care (**Fig. 26**). By creating a defect in the structure of the cast, the pressure applied to skin in contact with the edges of the window will be increased and edema may occur in the soft tissues, even if the piece of cast is replaced and tightly maintained with strong tape into the defect. After fenestration there is more movement at the fracture site, increasing the chance of delayed union. Fenestrated cast, although appealing, is difficult to manage and should be used as a last resort.

Prognosis of open fracture is poor and the cost of the treatment is elevated. The sum of costs of a treatment with external immobilization may also be equivalent to the amount of investment for the use of external fixators, without the opportunity to provide the same level of fracture stability and wound care. On a retrospective study of 20 fractures of the metacarpus and metatarsus III–IV, Ravary and Desrochers reported a success rate of 50% of the open fracture treated with a cast.[19]

USE OF MODIFIED THOMAS SPLINT

Fracture of the tibia and the radius cannot be treated effectively with simply a full limb cast because the proximal joint cannot be immobilized. The use of a modified Thomas splint allows not only the loading forces to be transmitted from the distal aspect of the splint to the shoulder or the hip in forelimb or hind limb, respectively, but also the limb is kept in full extension, thus maintaining the alignment of the bone fragments. Further application and technical information is covered in the article in this issue by xxx.[22–24]

SUMMARY

External coaptation remains the most widely used means of fracture treatment in bovine orthopedics based on its affordability and the excellent prognosis of healing carried for closed fracture. Casting techniques are indicated for distal limb closed fractures, mainly metacarpal-tarsal III–IV but also phalanges. Whether a full limb cast, half limb cast, or a cast associated with transfixation pins should be applied to stabilize the fracture depends only on the nature of the fracture. All minor acute changes in the comfort of the animal or modification of the gait during weight-bearing should alert the owner and the clinician of an ongoing complication of the limb and the cast should be removed for a thorough assessment of the entire limb as well as of the fracture site by 2 orthogonal radiographic views. Open fractures type 1 should be carefully evaluated and other treatment options, such as external skeletal fixation devices, should be favored before embedded them in a cast. Prognosis of type 1 open fracture has been reported to be around 50%. Calving chain injuries occur on a regular basis during forced extraction. Prognosis is excellent with external fixation; however, a cast change every 3 to 4 weeks is mandatory to avoid severe complications. Alteration of the distal blood vessels needs to be discussed with the owner at the time of treatment choice because distal skin necrosis may be present at the time of cast change.

SUPPLEMENTARY DATA

Supplementary data related to this article can be found online at http://dx.doi.org/10.1016/j.cvfa.2013.11.007.

REFERENCES

1. Tulleners EP. Management of bovine orthopedic problems. Part I. Fractures. Comp Cont Educ Pract 1986;8(2):S69–79.
2. Cadiot et Almy. Affection du canon et des tendons. Traité de thérapeutique chirurgicale des animaux domestiques Tome, vol. 2. Paris: Asselin et Houzeau ed; 1901. p. 523–55.
3. Hara S, Kawamoto Y, Nuta S, et al. Mechanical strength of synthetic casting tape for application to fracture treatment of farm animals. Vet Comp Orthop Traumatol 1996;9:79–83.
4. Berman AT, Parks BG. A comparison of the mechanical properties of fiberglass cast materials and their clinical relevance. J Orthop Trauma 1990;4(1):85–92.
5. Wilson DG, Vanderby R. An evaluation of fiberglass cast application techniques. Vet Surg 1995;24:118–21.
6. Auer JA, Steiner A, Iselin U, et al. Internal fixation of long bone fractures in farm animals. Vet Comp Orthop Traumatol 1993;6:36–41.
7. Pacholek X, Déry M. Étude rétrospective des fractures obstétricales chez le veau. Med Vet Québec 1991;21:175.
8. Steiner A, Iselin U, Auer JA, et al. Shaft fractures of the metacarpus and metatarsus in cattle. Vet Comp Orthop Traumatol 1993;6:138–45.
9. Steiner A, Iselin U, Auer JA, et al. Physeal fractures of the metacarpus and metatarsus in cattle. Vet Comp Orthop Traumatol 1993;6:131–7.
10. Mulon PY. Correction of a severe torsional malunion of the metacarpus in a calf by transverse osteotomy, transfixation pinning and casting. Vet Comp Orthop Traumatol 2010;23:62–5.
11. Edinger H, Kofler J, Ebner J. Angular limb deformity in a calf treated by periosteotomy and wedge osteotomy. Vet Rec 1995;137:245–6.
12. Tulleners EP. Metacarpal and metatarsal fractures in dairy cattle: 33 cases (1979-1985). J Am Vet Med Assoc 1986;189:463–8.
13. Crawford WH, Fretz PB. Long bone fractures in large animals: a retrospective study. Vet Surg 1985;14:295–302.
14. Martens A, Steenhaut M, Gasthuys F, et al. Conservative and surgical treatment of tibial fractures in cattle. Vet Rec 1998;143:12–6.
15. Brianza S, Brighenti V, Boure L, et al. In vitro mechanical evaluation of a novel pin-sleeve system for external fixation of distal limb fractures in horses: a proof of concept study. Vet Surg 2010;39:601–8.

16. Brianza S, Vogel S, Rothstock S, et al. Comparative biomechanical evaluation of a pin-sleeve transfixation system in cadaveric calf metacarpal bones. Vet Surg 2013;42(1):67–74.

17. St-Jean G, Clem MF, DeBowes RM. Transfixation pinning and casting of tibial fractures in calves: five cases (1985–1989). J Am Vet Med Assoc 1991;198: 139–43.

18. St-Jean G, DeBowes RM. Transfixation pinning and casting of radial-ulnar fracture in calves: a review of three cases. Can Vet J 1992;33:257–61.

19. Ravary B, Desrochers A. Vingt fractures du canon chez des bovins adultes. Le Point Veterinaire 2003;235:64–7.

20. Desrochers A. Les fractures des membres chez les bovins adultes. Le Point Veterinaire 2003;232:50–4.

21. Mulon PY. Management of long bone fractures in cattle. In Pract 2013;35:265–71.

22. Ferguson JG. Management and repair of bovine fractures. Comp Cont Educ Pract 1982;4:S128–35.

23. Anderson DE, St-Jean G, Vestweber JG, et al. Use of a Thomas splint-cast combination for stabilization of tibial fracture in cattle: 21 cases (1973-1993). Agri-Practice 1994;15:18–23.

24. Gangl M, Grulke S, Serteyn D, et al. Retrospective study of 99 cases of bone fractures in cattle treated by external coaptation or confinement. Vet Rec 2006;158: 264–8.

Use of the Thomas Splint and Cast Combination, Walker Splint, and Spica Bandage with an Over the Shoulder Splint for the Treatment of Fractures of the Upper Limbs in Cattle

Aubrey Nicholas Baird, DVM, MS*, Stephen B. Adams, DVM, MS

KEYWORDS

- Thomas splint • Walker splint • Spica bandages • Fractures

KEY POINTS

- The use of splints has been a part of food animal practice for decades.
- Many proximal limb fractures can be successfully treated with splints in food animals.
- Thomas splint-cast combinations and Walker splints can be used in the field without specialized equipment.

INTRODUCTION

A review of records of cattle admitted to 10 veterinary medical schools for years 2003 up to and including 2012 discovered that 778 (2.3%) of 23,754 cattle were presented for fractures. There were 91 (11.7%) tibial fractures and 29 (3.7%) fractures of the radius (The Veterinary Medical Database [VMDB]. http://www.vmdb.org/. The VMDB does not make any implicit or implied opinion on the subject of this article.) These percentages are similar to those reported from a database review between 1985 and 1994.[1] Many methods have been reported for the treatment of cattle with fractures of the tibia that include casts, various splint-cast combinations, external fixation with transfixation pins, and internal fixation with orthopedic implants.[2–9] Likewise, radius-ulna fractures have been reported to be treated by many of the same

Department of Veterinary Clinical Sciences, Purdue University School of Veterinary Medicine, 625 Harrison Street, West Lafayette, IN 47907, USA
* Corresponding author.
E-mail address: abaird@purdue.edu

Vet Clin Food Anim 30 (2014) 77–90
http://dx.doi.org/10.1016/j.cvfa.2013.11.012
0749-0720/14/$ – see front matter © 2014 Elsevier Inc. All rights reserved.

techniques.[2–8,10] The treatment methods for tibial and radial-ulnar fractures overlap because the tibia and the radius are similar-sized bones and similarly located in the upper limb near thick muscle coverage.[1]

For many years, splints, including the TSCC and Walker splints, have been an integral component of the bovine veterinarian's practice for treating orthopedic conditions in cattle. The TSCC and Walker splints have been used primarily for treatment of radial-ulnar and tibial fractures. Although the splints for large cattle can be technically challenging to construct and apply and some cattle wearing the splints may be difficult to manage, the splints have been used successfully in many cattle and small ruminants. Combined data from 3 separate studies evaluating the use of the TSCC for treatment of tibial fractures showed an 82% success rate in returning the cattle to production.[3,4,11] This success rate compares favorably to the success rates for both internal fixation and external fixation with transfixation pins and casts. A search of the literature shows a lack of citations for the use of splints for fracture repair in cattle in the last decade (or two). This lack may not only reflect that methods of splint application have not changed, but also coincides with an increased emphasis on internal fixation for lighter cattle and small ruminants and increased use of transfixation pin techniques and stronger casting materials eliminating the need for a metal splint in lighter animals. Current casting material have enough strength to be placed up to the axilla or groin to provide support much like the ring of the TSCC and Walker splints for cattle, calves, and small ruminants weighing less than 200 kg, which simplifies application of external coaptation because a separate splint does not have to be constructed. Cast application and subsequent management can be less complicated and less expensive than some of the splint-cast combinations for selected cases. The use of transfixation pins with casts may provide a more stable construct than the TSCC or Walker splint but requires general anesthesia for pin insertion, technical expertise for pin application, and intraoperative imaging. Costs for treatment of fractures with transfixation casts are generally much higher as compared with treatment with a TSCC or Walker splint. Internal and external fixation techniques for repair of upper limb fractures are generally done in referral hospitals. Application of TSCC, Walker splints, and spica bandages and splints can be done in field situations. Splint-cast combinations are the treatment of choice for heavy cattle with fractures of the tibia, radius-ulna, or olecranon. These combinations are used in cases in which the animal is too heavy for current internal fixation techniques and/or the fracture is too high to be stabilized by cast or transfixation pin cast. Splint-cast combinations are also useful for treatment of highly comminuted fractures that would be difficult to reconstruct with internal or external fixation. The splint-cast combinations are also a good choice for cattle and small ruminants of all sizes when costs need to be minimized.

ASSESSMENT OF THE PATIENT AND FRACTURE

All ruminant orthopedic patients should be examined carefully to determine the nature and extent of all the injuries before starting treatment. The veterinarian should be sure not to apply a splint on a recumbent ruminant with an obvious tibia fracture only to learn later that the animal also has some orthopedic condition of another limb. Cattle are seldom able to stand and move around with a specialized splint if they were not standing on 3 sound legs before splint application. Mature animals, especially, may have difficulty standing up in a splint if they are recumbent before application of a splint. One rule of thumb to reduce complications after any splint application is that ruminant fracture patients should be able to stand on the other 3 legs and ambulate before splint application. Most cattle that can ambulate before splint application learn to stand up, lie down, and ambulate in a splint. This process may take several days, and during this time, daily assistance to stand could be required. The exception to this may be the newborn that has suffered a fracture during delivery. This animal has never learned to walk on 4 normal limbs. Learning to walk with 3 normal limbs and a splint presents a special challenge to the newborn animal and requires dedicated nursing care from the veterinarian or owner.

The characteristics of the fracture are important, including its location, configuration, and whether it is open or closed. Fracture assessment should also provide the information needed for determination of the proper method of treatment, prognosis, and estimated costs. Young cattle and calves, because of their small size, are better orthopedic risks than adult cattle. Casts and splints are more easily constructed and applied to the smaller animal and are less likely to break. Fractures in younger cattle may heal more rapidly than in older animals. Young animals are also easier to manage during the convalescent period.

Cattle are surprisingly adept at managing casts or Thomas splint-cast combinations after their application once they learn to lie down and stand while in the splint. The well-broke, haltered cow, in contrast to the wild range cow, should be a superior orthopedic patient. Animal disposition varies among breeds and individuals, and it is difficult to predict how a certain animal will behave after application of a splint. However, even unhandled cattle may become an acceptable orthopedic patient when placed in a TSCC if left undisturbed in a stall.

There is no substitute for a thorough physical examination. The veterinarian should look closely near the fracture site for small puncture wounds of the skin or for skin abrasions. Running a hand over the fracture and checking for wet spots of blood or serum is helpful. Any fracture with an associated skin wound must be considered open, even if the wound does not extend directly to the fracture site. The dermis provides a natural barrier to infection, and loss of dermis destroys that barrier.

Radiographs of fractures are extremely useful for determining configuration if the equipment is available. Multiple radiographic views allow the veterinarian to determine the numbers and position of fragments, involvement of joints, and the presence of gas in tissue planes. Gas indicates infection or an open fracture. Fractures near or extending into joints carry a poorer prognosis than fractures in the middle of long bones. Absence of radiographs should not preclude application of a TSCC in field situations. Successful repair is still possible. Open fractures are more difficult to manage than closed fractures. Young cattle seem more likely to develop osteomyelitis after open fractures than older cattle.[2] Open fractures in any size animal that cannot be immobilized have a poor prognosis.

Fractures of forelimbs are easier to treat with external coaptation than fractures of the rear limbs. Cattle tolerate casts on the forelimbs better than on the rear limbs. Full-limb casts or splints can usually be made to fit the straight forelimb better than the angulated rear limb. Many adult cattle are heavily muscled and have short, thick gaskins, large udders, or pendulous scrotums that compound the difficulty of fitting a rear full-limb cast or splint. Fracture immobilization in the forelimbs is usually superior to that of the rear limbs because a better-fitting nonangulated TSCC can be applied.[1]

Delay in fracture repair results in additional soft-tissue and bone damage and increases the risk of infection. Extensive soft-tissue swelling after a long delay in fracture immobilization may make cast or splint change necessary 4 to 7 days after the initial fixation. This change adds to the cost of treatment and the risk of the fracture becoming open. Long delays between injury and evaluation by the veterinarian should not preclude fracture repair with external fixation. Fractures of the radius-ulna or tibia greater than 72 hours have been managed successfully with immobilization in the TSCC.[3]

THOMAS SPLINT-CAST COMBINATION
Application of the Thomas Splint-Cast Combination

The application of Thomas splint and cast combination is suitable for all closed radial fractures except those in the most distal aspect of the radius. Distal fractures can often be managed with a cast or transfixation pin and cast combination. The TSCC is also useful for most tibial fractures. In the authors' opinion, the TSCC is the method of choice for severely comminuted tibial and radial-ulnar fractures in all cattle and for fractures in cattle weighing more than 400 kg in which internal fixation may be disrupted by the weight of the patient.[1] The TSCC has been used to treat radial-ulnar fractures in cattle weighing up to 545 kg and tibial fractures in cattle weighing up to 1000 kg.[3,4]

Methods of TSCC application

Methods for TSCC application to cattle have not changed during the last 30 years except for the current use of fiberglass casting tapes instead of plaster casting tapes. Descriptions of splint application have been published in past years.[1–4] The following description of TSCC application from 1996[1] is repeated in this article for the reader's convenience (**Figs. 1–5**). The splint can be constructed of either steel rods or conduit (**Table 1**). It consists of a ring in the axilla or inguinal area, which is large enough not to contact osseous protuberances such as the shoulder, elbow, greater trochanter, tuber coxae, or tuber ischii. The vertical rods are continuous from the ring to the ground with one cranial and the other caudal to the limb. They are straight for front limbs or bent to match the angle of the hock in hind limbs. The rear limb splints for heavy mature cattle may be left straight for greater strength. The splint is completed by bending another piece of rod into a "U" shape with the length equal to the vertical rods from the ring. The 2 pieces fit together so the vertical component of the splint comprises double rods that are taped together. The animal is positioned in lateral recumbency with the affected limb up. This recumbency can be achieved by sedation or rope casting, depending on the temperament of the patient. General anesthesia is rarely needed. The limb is covered with a double layer of stockinette. Holes are drilled in the hoof

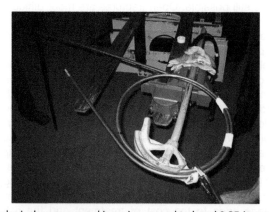

Fig. 1. A pipe bender is shown secured in a vise as used to bend 0.25-in steel bar to make the ring and proximal leg rods for the TSCC. A section of equine stomach tube was placed in the calf's axilla to determine the appropriate ring size and used as a template for bending the bar.

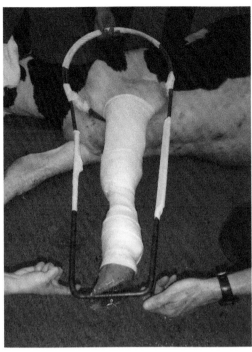

Fig. 2. The calf has been restrained in lateral recumbency. The lower U-shaped bar has been taped to the proximal leg extension from the ring. The limb is covered by a double layer of stockinette over cast padding around the dewclaws. Cotton is placed between the toes, which are wired to the bottom of the splint.

wall for wires that secure the hoof to the bottom of the splint. The splint is placed over the limb and the foot is secured to the splint. A cast is placed on the limb within the splint; then the cast material is placed around the splint as well. Tape or acrylic is used to cover the bottom of the splint to prevent wear. The limb should be in enough traction to prevent overriding of the fracture ends but no more tension than necessary, as this makes rubs in the axilla or inguinal region worse.[1] Alternatively, one may place a cast from the axillary or inguinal region distally to the mid-cannon bone before applying the splint. Additional cast material is then applied over this cast and cast around the splint.[4] Cast application before incorporation in the splint is most useful when fracture fragments are not markedly displaced or overriding and traction is not needed to realign fragments.

Management of Cattle Wearing Modified Thomas Splint-Cast Combinations

Patients should be monitored closely for integrity of the splint-cast or pressure sores, as well as general ambulation and comfort in the coaptation device. It may take several days for the animals to acclimate to using the splint. Some may require help to stand initially. Stalls should be bedded with absorbent material to help keep the splint clean and dry. Do not bed the stall deeply with straw as this may make movement of the limb more difficult. The cast or splint-cast combinations should be inspected daily for cracks, breakage, or protrusion of the foot through the bottom of the cast or splint-cast combination. Broken casts should be replaced immediately. Cracked casts may be patched with additional fiberglass casting tapes. Pressure sores or rubbing

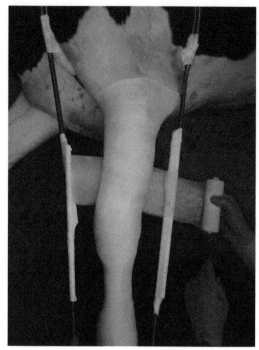

Fig. 3. Fiberglass cast tape has been applied to the leg from the elbow to the coronary band. Now a piece of cast tape is placed around the splint on the medial side of the limb to provide medial support and help keep the limb aligned in the splint. The remaining section of the tape is used to wrap around the entire splint and limb.

sores may be difficult to identify under fiberglass casts. Cattle that become increasingly reluctant to use the immobilized limb and spend increasingly longer periods of time lying down may be developing sores. Pressure sores or rubbing sores develop most commonly at the bulbs of the heel, the plantar or palmar aspect of the fetlock, over the accessory carpal bone, at the point of the hock, at the top rim of the cast, or under the ring of the modified Thomas splint. Visual inspection may reveal sores at the last point.

Support wraps may be applied to the contralateral limb to prevent tendon strain and limb abrasions. The bony protuberances of all noncast limbs should be wrapped with elastic adhesive tape to prevent skin abrasions from the floor or from attempts to rise.

Removal of Thomas Splint-Cast Combinations

Thomas splint-cast combinations may need to be changed after 4 to 7 days in those cattle with extreme swelling at the time of initial immobilization. Reduced limb size when swelling subsides causes the splint-cast combination to become loose and fit poorly.

Thomas splint-cast combinations should be changed every 3 weeks in the young, rapidly growing calves to accommodate the increased limb length. Adult cattle may wear the TSCC up to 6 weeks, providing no complications occur. Few noncomplicated radial-ulnar fractures need immobilization beyond 6 weeks, however. The mean time of fracture immobilization of radial-ulnar and tibial fractures in modified

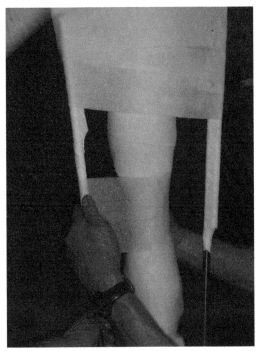

Fig. 4. Cast tape is being applied around the proximal cannon bone, then to the dorsal leg bar before encircling the entire splint to help secure the limb position.

Thomas splint-cast combinations from one study was 5.5 and 7.3 weeks, respectively.[3] In another study, the mean time of splint-cast immobilization was 8.4 weeks for tibial fractures.[4]

Fractures do not need to be immobilized until there is radiographic evidence that bone union has occurred. Palpable callus and clinical stability are significant

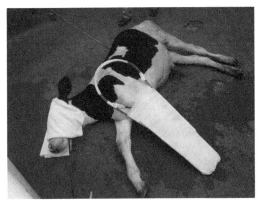

Fig. 5. The calf is shown in lateral recumbency with the aid of a flank casting rope. The halter is tied and the eyes are covered to limit stimulation. The TSCC could have hoof acrylic or inner tubing applied to the bottom of the splint to prevent wear.

Table 1
Proper size of steel rod for construction of modified Thomas splints for cattle

Forelimb		Rear Limb	
Weight (kg)	Rod Size (in)	Weight (kg)	Rod Size (in)
<225	3/8	<180	3/8
225–450	1/2	180–360	1/2
>450	5/8	360–540	5/8
		>540	1-in conduit pipe

From Adams SB. The role of external fixation and emergency fracture management in bovine orthopedics. Vet Clin North Am Food Anim Pract 1985;1:109; with permission.

indications that immobilization can be stopped. These clinical signs usually occur before radiographic evidence of bone union is present.

Thomas splint-cast combinations should be cut with an oscillating saw for removal. The limb should be supported with wraps or a temporary splint after removal of the TSCC, and the animal should be confined to a stall or small paddock for an additional 3 to 6 weeks. Exercise should be increased gradually until normal ambulation returns. This period of confinement is generally sufficient for resolution of decubital sores and ligamentous laxity. Poorly aligned fractures often remodel to a more normal configuration during a 6- to 18-month period.

Complications and Prognosis

Complications from treatment of tibial or radial-ulnar fractures by modified Thomas splint-cast combinations include development of pressure sores, closed fractures becoming open, chronic recumbency, distal physeal fractures, delayed union, poor fracture alignment after healing, ligamentous laxity after splint-cast removal, breakage or damage to the splint-cast, and chronic lameness after healing.[3,4] Complications occur with greater frequency in older heavier cattle. Cattle with tibial fractures that weigh more than 800 kg have a poor prognosis.[4] Most complications can be treated satisfactorily and do not preclude the animals being used for breeding or milking.

WALKER SPLINTS

The construction and application of a splint designed specifically for use on the hind limb of cattle was described by Walker in 1979.[9] This splint is intended primarily for treatment of tibial fractures but has been used for cruciate and meniscal injuries in cattle as well. This splint provides medial support for tibial fractures to prevent medial deviation of the fractured bone by having the leg pieces of the splint on the medial aspect of the limb and slightly bent to conform to the fractured limb. The splint also consists of a footplate on threaded rods that allow for a mechanical advantage to apply traction to the limb. However, this splint can be difficult and frustrating to build, and most practitioners need to enlist the assistance of an accomplished pipe bender and welder. Walker splints may be used several times, so the authors recommend making several different sizes of splints before need arises for fracture stabilization in those practices anticipating periodic use of the splints. This practice makes the splint readily available when needed for immediate application. However, custom-sized Walker splints can be made for a specific animal. The authors have summarized the steps in building and applying the Walker splint to save the reader from searching archives to find the original article.

Construction and Application of the Walker Splint

The materials and measurements for Walker splint construction are given in **Box 1**. The ring is made from a 10-ft piece of conduit, which is cut into 2 pieces and welded back together. A 110° bend is made about 36 in from the end of the conduit. The second bend is of 80° perpendicular to the first and as close to the first bend as possible. The third bend is 110° in the same plane and a mirror image of the first bend. The resultant distance between the first and third bends should equal the previously measured cranial to caudal length of the leg at the level of the patella. The fourth bend is the counterpart of the previous 80° bend. Both ends of the pipe are then cut with a hacksaw on a horizontal line immediately adjacent to the second and fourth bends. This part is the ventral component of the ring, which goes into the inguinal region of the animal.

The dorsal part of the ring is made by bending one end of the remaining conduit to make a half circle with the distance between the ends of the conduit equal to the cranial to caudal measurement of the limb at the level of the stifle. This half circle is matched to the ends of the ventral component to determine the correct angle and location to cut this piece. These pieces are then welded together to form the ring (**Fig. 6**). As a tip, short sections of water hose may be fit snugly into this conduit to hold it together for welding.

From the remaining conduit, 2 pieces approximately 2 in shorter than the length of the leg measured earlier are cut. Identical bends of 15° are made in one end of the 2 leg pipes. This bend is at the proximal end of the leg pieces welded to the flat part of the ventral aspect of the ring and supplies the medial support for the limb. This weld is at a 45° angle to the ring. The leg pieces should be 6 to 8 in apart at the weld and converge to be about 3 in apart at the bottom. This weld should be reinforced with a rectangular piece of strap iron on the concave side. For extra strength in mature animals, a 10-in piece of conduit curved in a quarter circle is welded between the ring and leg pieces cranially and caudally (**Fig. 7**).

The footplate is made by cutting a piece of boiler plate to 4.5 in wide by 6 in long with rounded corners and a flange 3 in long on one of the 6-in sides that is 2.5 in wide. The boiler plate is heated to bend the flange to 90° to the rest of the plate. Holes are drilled in the plate for placing wires that secure the foot to the plate. The edges of the drill holes should be smoothed with a punch to decrease the chance of the wires being cut by the plate.

Box 1
Materials and measurements needed for construction of the Walker splint

One-inch electrical conduit—approximately 15 ft (0.75 in can be used for animals less than 700 lb [about 320 kg])

Sand to fill the conduit for bending to prevent kinking

One-fourth-inch-thick boiler plate—6 in by 7 in

Five-eighth-inch threaded rod—30 in long

Refrigeration insulation tubing (1 in or 0.75 in to match the conduit size)

Measure the length of the limb from the perineum to the ground

Measure the cranial to caudal width of the leg at the level of the patella

These measurements are used to assure the ring is big enough and the overall length of the splint is appropriate.

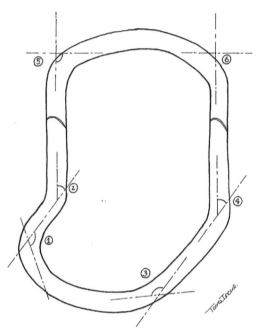

Fig. 6. Line drawing of the ring or crutch part of the Walker splint including the location of the different bends needed to shape the ring. The bends numbered 1 through 4 correlate with the text description. Bends 5 and 6 are the two 90° bends that make the half circle for the dorsal part of the ring. (*Courtesy of* Dr Tomo Inoue, DVM, Purdue University.)

Two sections of 14-in length 5/8-in diameter threaded rod are then welded to the side of the flange, which has been bent opposite the footplate 3 in apart. Two nuts should be threaded down each rod to the level of the footplate. Then an 8-in-long piece of 0.75-in conduit is placed over the rods. These pieces of conduit go into the distal leg pieces to make rods more stable in the leg section.

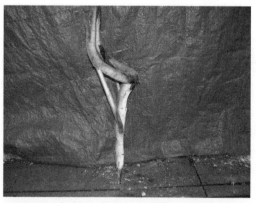

Fig. 7. The proximal part of a Walker splint without the footplate. Notice the bend in the proximal part of the leg bars. This ring is welded to the leg bars, to fit the patient it was used on, at a sharper angle than the suggested 45° that fits most cattle best. (*Courtesy of* Dr Dwight Wolfe, DVM, MS, Auburn University.)

The splint is then padded with refrigeration insulation of appropriate size for the conduit. The insulation is split and secured over all the conduit of the splint with 2-in adhesive tape.

The animal is restrained appropriately for the application of the splint. Some animals require heavy sedation or even anesthesia, whereas others do well with casting and rope restraint alone. The animal should be placed in lateral recumbency with the affected limb up. Animals that can have the Walker splint applied safely with physical restraint alone stand in the splint much easier than ones that must recover from sedation or anesthesia with the splint in place.

Four holes are drilled in the hoof wall of each digit so wire can be looped through the hoof to anchor it to the footplate. The limb is placed into the splint. An assistant is made to hold tension on the dorsal part of the ring so it sits tightly in the inguinal region. The threaded rods welded to the footplate are placed within the leg supports without tension. The free ends of the wire loops near the toe of the claws are placed through holes in the footplate. Using pliers, the wires are pulled so the toe is in contact with the footplate. The wires are then twisted and bent against the bottom of the plate. The wires closer to the heel or quarter of the claw are tightened in a similar fashion, but the heel may be an inch or so off the plate. One can cover the wire twist with acrylic to prevent wearing and premature breakage. Next, the nuts are tightened to the end of the leg supports to apply traction to the limb and better align the fracture.

Dr Walker's original description used plaster cast from above the hock down to the hoof incorporating the leg supports of the splint without any padding.[9] Today, fiberglass casting tapes are used, over stockinette, because they are much lighter and stronger than plaster (**Fig. 8**). Some animals adapt to the splint more quickly than others. Some have to be rolled when they chose to lie on the splinted leg. The splint should be worn 5 to 6 weeks, during which time the patient develops a pressure sore and even skin necrosis in the inguinal regional; this heals once the splint is removed.

SPICA BANDAGES AND SPLINTS

The spica bandage as described for small animals[12] consists of a splint (or cast) from the elbow to the ground. Roll gauze plus cotton for padding is wrapped around the body in a figure eight fashion at the level of the thoracic limb crossing the material between the legs ventrally; this may be used in the hind limb as well, but one must be careful in male animals not to incorporate the testicles or obstruct urine flow. If one looks at the wrap from the side, it appears "V-shaped." Cast material is then applied laterally from the ground to the dorsal midline conforming to the bandage. Metal rods may also be included for added strength. The conformed cast is then secured to the patient with more bandage material. The spica bandage/cast provides stability against rotational and bending forces on the fractured humerus. This type of bandage/cast is used to treat humeral fractures of small ruminants.

The spica bandage combined with a specialized splint may be used to treat humeral fractures in young calves and as first aid to temporarily immobilize tibial and radial-ulnar fractures (Dr David E. Anderson, personal communication, University of Tennessee). This technique is difficult to apply in mature cattle. For humeral fractures in young cattle or small ruminants, internal fixation achieves better stability, quicker healing, and fewer complications caused by excessive weight bearing on the healthy contralateral limb as compared with the spica bandage and splint. However, internal fixation is much more expensive than splint application and may not be feasible for many owners.

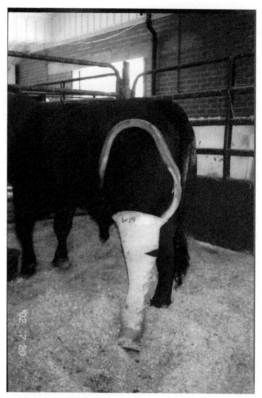

Fig. 8. A bull with a tibial fracture standing in a Walker splint. (*Courtesy of* Dr Dwight Wolfe, DVM, MS, Auburn University.)

Spica bandages are often combined with lateral splints to increase fracture stabilization. One type of splint that may be used on ruminants of all sizes is the a lateral splint that extends from the ground past the elbow up to the top of the shoulder at the level of the withers. The lateral extension can be as simple as a board (1 in × 4 in or 2 in × 4 in) or metal rods. This splint is incorporated into the spica bandage or cast from the elbow to the ground and padded proximally along the shoulder to minimize rub sores. The board will prevent abduction of the distal limb. The animal may be able to bear some weight on the limb because the carpus is locked in extension. Although some humeral fractures can heal with just stall rest and time, the combination of the spica bandage or cast with a lateral splint allows some stability and weight-bearing ability that makes the patient more comfortable during the healing process. It also minimizes joint contracture, which occurs if the carpus is allowed to stay in a flexed position.

A modification of the lateral splint has been developed to increase humeral fracture stability in calves and small ruminants (Dr David E. Anderson, personal communication, University of Tennessee, 2013). These splints are useful in small-frame, lightweight livestock (<150 kg). This lateral splint is placed over the dorsum of the affected limb and down the contralateral shoulder and may be used for partial immobilization of humeral fractures when surgical repair is not an option. These splints are appropriate for injuries of the forelimb only and cannot be adapted to the rear limb because the splint relies on the neck to help maintain proper positioning throughout the period

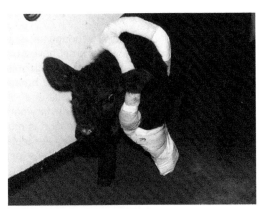

Fig. 9. A calf with a spica splint showing the padded bars continuing over the dorsal midline. (*Courtesy of* Dr David Anderson, DVM, MS, University of Tennessee.)

of coaptation. These fractures should be minimally displaced because the spica splint is unlikely to achieve fracture reduction. Spica splints are extremely difficult to properly conform and achieve rigidity in taller, larger livestock.

The over the dorsum modified splints are similar in concept to Thomas splints in that they are designed to allow tension to be applied to the limb as a means of stabilizing an injury. However, the splint is continued over the back and down the opposite side to the level of the shoulder or elbow (**Figs. 9** and **10**). As with Thomas splints, weight bearing can be achieved when proper fit to the limb is achieved. The splint should be conformed to the limb and thorax as closely as possible to secure the limb to the thoracic region as a rigid frame.[13–15] Proximal fractures require that the splint be fitted with the limb in full extension. Inadequate tension of the limb results in complications, including displacement of the fracture, nonunion, delayed union, malunion, creation of an open wound, and/or pressure sores. Although rarely used, over the dorsum modified splints may offer a better prognosis than surgical repair in small ruminants and calves for minimally displaced, spiral oblique fracture of the humerus (Dr David E. Anderson, personal communication, University of Tennessee, 2013).

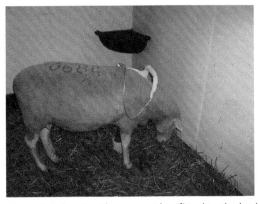

Fig. 10. A ewe in a spica splint showing the support bar fitted to the body on the side opposite to the fracture. (*Courtesy of* Dr David Anderson, DVM, MS, University of Tennessee.)

SUMMARY

Application of the TSCC, Walker splint, and spica bandage and splint for treatment of fractures of the tibia, radius-ulna, elbow, and humerus still have a place in bovine practice. The success rate for healing is good when compared with other methods of fracture repair. Cosmetic appearance of healed limbs may not be acceptable for show cattle. The splints are especially indicated for large cattle and for cattle with highly comminuted fractures that are not amenable to repair with internal fixation or external fixation with transfixation pins. Generally, splint application is much less expensive than other methods of treating fractures, and this makes the techniques particularly useful for commercial grade cattle that may not warrant the expense of other treatment methods.

REFERENCES

1. Adams SB, Fessler JF. Treatment of fractures of the tibia and radius-ulna by external coaptation. Vet Clin North Am Food Anim Pract 1996;12:181–98.
2. Adams SB. The role of external fixation and emergency fracture management in bovine orthopedics. Vet Clin North Am Food Anim Pract 1985;1:109–29.
3. Adams SB, Fessler JF. Treatment of radial-ulnar and tibial fractures in cattle using a modified Thomas splint-cast combination. J Am Vet Med Assoc 1983;183: 430–3.
4. Anderson DE, St. Jean G, Desrochers A. Use of a Thomas splint-cast combination for stabilization of tibial fractures in cattle: 21 cases (1973-1993). Agri-Pract 1994;15:16–23.
5. Denny HR, Sridhar B, Weaver BM, et al. The management of bovine fractures: a review of 59 cases. Vet Rec 1988;123:289–95.
6. Ferguson JG. Management and repair of bovine fractures. Compend Contin Educ Pract Vet 1982;4:S128.
7. St. Jean G, Clem MF, DeBowes RM. Transfixation pinning and casting of tibial fractures in calves: five cases (1985-1989). J Am Vet Med Assoc 1991;198:139–43.
8. Tulleners EP. Management of bovine orthopedic problems, Part I: fractures. Compend Contin Educ Pract Vet 1986;8:S69–79.
9. Walker D. Coaptation splinting of the bovine rear limb. Mod Vet Pract 1979;60: 629–33.
10. Baxter GM, Wallace CE. Modified transfixation pinning of compound radius and ulna fracture in a heifer. J Am Vet Med Assoc 1991;198:665–8.
11. Gangl M, Grulke S, Serteyn D, et al. Retrospective study of 99 cases of bone fractures in cattle treated by external coaptation or confinement. Vet Rec 2006; 158(8):264–8.
12. Arnoczky SP, Blass CE, McCoy L. External coaptation and bandaging. In: Slatter DH, editor. Textbook of small animal surgery. Philadelphia: W. B. Suanders Company; 1985. p. 1988–2003.
13. Holm LM. Management of humeral shaft fractures: fundamental nonoperative technics. Clin Orthop Relat Res 1970;71:132–9.
14. Pollock FH, Drake D, Bovill EG, et al. Treatment of radial neuropathy associated with fractures of the humerus. J Bone Joint Surg Am 1981;63(2):239–43.
15. Stewart MJ, Hundley JM. Fractures of the humerus: a comparative study in methods of treatment. J Bone Joint Surg Am 1955;37(4):681–92.

Plates, Pins, and Interlocking Nails

Karl Nuss, Dr Med Vet

KEYWORDS

- Cattle • Long bone fractures • Internal fixation • Locking plates
- Intramedullary nails

KEY POINTS

- Treatment decisions for repair of long bone fractures in cattle should ideally be made quickly using evidence-based criteria that promise the best outcome for the patient. Such criteria have not been established.
- Open reduction and internal fixation require surgical expertise and substantial input of time and finances to be successful. Plate osteosynthesis usually provides the most stable type of internal fixation in cattle.
- Recently introduced locking compression plates offer a wide range of treatment options; the type of plate can be selected to accommodate calves with relatively soft bones or heavy patients.
- Internal fixation may therefore be the treatment of choice not only for fractures in cattle of high economic value but also for certain types of fractures, in which rapid and uneventful healing can be better achieved through surgical intervention.

INTRODUCTION

This article provides farm animal veterinarians with an overview of newer implants (**Tables 1** and **2**) and established and newer methods of open reduction and internal fixation of long bone fractures in cattle. The results of surgical treatment of specific fractures in cattle from the literature are summarized (**Tables 3–9**), and the advantages and disadvantages of intramedullary fixation and plate osteosynthesis are discussed to provide information for decision making in clinical cases.

Prevalence

Long bone fractures are probably the most dramatic cause of lameness in cattle; a decision as to whether the patient should be euthanized, slaughtered, or treated must be made promptly. Because the value of individual cattle and treatment costs are

Conflicts of Interest: None.
Department of Farm Animals, Vetsuisse-Faculty, University of Zurich, Winterthurerstrasse 260, CH-8057, Zurich, Switzerland
E-mail address: knuss@vetclinics.uzh.ch

Table 1
Screws used for large animal fracture fixation[60],*

Screw Type	Cortex	Cortex	Cortex	Cancellous	Locking	Cannulated
Thread diameter (mm)	3.5	4.5	5.5	6.5	5.0	7.3
Glide hole diameter (mm)	3.5	4.5	5.5	4.5	None	7.3
Thread hole diameter (mm)	2.5	3.2	4.0	3.2	4.3	5
Core diameter (mm)	2.4	3.0	3.8	3.0	4.4	4.5
Tap diameter (mm)	3.5	4.5	5.5	6.5	Self-tapping	Self-tapping
Pitch (mm)	1.25	1.7	2	2.75	1	2.75
Drive type	2.5 Hexagonal	3.5 Hexagonal	3.5 Hexagonal	3.5 Hexagonal	T25 Stardrive	4 mm Hexagonal

The stardrive recess provides torque transmission to the screw, and a holding sleeve for the screw is not necessary.
* SYNTHES (USA), Paoli, Philadelphia.

increasingly divergent, it is unlikely that most cattle with a long bone fracture are referred to a clinic for therapy. The prevalence of long bone fractures in cattle is not known, because the available data originate from older or regional studies.[1–5] In more recent studies of causes of death in dairy cows, fractures are seldom listed.[6,7] The bones commonly fractured in cattle are the large metacarpal/metatarsal bones (21%–50% of cases), the tibia (12%–58% of cases), and the femur (15%–40% of cases); fractures of the humerus, the radius/ulna, and the calcaneus are less commonly reported.

Literature

The use of internal fixation of fractures in cattle started to increase in the 1950s; it was first reported in individual patients[8] and later progressed to studies of case series.[9,10] **Tables 3–9** summarize the literature and show the individual bones in which plates, pins, and intramedullary nails were used for repair of fractures in cattle. These tables are not meant to be complete; not all case series were published[11,12]: some appeared in conference proceedings[13,14] and others in dissertations that are not easily accessible.[1,10,15,16] Some studies[4,17–19] were not included in the tables because the results of the operations were not clear with regard to the type of repair, type of bone repaired, or individual animal operated.

Methods

The choice of type of surgical treatment in bovine fracture patients depends on many factors. Instruments and implants are expensive, and most clinics do not have all types of instruments at their disposal; this limits the number of repair methods that can be used. It can be assumed that for this reason, a particular repair technique is preferred by a clinic,[3,20–24] although many fractures can be treated with equal success using a different technique. Because fracture repair is uncommon in cattle, it is difficult to gather sufficient information on all repair methods. Some fractures are more commonly treated because certain breeds tend to incur a particular type of fracture, for example tibia fractures in Belgian blue cattle.[5,24,25] Individuals of this breed are

Table 2
Plates used for large animal fracture fixation[60],*

Name	LC-DCP 4.5 Standard	LC-DCP 4.5 Broad	DCP 4.5 Broad	DCS Plate	LCP 4.5 Narrow	LCP 4.5 Broad	Equine LCP 5.5 Broad
Width (mm)	13.5	17.5	16	16	13.5	17.5	17.5
Thickness (mm)	4.2	5.2	4.8	5.4	4.2	5.2	6
Length (mm)	34–394	106–394	103–359	114–370	66–287	116–440	188–440
Number of holes	2–22	6–22	6–22	6–22	3–16	6–24	10–24
Screw size (LS = locking screws)	4.5, 5.5 (6.5)	4.5, 5.5 (6.5)	4.5, 5.5 (6.5)	4.5, 5.5 (6.5)	4.5, 5.5 (6.5), 5.0 LS	4.5, 5.5 (6.5), 4.0/5.0 LS	4.5, 5.5 (6.5), 4.0/5.0 LS
Hole arrangement	Straight	Staggered	Staggered	Staggered	Straight	Staggered	Staggered
Hole spacing	18	18	16	16	18	18	18
Hole design	DCU	DCU	DCP[a]	2 Round, rest DCP, combi hole	Combi hole[b]	Combi hole	Combi hole

Abbreviations: DCP, dynamic compression plate; DCS, dynamic condylar screw; DCU, dynamic compression unit (bilateral compression); LC-DCP, low contact dynamic compression plate; LCP, locking compression plate.
[a] Unilateral compression.
[b] Combi hole: dynamic compression plate part beside threaded part.
* SYNTHES (USA), Paoli, Philadelphia.

Table 3
Internal fixation in humerus fractures: overview of the literature

No. of Animals Treated	Body Weight or Age	Segment[a]	Implants	Outcome	Reference
1	9 mo	2	1.3-cm (0.5-in) stainless steel intramedullary pin	1/1 excellent 1 y postoperatively	9
1	No information	—	Intramedullary pins	No information given	17
1	2.5 y	2	Küntscher nail	1/1 sound	85
3	3–8 y	—	14 mm intramedullary Küntscher nail	2/3 cured, 1 died (osteomyelitis)	80
1	275 kg	2	9.5-mm threaded stainless steel pin for 5 wk	1/1 healed	86
1	7 mo	2	10-hole broad DCP cranially	1/1 sound at 22 mo	79
1	18 mo	2	12-hole broad DCP cranially, 9-hole broad DCP laterally	1/1 sound 1 mo postoperatively	
1	4 y	3	12-hole broad DCP cranially, 10-hole broad DCP laterally	1/1 fracture of os femoris at day 13, euthanized	
1	250	2	10-hole DCS plate	1/1 slaughter	21
1	90	2	7-hole broad 3.5-mm DCP, 2 lag screws 3.5 mm	1/1 slaughter	
1	200 kg	—	14-hole bone plate	1/1 good after 37 d	57
3	300–450	2	2 clamp rod internal fixators, lag screws	1/3 successful, 2 implant breakdowns	55
1	2 d	2	Narrow 4.5 DCP	1/1 instability, euthanasia	31

Abbreviation: DCP, dynamic compression plates.
[a] Segment: 1, proximal epiphysis/metaphysis; 2, diaphysis; 3, distal epiphysis/metaphysis.

Table 4
Radius-ulna fractures in bovines treated by internal fixation: overview of the literature

No. of Animals Treated	Body Weight or Age	Segment[a]	Implants	Outcome	Reference
1	3 d	2	Eggers-type stainless steel plate, plaster cast	1/1 limb deformity	9
1	2 d	2	Venable-type stainless steel plate	1/1 normal leg use	
1	9 y	2	Venable-type stainless steel plate, plaster cast	1/1 implant failure 2 d postoperatively	
1	5 y	1	Intramedullary nail	1/1 healed, contracted tendons and slaughter 15 mo postoperatively	64
1	240 kg	3	2 Rush pins (2/B)	1/1 sound 10 mo postoperatively	10
1	2 d	2	4-hole DCP	1/1 sound 1 y postoperatively	87
1	7 d	3	2 plates	1/1 normal walk 8 wk postoperatively	88
1	18 mo	2	Broad 4.5-mm DCP	1/1 successful	72
1	620 kg	2	12-hole DCS plate, 10-hole broad 4.5-mm DCP, 2 lag screws 5.5 mm	1/1 excellent	21
1	450 kg	2	14-hole broad 4.5-mm DCP, 12-hole broad 4.5-mm DCP	1/1 implant failure, reoperation, then excellent	
1	480 kg	2	10-hole DCS plate, 12-hole 4.5-mm DCP		
	110 kg	2	8-hole broad 4.5-mm DCP, 5-hole small 4.5-mm DCP	1/1 excellent	
1	823 kg	3	14-hole DCS plate and 12-hole DCP, plate luting, full limb cast, Thomas-Schroeder splint	1/1 good	34
1	1018 kg	1 (olecranon)	10-hole broad 4.5-mm DCP, 5.5-mm cortical screws, plate luting with polymethylmethacrylate	1/1 sound 8 mo postoperatively	81
1	300 kg	2	2 10-hole bone plates	1/1 sound 3 y postoperatively	57
6	299 kg (mean)	2	2 clamp rod internal fixators	5/6 sound, 1 failure (534 kg cow)	55
6	1–14 d	2	1 DCP	5/6 sound, 1 died 5 d postoperatively	31

Abbreviation: DCP, dynamic compression plates.
[a] Segment: 1, proximal epiphysis/metaphysis; 2, diaphysis; 3, distal epiphysis/metaphysis.

Table 5
Metacarpal bones in bovines treated by internal fixation: overview of the literature

No. of Animals Treated	Body Weight or Age	Segment[a]	Implants	Outcome	Reference
1	85 kg	1	2 Rush pins (3/D), plaster cast	1/1 sound 5 mo postoperatively	10
1	3 wk	Open fracture since birth	2 plates, plaster cast	1/1 infection persisted, euthanasia	88
1	6 mo	2	Broad 4.5-mm DCP	1/1 successful	72
1	>24 mo	2	DCP	1/1 successful	33
2	6 mo	3	2 pins (physeal fracture)	2/2 successful	
1	260 kg	2	10-hole broad 4.5-mm DCP, 3 lag screws 4.5 mm	3/3 excellent	21
1	360 kg	1	10-hole broad 4.5-mm DCP		
1	228 kg	2	9-hole broad 4.5-mm DCP, 2 lag screws 4.5 mm		
1	50 kg	3, open	Broad 6-hole DCP	1/1 not successful, osteomyelitis	89
6	217–450 kg	1, 2	5 animals 1 DCP and locking screws, 1 animal 1 DCP and 1 DCS plate	4/6 healed long-term	63
3	Not specified	Not specified	Clamp rod internal fixator, lag screws	3/3 healed long-term Good long-term result, exuberant callus formation	55

Abbreviation: DCP, dynamic compression plates.
a Segment: 1, proximal epiphysis/metaphysis; 2, diaphysis; 3, distal epiphysis/metaphysis.

Table 6
Metatarsal bones in bovines treated by internal fixation: overview of the literature

No. of Animals Treated	Body Weight or Age	Segment[a]	Implants	Outcome	Reference
1	315 kg	1	12-hole broad DCP	1/1 sound 6 mo postoperatively	90
1	13 mo	3	Broad 4.5-mm DCP	1/1 successful	72
1	Heifer	2	10-hole 4.5-mm DCP	1/1 sound 4 y postoperatively	33
1	409 kg	2	12-hole broad 4.5-mm DCP, 7-hole broad 4.5-mm DCP	1/1 excellent	21
1	300 kg	2	12-hole broad 4.5-mm DCP, 3 lag screws 5.5 mm	1/1 fair	
1	350 kg	2	10-hole broad 4.5 mm DCP, 6-hole small 4.5 mm DCP	1/1 excellent	
1	9 mo	1	8-hole plate	1/1 successful	71
4	250–409 kg	2	2 animals with 1 DCP and lag screws, 2 with 2 DCP, and splint bandage	3/4 successful, 1 implant failure with bowing of leg (1 DCP)	63
5	—	—	2 clamp rod internal fixators	5/5 good long-term result, exuberant callus formation	55

Abbreviation: DCP, dynamic compression plates.
[a] Segment: 1, proximal epiphysis/metaphysis; 2, diaphysis; 3, distal epiphysis/metaphysis.

Table 7
Os femoris fractures in bovines treated by internal fixation: overview of the literature

No. of Animals Treated	Body Weight or Age	Segment[a]	Implants	Outcome	Reference
1	40 kg	3	2 Steinmann pins	1/1 normal leg use 8 wk postoperatively	10
2	40-45 kg	3	1 Küntscher nail	2/2 failures 1 infection, slaughtered 6 mo postoperatively, 1 migration of nail, euthanasia postoperatively, 1 recumbent, euthanasia	91
1	180 kg	1	Intramedullary pins	—	
2	3-8 y	2	14-mm intramedullary Küntscher nail	2/2 sound 1 y postoperatively	80
4	—	2	Intramedullary nail	2/4 calves died of pneumonia	92
4	—	2	6-hole plates	4/4 healed	
8	—	3	Condylar plates	7/8 healed, 1 not healed	13
1	—	—	Plate	1/1 not successful	15
3	Not given	Not given	Intramedullary pins (2), double plating (1)	1/3 double plating successful, 2 pin migration and infection	43
5	5 aged 2 d to 3 mo	2	Broad 4.5-mm DCP	5/5 successful	72
1	200 kg	3	Cobra head plate	1/2 mild intermittent lameness 4.5 y postoperatively, 1/2 sound 1 y postoperatively	93
1	60 kg	3			
5	1-9 d	3	90° blade plate	3/5 alive, 2 in reproductive use	14
12	≤1 mo	2	2 or 3 intramedullary pins and cerclage wires (7 animals)	10/12 successful	39
Several	Neonatal calves	—	Interlocking nail	Successful clinical outcome	12
2	Not given	2	Clamp rod internal fixator, lag screws	1/2 sound, 1 failure	55
5	3 mo	2	Polyacetal intramedullary interlocking nails	4/5 failed after 14 d	78
4	3 mo	2	Polyamide intramedullary interlocking nails	2/4 nails implanted after polyacetal nail failures, failed after 14 d	
3	45 kg	2	Stack pinning, 1 with cerclage wires	2/3 sound, 1 died of enteritis	76
2	34 kg	3	Intramedullary interlocking nail	2/2 euthanized	
1	39 kg	3	Rush pins	1/1 euthanized	
27	Calves 1-14 d old	1, 2, 3	1 DCP to 2 DCP	18/27 sound, 2/27 lameness	31
4		3	Steinmann pins	4/4 failures	
2		3	Rush pins	2/2 failures	
1		2	1 clamp rod internal fixator	1/1 sound	
25	Calves 1-6 d old	2	Custom-made intramedullary interlocking nail	15/25 sound, 3/25 persistent lameness	40

Abbreviation: DCP, dynamic compression plates.

a Segment: 1, proximal epiphysis/metaphysis; 2, diaphysis; 3, distal epiphysis/metaphysis.

Table 8
Femoral capital physeal fractures in bovines treated by internal fixation: overview of the literature

Animals Treated	Body Weight or Age	Implants	Outcome	Reference
3	4, 25, and 30 d	2–3 pins	2/3 euthanized because of femoral nerve in degeneration contralateral limb, 1/3 able to walk 6 wk after surgery	84
10	16.9 mo (means, range 4–28 mo, or 419 kg)	5.1–8.3 cm (2–3.25 in) Steinmann pins	4/10 functional >6 mo postoperatively, 3 unsuccessful, 3 unknown	26
5	7–24 mo old, 420–690 kg	3 cannulated 7.0-mm screws	5/5 lived >7 mo, 1 slight lameness	27
8	10–26 mo	2–3 Steinmann pins	4/8 lived >8 mo, 3 in bull stud	28
4	1–4 mo	6.5-mm partially threaded cancellous bone screws	3/4 lived >6 mo, 1 unknown	28
20	19 mo and 513 kg (means)	2–3 cannulated 7.0-mm screws	14/20 bulls serviceable, 11 of them lame (grade 1–3/5)	29

Table 9
Tibia fractures in bovines treated by internal fixation techniques: overview of the literature

Animals Treated	Body Weight or Age	Segment[a]	Implants	Outcome	Reference
1	13 mo	Os calcis	2 stainless steel plates	Serviceable 4 mo postoperatively	8
1	2 d	2	Stainless steel Sherman plate	1/1 died 2 d postoperatively	9
1	3 d	2	Venable-type stainless steel plate	1/1 sound	
1	9 mo	1		1/1 sound	
1	6 mo	1	3/8 stainless steel intramedullary pin	1/1 unable to stand, destroyed 3 d postoperatively	
2	190/425 kg	1	2 Rush pins plus Thomas splint	1/2 sound 18 mo postoperatively, 1 pin migration and infection/euthanasia	10
10	92 kg (minimum 47 to maximum 200 kg)	2	Experimental study. 2 to 3 Rush pins 3–4 mm thick	6/10 healed, 2 infections, 2 instability	75
1	1 d	2	4.76-mm threaded stainless steel pin for 5 wk	1/1 alive 9 mo postoperatively	86
12	80–150 kg	2	Experimental study. Küntscher nails 12–14 mm in diameter	12/12 complete healing at week 12 postoperatively	62
12	80–150 kg		Experimental study. 1 longer stainless steel plate medially, 1 shorter cranially		
4	Not given	Not given	Intramedullary pins (2), double plating (2)	4/4 dead: pins angular limb deformity (1), pneumonia (1). Plate breakage (1), bloat (1)	43
2	2 y	2	Broad 4.5-mm DCP	1/2 sound, 1 refracture	72
1	6 wk	Os calcis	Kirschner pins, tension band wire	1/1 union complete after 8 wk, implant removal	
1	220 kg	2	14-hole broad 4.5-mm DCP, 9-hole broad 4.5-mm DCP	1/1 sound	21
1	350 kg	2	12-hole broad 4.5-mm DCP, 8-hole broad 4.5-mm DCP, 1 lag screw 5.5 mm	1/1 sound	
1	50 kg	1	Rush pins	1/1 euthanasia	
1	45 kg	1	Steinmann pins	1/1 euthanasia	
3	Not specified	Not specified	Clamp rod internal fixator	3/3 sound	55
22	1–14 d	1–3	DCP	12/22 sound, 10 failures	31
7		1	Rush pins	3/7 sound, 4 failures	
3		1	Steinmann pins	1/3 sound, 2 failures	
1		2	Clamp rod internal fixator	1/1 sound	

Abbreviation: DCP, dynamic compression plates.

a Segment: 1, proximal epiphysis/metaphysis; 2, diaphysis; 3, distal epiphysis/metaphysis.

valuable and are therefore usually treated, which aids in gathering larger amounts of data for a particular repair technique. A few operations, such as fixation of slipped capital femoral fracture, are rarely performed.[26–29] Because of these factors, decisions about whether a bovine fracture patient should be treated conservatively or surgically are not necessarily made using evidence-based criteria. In addition, because only a few cattle have been treated by means of internal fixation, it is difficult to accurately evaluate the prognosis and success rate for this treatment in cattle.[21]

GUIDELINES FOR SELECTION OF PATIENTS FOR INTERNAL FIXATION

Guidelines for determining the optimal technique for repair of fractures in ruminants have not been determined.[12] Many fractures can be successfully repaired with either external or internal fixation,[3,5] and often the seemingly less expensive conservative approach is chosen.

The cost of internal fixation is considerable when preoperative, intraoperative, and postoperative radiographs, implants, the number of surgeons and anesthetists, anesthesia, surgery time, medical treatment, complications, prolonged hospitalization, cast changes, and rehabilitation measures are taken into account. All expenses need to be discussed with the client before treatment is initiated.

The costs of conservative treatment alone should certainly not be underestimated. Conservative treatment is often the less optimal choice, because of multiple cast changes and a lengthy rehabilitation period. In heavy patients, fracture fragments are more likely to shift, pressure sores or open fractures may develop, and pain results in increased recumbency, with rapid development of decubital ulcers.[5] Calves are prone to increased recumbency, which may lead to secondary disorders, including bronchopneumonia, diarrhea, and omphalitis. Concomitant disease substantially reduces the chances of healing[5,30,31] and simultaneously increases the expense and duration of treatment. In high-producing dairy cows, milk production decreases in the postoperative phase, and pain leads to reduced feed intake, with resultant metabolic disease and weight loss.

Internal fixation is usually the treatment of choice for fractures in valuable patients or show cattle,[32] but may also be the best option for certain fractures that are known to heal better and faster after surgery. Cattle are usually able to compensate well for mild angular deformities that may occur during fracture healing.[33]

Mature Cattle

When an owner requests internal fixation for their animal, the clinician must consider the fracture configuration and prognosis for the bone in question (see **Tables 3–9**) to plan the best possible treatment. Radiographs of the entire bone(s) must be taken in 2 planes to ensure that fragments are clearly visible and fissures or multiple fractures, for example fracture of the olecranon together with a diaphyseal fracture of the radius/ulna, are not missed. It may be necessary to take 4 to 5 radiographic views of a bone in mature cattle with fractures of the radius/ulna, tibia, or femur.

Older cattle often have a guarded to poor prognosis, because special implants designed for heavy animals with large bones are not available. Fractures of long bones proximal to the carpus or tarsus in heavy cattle are rarely treated.[21,34] Likewise, in the adult horse, comminuted diaphyseal fractures of the radius and tibia are considered to have a poor prognosis, even if modern implants and techniques are used.[35,36] Implants must be strong enough to sustain the weight of the patient during rising and lying down, which is often not the case with fractures of the tibia (**Fig. 1**), humerus, or femur.

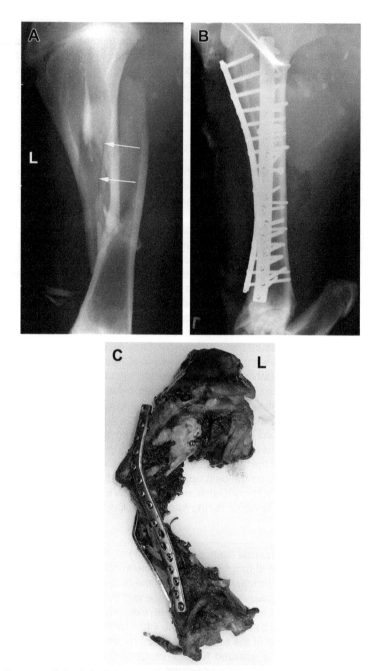

Fig. 1. Fracture of the left tibia in a 500-kg cow. (*A*) Preoperative lateromedial radiograph shows that the fracture consists of 2 main fragments and many small fragments; a fissure is also visible (*arrows*). (*B*) Mediolateral intraoperative radiograph shows that good repositioning of the fragments was achieved with 4.5-mm lag screws and fixation with 2 staggered long broad DCP. (*C*) Postmortem specimen shows failure of the implant, which occurred when the cow attempted to rise after anesthesia. Craniolateral view of the bone showing that the plates are still attached proximally and distally, but both are bent and there are multiple diaphyseal fractures.

Fractures in mature cattle are usually the result of massive trauma and therefore severely comminuted, which makes repair difficult, because there is insufficient bone to provide stability. In heavy cattle, the bone fragments must be aligned so that they support one another to maintain the fixation, because plates and screws alone do not provide enough strength, even when 2 strong plates are used.

Calves

The most common cause of fractures in newborn calves is excessive traction during assisted parturition.[19,31,37–40] Forced extraction of calves often leads to other injuries, such as rib and vertebral fractures,[41,42] and inadequate colostrum intake results in weakened immunity and secondary infection. Newborn calves do not know how to stand and initially bear weight on a fractured limb rather than favor it. Umbilical infection often develops in the first few days after fracture treatment as a result of increased recumbency. Omphalitis may require surgical treatment later on to prevent hematogenous spread of infection, with resultant osteomyelitis.[30,31,43]

In addition to these general risks, the bone structure in calves poses problems. Only the central part of the diaphysis has cortical bone that is thick enough to hold screws. The cancellous metaphyseal region is a predilection site for fractures. In newborn calves, 60% of femur and tibia fractures occurred in the metaphyseal region near the stifle and only 25% were seen in the diaphyseal area.[31] It is difficult to find sufficient bone in short metaphyseal-epiphyseal fragments containing a growth plate.

Screws cannot be inserted securely into thin and soft cortical bone, and plate fixation often fails at the bone-screw interface.[19,44–46] A high insertion torque does not necessarily produce significantly higher push-out forces on the screws.[47,48] However, an insertion torque greater than 3 Nm is necessary to achieve adequate stability in compression of the plate to the bone and to prevent movement between the components of an osteosynthesis.[49–52] When this goal is not achieved, movement of the plate results in loosening of the screws and shearing of the bone directly engaged by the screw heads, subperiosteal saucer fractures in the near (cis) cortex, and subendosteal saucer fractures in the far (trans) cortex.[53]

Results of in vitro studies in bones of young calves have shown that 6.5-mm cancellous screws have greater holding power in the metaphysis than 4.5-mm and 5.5-mm cortical screws.[44,45,54] For that reason, 6.5-mm cancellous screws should be preferred for use in the metaphysis of young calves.

GENERAL CONSIDERATIONS OF INTERNAL FIXATION
Anesthesia and Surgery Time

General anesthesia is generally required for open reduction and fixation of fractures, except for those of the growth plate of the metacarpal and metatarsal bones (**Fig. 2**), which can sometimes be repaired with pins and local anesthesia.

Several hours should be planned for internal fixation of long bone fractures. A mean anesthesia time of approximately 4.55 hours ± 60.5 minutes was reported for the repair of fractures with clamp rod internal fixators. The mean surgical time for metacarpal/metatarsal bone fractures was approximately 3.4 hours ± 33.2 minutes and approximately 4 hours ± 53.5 minutes for fractures proximal to the carpus/tarsus.[55] Duration of open reduction and intramedullary pinning of femur fractures in calves ranged[39] from 50 minutes to 3.8 hours (mean, 2.1 hours). Bellon and Mulon[40] required 1 hour and 15 minutes to 2 hours and 30 minutes (median 90 minutes) for insertion of intramedullary interlocking nails.

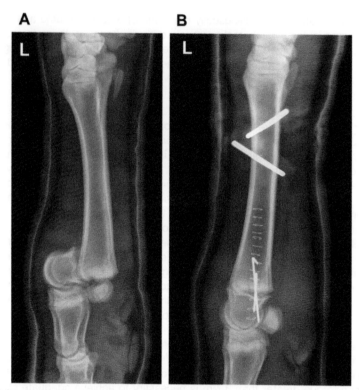

Fig. 2. Salter-Harris I fracture of the left metacarpal bone in a 400-kg heifer. (*A*) The fracture became again displaced despite correct reduction and stabilization with a fiberglass cast. (*B*) Healing was achieved using a fixation with Kirschner wires and additional stabilization with a transfixation pin cast.

The long operation time increases the risk of pressure-related injury as well as infection. Careful positioning of cattle on the operating table is critical for prevention of nerve and muscle damage.[12] Thus, preoperative planning must ensure that the appropriate implants are ready and the surgery team has been properly trained to minimize the operation time.[56] Recently developed cortical screws and locking screws (see **Table 1**) are self-threading, which reduces the intraoperative time considerably. However, locking screws are expensive and therefore not commonly used in cattle.

Methods for Simplifying Fracture Reduction

Traction is routinely applied to the limb to reduce fractures of the metacarpal/meta-tarsal bones and radius/ulna once the patient has reached a sufficient plane of anesthesia. Fixation of the limb with the help of a hoist also allows optimal surgical preparation of the suspended limb. The rope can be secured to various aspects of the pastern (dorsal, lateral, or palmar/plantar) to alter the direction of pull, thus facilitating reduction of the fracture. A combination of traction and release events is helpful for reduction in these axially loaded bones. In fractures of the humerus, femur, and tibia, traction on the limb often leads to overriding of the fracture fragments and hinders repositioning efforts. However, this blockade effect, for example, the reciprocal apparatus on the tibia, can be overcome when the pull on the rope is changed to cranial or caudal. Other measures to aid reduction are the use of local anesthesia, a deeper plane of anesthesia, and less frequently, muscle relaxants and fragment distractors.[57] Tenting of the fragments should be performed cautiously, because it can exacerbate fissures or lead to chip fractures.

Aims of Internal Fixation

The goal of fracture repair is to produce an anatomically correct and stable fixation, which allows rapid and pain-free use of the limb. However, the principal goal is no longer primary bone healing using compression plating or neutralization plating, because these techniques can impair blood supply, resulting in delayed union, nonunion, refracture, and infection.[58] Relative stability and secondary bone healing are preferred. Secondary bone healing occurs when strain at the fracture gap is maintained at 2% to 10%. Splints, casts, locked plates, and external fixators can provide this relative stability.[59]

In heavy and mature cattle, correct anatomic reconstruction and compression plating are still indispensable, because of high loading forces. In large animals, fragments must be repositioned correctly to facilitate plate fit, which together with the bone provides most support.[60] Because of the nature of the injury, the periosteum is frequently detached from the fracture site and cannot be sutured and preserved. When freeing the periosteum for fragment repositioning, blood vessels and nerves can be protected by keeping them out of the surgical field.[56] Methods that are deemed minimally invasive for plate application may also damage nerves and blood vessels.

Sometimes, internal fixation alone does not provide sufficient stability in adult cattle, and external coaptation or transfixation pin casts are added to protect the bone-implant unit.[21,61–63]

Postoperative Phase

Cattle are usually less prone to implant failure and refracture during the anesthesia recovery phase than horses, although considerable risk is associated with internal fixation of fractures of the humerus, femur, and tibia. In addition, acute laminitis of the claws of the contralateral limb is seen less frequently, because cattle lie down more often than horses. However, with inadequate fixation or with complications during fracture healing, considerable deformation (bending) of the contralateral limb occurs in young animals, and decubitus ulcers are seen in cattle of all age groups. During the postoperative period, the owner must be prepared to house the patient alone in a box stall for 3 to 4 months. The plates are usually not removed after fracture healing in cattle. However, they may become incorporated into the bone, forming a weak point, possibly resulting in refracture years after fixation (**Fig. 3**).

IMPLANTS AND TECHNIQUES

The materials used for fracture reduction and internal fixation include Rush pins, intramedullary Steinmann nails, or interlocking nails and plates of various shapes and sizes (see **Table 2**). There are few implants designed specifically for cattle[40,64] and few studies on implants for use specifically in cattle.[46,65] Implants have been modified considerably over the years, and ones such as the clamp rod internal fixator[55] are no longer readily available for large animals. New implants such as locking compression plates (LCP)[66] or custom-made implant systems[40] have been successfully introduced. No extensive studies have been published on the new locking plate system in cattle. A particularly strong plate developed for fractures in horses called the Equine

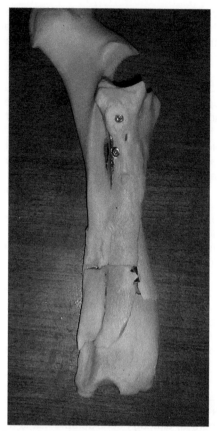

Fig. 3. Postmortem specimen of the right radius/ulna of a cow, recovered 4 years after repair of a radius/ulna fracture with a single DCP at the age of 1 month. During growth of the bone after surgery, the DCP was incorporated into the bone, and its distal end became located in the diaphysis. This situation likely posed an area of stress concentration, resulting in refracture.

5.5 broad LCP can also be used in cattle. It has a rounded end, which makes it easier to place near joints.[60]

Plates and Screws

Plating provides the most rigid form of internal fixation in ruminant orthopedics.[12] Conventional dynamic compression plates (DCP) and cortical and cancellous screws are being replaced with LCP with locking screws (see **Tables 1** and **2**). LCP have combi holes and, therefore, are compatible with conventional as well as locking screws, which means that they can be used in dynamic compression and locking fashion.

Dynamic compression plating can function well only when there is no or only minimal motion between the plate and bone. A DCP must be contoured precisely and attached firmly to the surface of the bone for ideal friction. When the plate is not contoured accurately, the fragments can move during cortical screw insertion, which leads to primary loss of reduction. With optimal reduction, cyclic loading forces encountered during standing and movement can lead to loosening, bending, or breakage of the (conventional) screws and resultant displacement of the plate and fragments. This process is called secondary loss of reduction.

Locking plates and screws prevent primary as well as secondary loss of reduction. Primary dislocation of fragments is not possible, because the thread in the screw head is inserted in the thread of the plate and the bone is not pulled toward the plate. A strong unit is created after insertion of the screw head in the locking plate, which accounts for the lack of movement between the plate and screws, even under load.

The fracture configuration, possible approach(es), and presumed tension side of the bone(s) are considered before application of the plate(s) to the bone surface. The fragments are repositioned and held in place with large pointed reduction forceps. Several 3.5-mm cortical screws are placed, usually in a lag screw fashion, to maintain the position of the fragments temporarily. The reduction forceps are removed so that they do not interfere with plate application. In cases in which the 3.5-mm positioning screws are not removed, the screw head must be recessed into the cortex so the plate can be applied over it. Otherwise, the positioning screws are removed once the larger (lag) screws in the plate have stabilized the bone. Multiple fragments are repositioned and held in place with lag screws to compose 2 main fragments (**Fig. 4**) and then adapted as described earlier.

Double plating is recommended for most long bone fractures in mature cattle; 1 plate is placed on the tension side of the bone and the second at a plane rotated

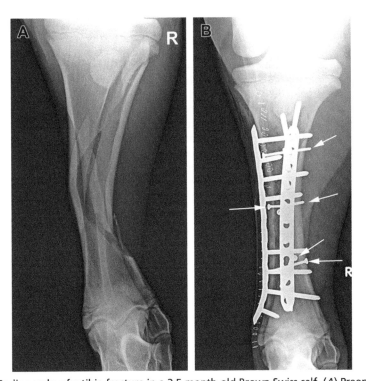

Fig. 4. Radiographs of a tibia fracture in a 3.5-month-old Brown Swiss calf. (*A*) Preoperative craniocaudal view shows a long oblique tibia fracture with a large fragment situated medially. (*B*) Radiographic view taken immediately postoperatively show adaptation of the fragments, which was performed in a stepwise fashion using 3.5-mm lag screws (*arrows*), and fracture fixation using a standard LCP placed cranially and a wide LCP placed medially. The patient was able to bear weight well at the time of discharge 4 weeks postoperatively and was completely healthy according to the owner 1 year after surgery.

by 90° relative to the first.[21,56,67] This technique strengthens the torsional and bending strengths of the constructs considerably. To avoid stress concentration in the diaphysis, where secondary fracture is more likely, the plates should begin and end in the metaphysis and be staggered in their relative proximal and distal orientation.[35] Staggering prevents stress concentration at the plate ends and facilitates screw placement.[12] Screws should be placed in all of the plate holes, because empty screw holes present a site of weakness that breaks under load. In cattle heavier than 200 kg, 5.5-mm cortical screws are recommended.[21]

Locking or locked plates act as rigid internal fixators, because of their proximity to the bone and fracture site. They are more resistant than compression plates, because they convert shear stress to compressive stress at the screw-bone interface. For these reasons, locking plates cannot be used as buttress plates; cyclic compressive loading with a fracture gap leads to plate fatigue and breakage. The stability of the LCP corresponds to that of the DCP only when its distance is less than 2 mm from the bone.[68]

The combi holes in the LCP mean that it can be compressed to the bone first using cortical screws and then secured with locking screws. The combi hole allows interfragmentary compression, compression plating, and internal fixation to be combined (hybrid modus). Placement of cortical screws at the plate ends provides the desired reduction in stiffness of locked plating constructs and retains construct strength.[69] Whenever cortical screws are used, they must be placed before the locking screws to prevent them from pulling out.

Similar to low contact DCP (LC-DCP), locking plates have a low contact surface, which serves to protect blood vessels and can be applied in a minimally invasive fashion, because of their pointed ends. The LCP are particularly suited for osteopenic or osteoporotic bone. This feature should provide better stability in the long bones of newborn calves.[46,70] A disadvantage of locked screws is that they cannot be inserted on an angle, for example, across a fracture line or to avoid a joint or the screws of another plate in double plating techniques. For those circumstances, shorter locking screws or cortical screws should be used. A torque limiting attachment is used on the screwdriver for locking screws to ensure that the appropriate amount of torque (4.0 Nm) is applied. Hand tightening of locking screws is recommended in large animals to ensure that the head thread is tightened sufficiently.[60]

Pins and Intramedullary Nails

Kirschner pins, Rush pins, Steinmann nails, or intramedullary interlocking nails are inexpensive for use in fracture fixation. Kirschner pins can be used to adapt and fix fragments associated with epiphyseal fractures. They are especially suited for growth plate fractures (see **Fig. 3**), particularly of the cannon bone[33,71] as well as the radius and tibia. Kirschner wires are used together with cerclage wires on apophyseal fractures, for example the calcaneus,[72] but additional external stabilization is usually required.

Küntscher nails, Steinmann pins, Rush pins, and interlocking nails are used for intramedullary fixation. The V-shaped and cloverleaf-shaped Küntscher nails[62] have largely been replaced by different variations of interlocking nails.[73,74] The Rush pin system is still available, although seldom used. Although it can be difficult to carry out accurately, it is an elegant technique used mainly for repair of fractures of the proximal metaphysis of the tibia in calves,[31,75] which occur commonly. It has also been effective for repair of fractures of the radius and metacarpal bones.[10] Frequent complications, including instability and infection, have been reported with the use of Rush pins in the femur of calves, partly because this system requires strong cortical bone, which in young animals occurs only in the mid-diaphyseal region.

The 2 greatest disadvantages of intramedullary pins are poor torsional stability and lack of resistance to collapse in oblique and comminuted fractures. Steinmann pins are used most commonly, particularly in calves for fractures of the humerus or femur (see **Tables 3** and **7**). Steinmann pins have a diameter of up to 6.35 mm and are available with or without a threaded end.[76] Primary bone healing is not achieved after intramedullary pinning, because considerable callus formation is seen. This type of fixation is unstable and painful until callus has developed.[39,56,62] In some cases, cerclage wire is used for additional support.[11,74] Migration of pins is associated with damage to the intramedullary cavity and physeal cartilage and subsequently can result in infection.[18,39,76]

The use of multiple pins (stack pinning) in the medullary cavity increases the contact area between the implants and cortex, thereby improving resistance to torsion and bending.[12,73] Pins should occupy 60% to 75% of the narrowest region of the medullary cavity.[74] Threaded Steinmann pins have been recommended for fixation of fractures in newborn calves so that they are less prone to migration.[12]

The interlocking nail decreases torsional instability and has been shown to prevent collapse of comminuted fractures caused by weight bearing and migration of the pins. However, the compressive stiffness of interlocking nails was reported to be only 15% of intact bone after a gap of 1 cm had been created, which is important in unsupported fractures, such as those that commonly occur in the femur.[65] Interlocking nails have a diameter of up to 13 mm, which is adequate for the medullary cavity of the femur in calves, and screw holes placed 16.5 mm apart along the entire length of the nail or only 2 screw holes on either side of the fracture. The screws are inserted using an aiming device, which is secured to the pin and ensures accurate drilling and placement of the screws. Empty screw holes present a point of weakness, which is the first part of the pin to fail under load. Solid interlocking nails have been shown to be markedly more resistant than tubular interlocking nails.[65]

Bellon and Mulon developed a special intramedullary nail for repair of femoral fractures, which was clinically used in 25 Charolais calves. The custom-made stainless steel interlocking nail was 190 mm long and 10 mm in diameter and had 4 divergent pins at the distal end. After insertion of the nail, these 4-mm pins became seated in the distal fracture fragment: 2 pins in the trochlea and the other 2 in the femoral condyle. This strategy prevented rotation of the pin, and the nail was usually locked only in the proximal fracture fragment with cortical screws.[40]

Various polymers have been tested for use as interlocking intramedullary nails for repair of fractures of the humerus and femur in calves as well as in a computer model, because these materials are light, inexpensive, and, purportedly, biocompatible.[77,78] They also result in less stress protection, and an aiming device is not needed for insertion of the interlocking screws. The results in fractures of the humerus have been encouraging, but in the femur, intramedullary interlocking nails made of polyacetal or polyamid 6 provided insufficient stability during locomotion.[77]

Rarely is impairment of intramedullary blood supply discussed with the use of nails or when reaming of the medullary cavity is carried out.[12,40] Growth plate injury is not uncommon (just as it is with plate osteosynthesis) when migration of intramedullary pins occurs. This risk is enhanced by the recommendation that the nails be advanced into the subchondral bone.

FRACTURES OF SPECIFIC LONG BONES
Fractures of the Humerus

Access to the humerus for plate osteosynthesis is difficult because of the large muscle bellies and origins and insertions of tendons (see **Table 3**). The superficial and deep branches of the radial nerve that are encountered in the surgical field must be protected. These factors are slightly less of a problem when a cranial approach is used[79] rather than a lateral approach; however, the distal aspect of the humerus still cannot be clearly visualized or easily manipulated. Reduction of the fracture is difficult because of the musculature and fragmentation of the bone. Application of a lateral plate is problematic because of the shape of the humerus; a cranial plate must be heavily contoured to fit the radial fossa. When drilling the distal screw holes, one must be careful not to inadvertently place a screw through the olecranon fossa. Fixation of fractures of the humerus via plate osteosynthesis often fails (**Fig. 5**), because of the body weight in older animals and weak bone structure in younger animals, which impede fixation of the implants. Thus, the prognosis of plate osteosynthesis for repair of fractures of the humerus in cattle is guarded to poor.

Internal fixation using an intramedullary pin or interlocking nail seems to have a better outcome than other methods in calves and light cattle breeds.[11,80] Fractures of the humerus heal adequately with the use of intramedullary pins and confinement of the patient to a box stall. Healing is probably attributable to maintenance of axial alignment by the implant(s). A better outcome is more likely with intramedullary implants, because the surrounding musculature acts to compress the fracture fragments to a certain degree. Mild displacement of the nail is tolerated, if the bone axis is well maintained. Furthermore, cattle generally have good callus formation capabilities. Single

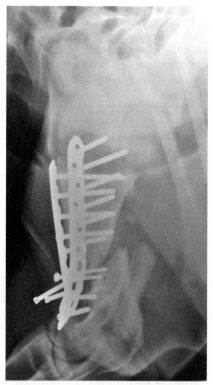

Fig. 5. Fracture of the humerus in an 8-month-old Holstein-Friesian heifer. Mediolateral radiographic view 5 weeks after fixation of an oblique fracture in the distal metaphysis/diaphysis using 2 narrow LCP. The 3.5-mm lag screws and the locking screws in the distal fragment have pulled out. The heifer was subsequently euthanized.

nails are usually not sufficient for heavy cattle, and stack pinning with Steinmann nails or an interlocking nail should be used.

Fractures of the Radius and Ulna

Internal fixation or conservative treatment with a cast or transfixation pin cast can be used for repair of fractures of the distal aspect of the radius. The ulna is also usually fractured but not always (**Fig. 6**). In cattle, fracture of the olecranon is rare.[81] Intramedullary nails are not as suitable for radius fractures as other methods of internal fixation,[12] although good outcomes have been achieved using these implants or Rush pins.[10]

A good outcome has been reported for the repair of radius/ulna fractures using plate osteosynthesis or the clamp rod internal fixator, even in heavy cattle.[21,34,55,81] The plate is applied to the cranial side of the radius, because this is the tension side. A single 4.5-mm DCP can be used in calves less than 200 kg (**Fig. 7**). In heavy patients, double plating should be carried out on the cranial, and lateral or medial side, depending on the fracture configuration (**Fig. 8**). The stronger Equine 5.5 broad LCP is available for this purpose (see **Table 4**).

Application of a cast from the claws to just below the elbow joint changes the side of tension of the radius to the caudal aspect.[82] In cattle, a high fiberglass cast can be extended above the olecranon, which stabilizes the elbow joint and provides better neutralization of forces (see **Fig. 8B**).

Fractures of the Large Metacarpal and Metatarsal Bones

Wound closure and plate coverage on the metacarpus and metatarsus are more difficult, because there is no muscle layer.[56] Plate fixation is not the treatment of choice for fractures of the metacarpal and metatarsal bones of very young calves, because of the lack of muscle and soft tissue cover for protection of the implants. In addition, screws have little purchase in the soft bone, which results in instability. Both these factors increase the risk of infection. Newborn calves are particularly at risk of infection, and therefore, a less invasive method or minimal osteosynthesis should be used (**Fig. 9**); adaptation of fragments using lag screws or T-plates is feasible. However, this type of fixation does not provide adequate stability, and additional external coaptation with a cast is necessary. Rapid callus formation and healing occur, because soft tissues and blood supply are protected.

Open reduction and internal fixation (**Fig. 10**), mainly with DCP or dynamic condylar screw, produced significantly better results than various types of external coaptation, including transfixation pin casts, especially in heavier animals.[63] The degree of fracture reduction was significantly correlated with short-term as well as long-term results. A single plate applied to the dorsolateral side of tension is adequate for fracture repair in older calves or young cattle in which the bone structure is more stable (see **Tables 5 and 6**). The use of a double plating technique was recommended specifically for animals weighing more than 250 kg (MT III/IV) or 400 kg (MC III/IV).[63]

Internal fixation of the large metacarpal and metatarsal bones in older cattle is usually supplemented by temporary external coaptation. A splint bandage or fiberglass cast with regular changes is recommended. External coaptation helps prevent edema, protects sutures, and stabilizes the fracture when sudden heavy loads are applied. A stepwise reduction in the support provided by the type of external coaptation is carried out as healing occurs; a cast is used for 2 to 4 weeks, a splint bandage for the next 2 to 4 weeks, and a light bandage for the last 2 to 4 weeks. This gradual change in support promotes regeneration of the bone, muscles, and tendons and prevents the development of abnormal postures.

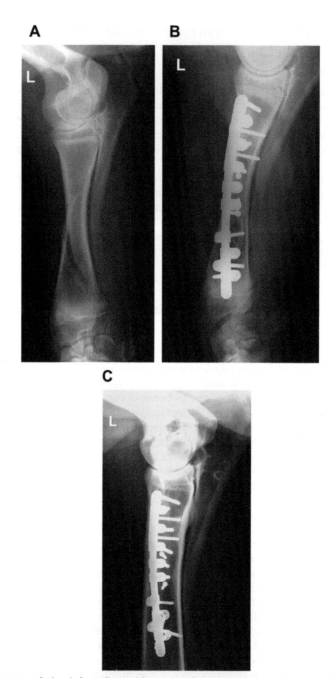

Fig. 6. Fracture of the left radius without involvement of the ulna in a 5-month-old Braunvieh heifer. The lameness score was 3/5. (*A*) Preoperative radiograph, mediolateral view. (*B*) Intraoperative radiograph of the same forearm after reduction of the fracture with 3.5-mm lag screws and fixation using a clamp rod internal fixator. The 4.5-mm cortical screws were inserted at different angles. (*C*) Lateromedial radiographic view 3.5 years postoperatively.

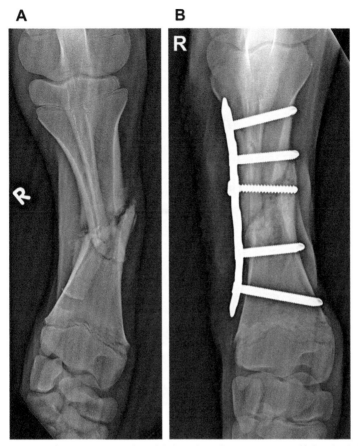

Fig. 7. Radius/ulna fracture in a 12-day-old, female Holstein-Friesian calf that had abnormal right forelimb posture since birth. Radiographs, craniocaudal views. (*A*) Fracture with deviation of the limb axis and callus formation. (*B*) Postoperative radiograph of correction of the malalignment and fixation using a narrow LCP with a 4.5-mm lag screw. Removal of immature callus and fragment repositioning were necessary before fixation. Locomotion was good immediately after surgery, and limb posture and use were normal at 12 months postoperatively.

In some complex fractures or fractures extending into the carpometacarpal or tarsometatarsal joint, a transfixation pin cast technique may be indicated to reduce the load transferred to the fractured bone.

Fractures of the Femur

Fractures of the femur (see **Table 7**) are common in newborn calves but less common in mature cattle, with the exception of femoral capital epiphyseal fractures (see **Table 8**). The most common cause of femoral fractures in calves is excessive traction during delivery, but trauma such as the dam standing on the calf has also been reported.[40] Femoral fractures occur most often in the proximal epiphysis and at the transition of the diaphysis to the distal metaphysis.[19,31,39,76] In a study of newborn calves, 28 of 50 femoral fractures (56%) were located in the region of the distal metaphysis.[31] Soft femoral bone and thin cortices are the major concerns for plate

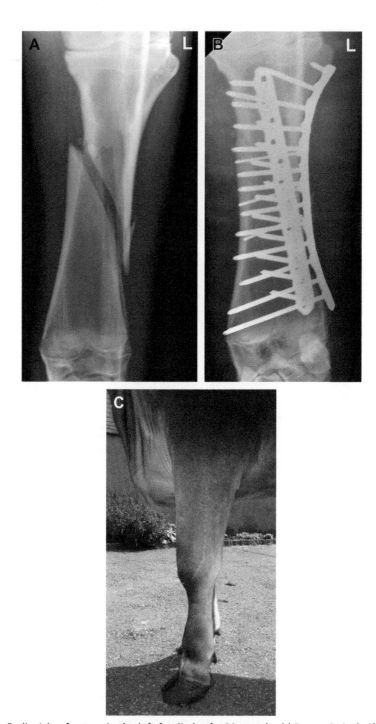

Fig. 8. Radius/ulna fracture in the left forelimb of a 20-month-old Brown Swiss heifer. Craniocaudal radiographs taken (*A*) at admission and (*B*) 2 weeks after fixation using 2 LCP, which were placed approximately 90° to one another. A cast that extended above the olecranon was applied postoperatively to protect the fixation. (*C*) The left forelimb of the same heifer 6 months postoperatively.

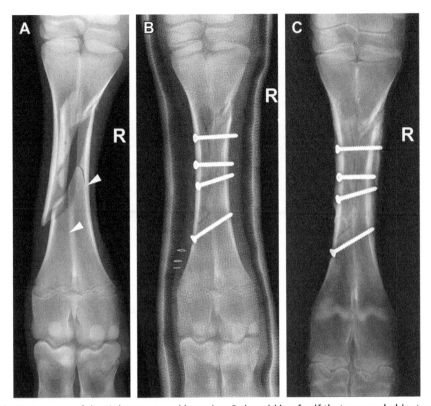

Fig. 9. Fracture of the right metatarsal bone in a 2-day-old beef calf that was probably stepped on by its dam. (*A*) A spiral diaphyseal fracture and fissures (*arrowheads*) are visible in the dorsoplantar radiographic view. (*B*) The fragments were adapted using 3.5-mm lag screws, and a high fiberglass cast provided additional stability. (*C*) After 5 weeks, callus formation and healing of the fracture are visible. The cast was replaced by a splint bandage, and no complications were encountered during further healing.

osteosynthesis in neonatal calves. Because the cortex becomes considerably thinner at the metaphysis, this part of the femur has only limited axial strength. Most femoral fractures in newborn calves are irregular transverse or oblique fractures. Gross displacement of the fragments, extensive stripping of the periosteum, and injury to adjacent tissues are typically seen.

Conservative treatment of femoral fractures is rarely successful, because the fractures are usually severely overridden and the fragment ends distracted. Internal fixation techniques have been recommended over a Thomas splint-cast combination in young calves and heavy animals because of treatment failures attributable to the formation of decubitus ulcers and slippage of splints. Poor outcomes predominated when conservative treatment was used for repair of fractures in the distal femur.[5] Rush pins also resulted in a poor outcome in the few cases in which they were used.[31,76]

The 2 most commonly used methods of open reduction and internal fixation in calves are plate osteosynthesis (**Fig. 11**) and intramedullary pinning; no other methods have shown better results. Although fixation of femoral diaphyseal fractures using Steinmann pins was associated with frequent pin migration and instability (in 50% of cases), 10 of 12 treated calves were ambulatory within a minimum of 6 months

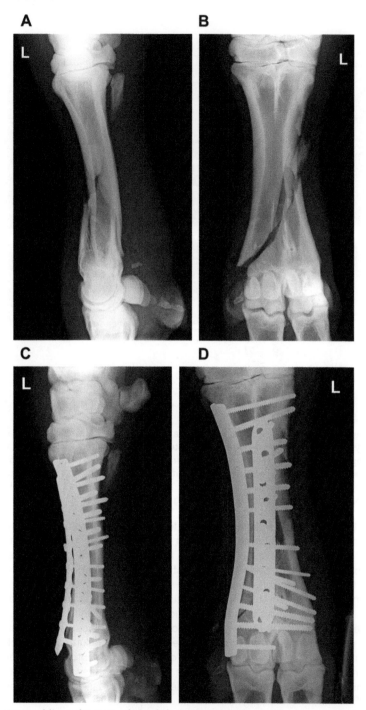

Fig. 10. Open oblique fracture of the left metacarpal bone with several fragments in a 2.5-year-old Simmental cow. (*A, B*) Preoperative radiographs showing fracture configuration and gas inclusions in the soft tissues. (*C, D*) A DCP was placed medially to prevent the proximal fragment from sliding distally. An LCP was placed dorsally. The pointed distal end of the locking plate protrudes slightly over the fetlock joint. A fiberglass cast and, after 2 weeks, a splint bandage were applied. The fracture healed without complications.

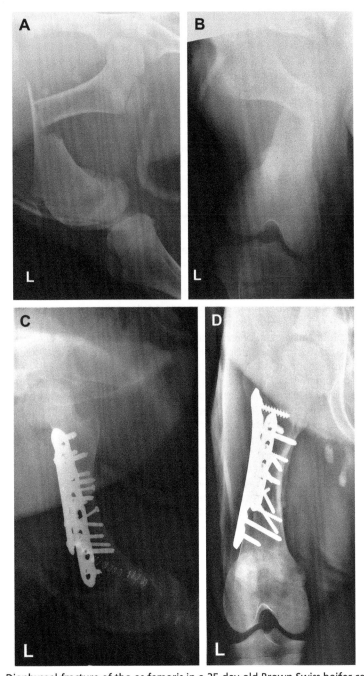

Fig. 11. Diaphyseal fracture of the os femoris in a 25-day-old Brown Swiss heifer calf. (*A, B*) Mediolateral and craniocaudal radiographic views. The fracture is not comminuted and only mildly displaced. (*C, D*) Radiographs taken 2 weeks postoperatively show callus formation caused by fixation with 3.5-mm lag screws and a lateral and cranial LCP (hybrid mode with 4.5-mm cortical screws and 5.0-mm locking screws). The cranial plate is short and prevents displacement of the fracture in craniocaudal direction. Long-term healing (>2 years postoperatively) was achieved.

postoperatively, with no complications.[39] However, a poor outcome has been reported for repair of fractures of the distal femoral metaphysis using intramedullary fixation.[76] Although 5 of 9 mid-diaphyseal fractures were successfully repaired with Steinmann pins and external fixation, the outcome was significantly worse for fractures in the distal metaphysis (0/6 cured).[76]

In contrast, the location of the fracture did not affect the outcome after plate osteosynthesis.[31] Two DCP in vitro femur constructs in immature horses provided superior strength and stiffness under bending and torsion compared with an intramedullary interlocking nail.[83] Angled blade plates were used to successfully repair fractures of the distal metaphysis of the femur in calves.[13,14] Likewise, when LC-DCP and LCP hybrid constructs underwent in vitro compression testing, LCP constructs were significantly more resistant to compression than LC-DCP constructs.[46]

Bridging of the growth plates by screws cannot always be avoided in fractures of the distal femoral metaphysis without severely compromising stability. In such cases, the implants should be removed as soon as possible once healing of the fracture is complete.[31,40]

A good outcome was achieved with the novel custom-made intramedullary interlocking nail[40] in 20 of 25 calves; 15 of the 25 calves that survived for more than 6 months postoperatively had no apparent growth retardation or lameness.[40] Distal diaphyseal fractures did not affect the outcome with this novel interlocking nail (see **Table 7**). Polymer interlocking nails broke 3 to 14 days after surgery in clinical cases as well as in a finite element analysis.[77,78]

Slipped capital femoral epiphysis (see **Table 8**) has been treated with open reduction using Knowles pins, multiple pins, or compression screws. Accurate and adequate pin placement is difficult in mature cattle.[26,84] For better interfragmentary compression, cannulated screws with a diameter of 7 mm and a length of up to 130 mm were used. Correct reduction is confirmed by placing guide wires and taking intraoperative radiographs; this may need to be repeated until correct repositioning is achieved.[27] Based on radiographs, this treatment led to healing of fractures in all of 5 bulls, 7 to 10 months postoperatively. Four bulls had a normal gait, and 1 bull had muscle atrophy and barely detectable lameness. In another study,[29] in which the mean age and body weight at the time of repair were 19 months (range, 11–27 months) and 513 kg (364–720 kg), 14 of 20 bulls were considered serviceable for semen collection postoperatively, but persistent lameness was evident in 11 of the 14 bulls. Mean duration for bulls to become serviceable was 5.5 months (range, 2–11 months). Six bulls remained severely lame and were euthanized. Age, weight, duration of injury at the time of repair, and degree of reduction did not significantly affect the success of surgical repair. A more favorable prognosis was given in cases in which early intervention had been carried out.[29]

Fractures of the Tibia

Fractures of the tibia (see **Table 9**) are usually located in the proximal epiphyseal region in calves and in the diaphysis in older animals. Comminuted fractures occur frequently (see **Figs. 1** and **4**; **Fig 12**). In calves, the proximal fragment is often too small to allow stable fixation (**Fig. 13**). Compared with fractures of the femur, infection occurred significantly more often in calves after repair of tibial fractures.[31] Because musculature with good circulation is not present on the medial side of the tibia, implants at this location have poor protection. Plates placed laterally on the tibia require more intense preparation to protect the lateral compartment of the femorotibial joint and the fibular nerve. Long-term healing was achieved using plate osteosynthesis in 12 of 22 (54%) calves.[31] There are only a few studies on the outcome of plate

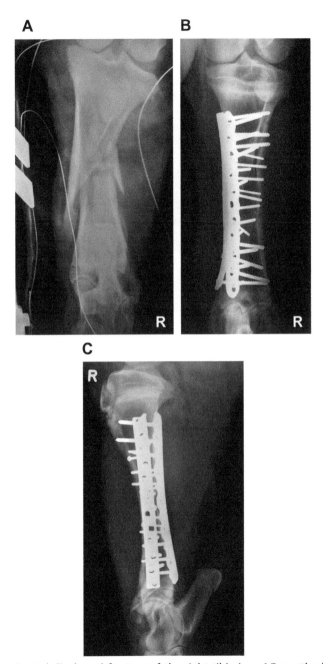

Fig. 12. Comminuted diaphyseal fracture of the right tibia in a 4.5-month-old Braunvieh heifer. (*A*) Caudocranial radiographic view. Cast fixation with implementation of metal bars had been used by the referring veterinarian for the transport. (*B, C*) Radiographs taken 12 days postoperatively show callus formation after double plating (1 medial DCP and 1 caudal LCP) for fracture fixation. Healing was uneventful.

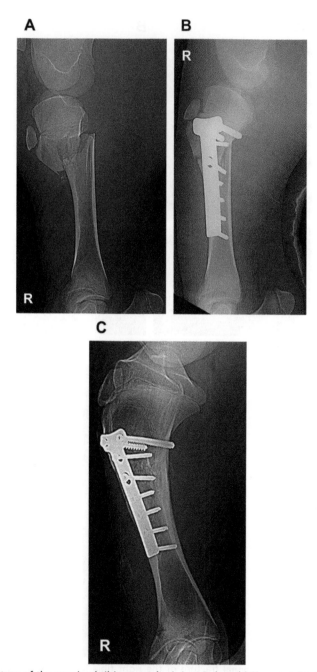

Fig. 13. Fracture of the proximal tibia metaphysis in a 2-day-old Simmental calf. (*A*) Medio-lateral radiographic projection shows an irregular oblique fracture with a small proximal fragment. (*B*) Fracture stabilization was achieved using T-plate, cancellous screws in the proximal fragment and a cast that extended above the stifle. (*C*) Radiograph on the right taken 12 months postoperatively. The patient had normal locomotion with no apparent postural defects.

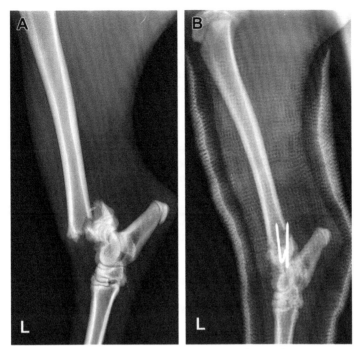

Fig. 14. Salter-Harris type II fracture of the distal physis of the left tibia in a 3-month-old dwarf goat. (*A*) Mediolateral radiographic view. (*B*) Postoperative radiograph of fracture fixation using Kirschner wires and a cast. Healing was uneventful, with a cast change and application of a splint cast.

osteosynthesis for repair of tibial fractures in older cattle, and most patients had a relatively light body weight[62] (see **Table 9**). Küntscher nails as well as plate osteosynthesis had a good outcome in that study.

Healing of fractures of the proximal tibial metaphysis occurred in a few animals treated with the Rush pin technique.[10,31,75] Although this implant does not always provide initial fracture stability, wedging of the fragments and formation of a stabilizing callus can occur, aided by muscle traction, especially in the proximal aspect of the tibia.

Fractures of the distal tibial physis in calves had a particularly poor prognosis.[31] The medial aspect of the distal tibia is covered only with skin and subcutaneous tissue. Often, the soft tissues in this region were severely injured and the fractures open. Also, growth plate fractures are difficult to stabilize, because of the small size of the distal epiphysis.[12,31] Bone fragments can be treated with Kirschner pins (**Fig. 14**), and a supportive transfixation cast is placed through the proximal metaphysis.

SUMMARY

Although intramedullary pins have a place in large animal orthopedic surgery, they are not designed for use in bovine long bones, and thus, the ideal intramedullary pin for cattle does not exist. However, it seems that intramedullary fixation is better than plate osteosynthesis for repair of fractures of the humerus in calves and mature cattle. In all other long bone fractures, plate osteosynthesis yields the same or better results than intramedullary pins, particularly in calves that weigh approximately 80 to 250 kg. In the future, locking plates, which are suitable for repair of soft bone, should allow successful management of long bone fractures in newborn calves as well as heavier cattle. In richly comminuted fractures in heavy animals, other methods of (external) fixation[20] may still be useful and indicated. Overall, the treatment options for repair of long bone fractures in cattle have improved, but as history has shown, the high cost and often guarded prognosis limit their application.

REFERENCES

1. Peitel M. Frequency of fractures of the extremities in horses and cattle and resultant economic loss. Wien Tierarztl Monatsschr 1971;58(4):158–63.
2. Ferguson J. Management and repair of bovine fractures. Pract Vet 1982;4: 128–35.
3. Adams SB. The role of external fixation and emergency fracture management in bovine orthopedics. Vet Clin North Am Food Anim Pract 1985;1(1):109–29.
4. Crawford W, Fretz P. Long bone fractures in large animals–a retrospective study. Vet Surg 1985;14(4):295–302.
5. Gangl M, Grulke S, Serteyn D, et al. Retrospective study of 99 cases of bone fractures in cattle treated by external coaptation or confinement. Vet Rec 2006;158(8):264–8.
6. Miller RH, Kuhn MT, Norman HD, et al. Death losses for lactating cows in herds enrolled in dairy herd improvement test plans. J Dairy Sci 2008;91(9):3710–5.
7. Thomsen PT, Dahl-Pedersen K, Jensen HE. Necropsy as a means to gain additional information about causes of dairy cow deaths. J Dairy Sci 2012;95(10): 5798–803.
8. Kirk H, Fennell C. Treatment of fracture of os calcis of a bull by plating. Vet Rec 1951;63(21):363–4.
9. Hickman J. The treatment of fractures in farm animals. Vet Rec 1957;69: 1227–36.
10. Verhaar W. Operative Fractuurbehandeling bij grote Huisdieren [Proefschrift]. Utrecht; 1965. [in Dutch].
11. Edwards R. Figures 11.2-1, 11.2-3, 11.2-4, 11.2-6, 11.2-7, 11.2-8, 11.2-9, 11.2-15, 11.2-18. In: Fubini S, Ducharme N, editors. Farm animal surgery. St Louis (MO): Saunders Elsevier; 2004. p. 290–315.
12. Trostle SS. Internal fixation. In: Fubini DL, Ducharme G, editors. Farm animal surgery. St Louis (MO): Saunders; 2004. p. 290–315.
13. Nemeth F. Treatment of supracondylar fractures of the femur in large animals. Proc. 12th World Buiatrics Congress. Amsterdam 1982, September 7-10: 791–793.
14. Ashworth C, Boero MJ, Baker GJ, Huhn J. Repair of distal femoral fractures in calves using a 90° blade plate. Scientific Meeting Abstracts — ACVS. Vet Surg 1990; 19 (1): 56.
15. Kahrs U. Vergleichende Untersuchungen über Gliedmaßenfrakturen und deren Therapie bei Rindern sowie über den Verbleib der Tiere [Inaugural Dissertation]. Hannover (Germany): Klinik für Rinderkrankheiten, Tierärztliche Hochschule; 1983 [in German].
16. Elma E. Frakturen beim Rind. Behandlung und Ergebnisse in den Jahren 1970–1987. [Inaugural Dissertation]. München (Germany): Veterinärmedizinische Universität; 1988 [in German].
17. Lundvall R. Fractures of the long bones. J Am Vet Med Assoc 1960;137(5): 308–12.

18. Mohanty J, Ojha SC, Mitra AK, et al. Treatment of fracture in cattle–an experimental and clinical study. Indian Vet J 1970;47(12):1118–24.

19. Ferguson JG, Dehghani S, Petrali EH. Fractures of the femur in newborn calves. Can Vet J 1990;31(4):289–91.

20. Adams SB, Fessler JF. Treatment of fractures of the tibia and radius-ulna by external coaptation. Vet Clin North Am Food Anim Pract 1996;12(1):181–98.

21. Auer J, Steiner A, Iselin U, et al. Internal fixation of long bone fractures in farm animals. Vet Comp Orthop Traumatol 1993;6:36–41.

22. Aithal HP, Amarpal, Kinjavdekar P, et al. Management of fractures near the carpal joint of two calves by transarticular fixation with a circular external fixator. Vet Rec 2007;161(6):193–8.

23. Aithal HP, Kinjavdekar P, Amarpal, et al. Management of tibial fractures using a circular external fixator in two calves. Vet Surg 2010;39(5):621–6.

24. Martens A, Steenhaut M, Gasthuys F, et al. Conservative and surgical treatment of tibial fractures in cattle. Vet Rec 1998;143(1):12–6.

25. Verschooten F, De Moor A, Desmet P, et al. Surgical treatment of tibial fractures in cattle. Vet Rec 1972;90(2):24–9.

26. Hull BL, Koenig GJ, Monke DR. Treatment of slipped capital femoral epiphysis in cattle: 11 cases (1974–1988). J Am Vet Med Assoc 1990;197(11):1509–12.

27. Wilson DG, Crawford WH, Stone WC, et al. Fixation of femoral capital physeal fractures with 7.0 mm cannulated screws in five bulls. Vet Surg 1991;20(4):240–4.

28. Ewoldt JM, Hull BL, Ayars WH. Repair of femoral capital physeal fractures in 12 cattle. Vet Surg 2003;32(1):30–6.

29. Bentley VA, Edwards RB 3rd, Santschi EM, et al. Repair of femoral capital physeal fractures with 7.0 mm cannulated screws in cattle: 20 cases (1988-2002). J Am Vet Med Assoc 2005;227(6):964–9.

30. Ferguson J. Special considerations in bovine orthopedics and lameness. Vet Clin North Am Food Anim Pract 1985;1:131–8.

31. Nuss K, Spiess A, Feist M, et al. Treatment of long bone fractures in 125 newborn calves. A retrospective study. Tierarztl Prax Ausg G Grosstiere Nutztiere 2011; 39(1):15–26.

32. Steiner A, Anderson DE. Fracture management in cattle. In: Anderson DE, Rings DM, editors. Current veterinary therapy food animal practice. 5th edition. St Louis (MO): Saunders Elsevier; 2009. p. 253–8.

33. Kostlin RG, Nuss K, Elma E. Metacarpal and metatarsal fractures in cattle. Treatment and results. Tierarztl Prax 1990;18(2):131–44.

34. Trostle S, Wilson D, Hanson P, et al. Management of radial fracture in an adult bull. J Am Vet Med Assoc 1995;206(12):1917–9.

35. Bramlage LR. Tibia. In: Auer JA, Stick JA, editors. Equine surgery. 4th edition. St Louis (MO): Elsevier Saunders; 2012. p. 1409–19.

36. Watkins JP. Radius and ulna. In: Auer JA, Stick JA, editors. Equine surgery. 4th edition. St Louis (MO): Elsevier Saunders; 2012. p. 1363–78.

37. Tulleners EP. Metacarpal and metatarsal fractures in dairy cattle: 33 cases (1979–1985. J Am Vet Med Assoc 1986;189(4):463–8.

38. Schuijt G. Leg fractures in newborn calves. Tijdschr Diergeneeskd 1991; 116(10):534.

39. St-Jean G, DeBowes RM, Hull BL, et al. Intramedullary pinning of femoral diaphyseal fractures in neonatal calves: 12 cases (1980–1990). J Am Vet Med Assoc 1992;200(9):1372–6.

40. Bellon J, Mulon PY. Use of a novel intramedullary nail for femoral fracture repair in calves: 25 cases (2008–2009). J Am Vet Med Assoc 2011;238(11):1490–6.

41. Mee J. Perinatal calf mortality–recent findings. Irish Vet J 1991;44:80–3.
42. Schuijt GD. Iatrogenic fractures of ribs and vertebrae during delivery in perinatally dying calves: 235 cases (1978–1988). J Am Vet Med Assoc 1990;197:1196–201.
43. Tulleners E. Management of bovine orthopedic problems. Part I. Fractures. Comp Cont Ed 1986;8(2):69–80.
44. Kirpensteijn J, Roush J, St-Jean G, et al. Holding power of orthopaedic screws in femora of young calves. Vet Comp Orthop Traumatol 1993;6:16–20.
45. Kirpensteijn J, St-Jean G, Roush J, et al. Holding power of orthopaedic screws in metacarpal and metatarsal bones of young calves. Vet Comp Orthop Traumatol 1992;5:100–3.
46. Hoerdemann M, Gedet P, Ferguson SJ, et al. In-vitro comparison of LC-DCP- and LCP-constructs in the femur of newborn calves–a pilot study. BMC Vet Res 2012;8:139.
47. Bufkin BW, Barnhart MD, Kazanovicz AJ, et al. The effect of screw angulation and insertion torque on the push-out strength of polyaxial locking screws and the single cycle to failure in bending of polyaxial locking plates. Vet Comp Orthop Traumatol 2013;26(3):186–91.
48. Tankard SE, Mears SC, Marsland D, et al. Does maximum torque mean optimal pullout strength of screws? J Orthop Trauma 2013;27(4):232–5.
49. Cornell CN. Internal fracture fixation in patients with osteoporosis. J Am Acad Orthop Surg 2003;11(2):109–19.
50. Gautier E, Sommer C. Guidelines for the clinical application of the LCP. Injury 2003;34(Suppl 2):B63–76.
51. Stoffel K, Dieter U, Stachowiak G, et al. Biomechanical testing of the LCP–how can stability in locked internal fixators be controlled? Injury 2003;34(Suppl 2):B11–9.
52. Korner J, Diederichs G, Arzdorf M, et al. A biomechanical evaluation of methods of distal humerus fracture fixation using locking compression plates versus conventional reconstruction plates. J Orthop Trauma 2004;18(5):286–93.
53. Fitch RB, Oliver JL, Hosgood G, et al. Fine morphological assessment of stripped screw sites in cortical bone. Vet Comp Orthop Traumatol 1999;12(1):20–5.
54. Blikslager A, Bowman K, Abrams C, et al. Holding power of orthopedic screws in the large metacarpal and metatarsal bones of calves. Am J Vet Res 1994; 55(3):415–8.
55. Gamper S, Steiner A, Nuss K, et al. Clinical evaluation of the CRIF 4.5/5.5 system for long-bone fracture repair in cattle. Vet Surg 2006;35(4):361–8.
56. Bramlage LR. Long bone fractures. Vet Clin North Am Large Anim Pract 1993; 5(2):285–310.
57. Ames NK, Belknap E, DeCamp C. Use of a fracture distractor in two cattle. J Am Vet Med Assoc 1995;207(4):478.
58. Frigg R. Development of the locking compression plate. Injury 2003;34(Suppl 2):B6–10.
59. Egol KA, Kubiak EN, Fulkerson E, et al. Biomechanics of locked plates and screws. J Orthop Trauma 2004;18(8):488–93.
60. Auer JA. Principles of fracture treatment. In: Auer JA, Stick JA, editors. Equine surgery. 4th edition. St Louis (MO): Elsevier Saunders; 2012. p. 1047–81.
61. Gertsen KE, Monfort TN, Tillotson PJ. Fracture repair in large animals. Vet Med Small Anim Clin 1973;68(7):782–90.
62. Vijaykumar DS, Nigham JM, Singh AP, et al. Experimental studies on fracture repair of the tibia in the bovine. J Vet Orthoped 1984;3:6–12.
63. Steiner A, Iselin U, Auer J, et al. Shaft fractures of the metacarpus and metatarsus in cattle. Vet Comp Orthop Traumatol 1993;6:138–45.

64. Voss HJ. Marknagelung am Unterarm einer Kuh. Dtsch Tierarztl Wochenschr 1961;68:134–6 [in German].
65. Trostle S, Wilson D, Dueland R, et al. In vitro biomechanical comparison of solid and tubular interlocking nails in neonatal bovine femurs. Vet Surg 1995;24: 235–43.
66. Frigg R. Locking Compression Plate (LCP). An osteosynthesis plate based on the dynamic compression plate and the point contact fixator (PC-Fix). Injury 2001;32(Suppl 2):63–6.
67. Florin M, Arzdorf M, Linke B, et al. Assessment of stiffness and strength of 4 different implants available for equine fracture treatment: a study on a 20 degrees oblique long-bone fracture model using a bone substitute. Vet Surg 2005; 34(3):231–8.
68. Ahmad M, Nanda R, Bajwa AS, et al. Biomechanical testing of the locking compression plate: when does the distance between bone and implant significantly reduce construct stability? Injury 2007;38(3):358–64.
69. Bottlang M, Doornink J, Fitzpatrick DC, et al. Far cortical locking can reduce stiffness of locked plating constructs while retaining construct strength. J Bone Joint Surg Am 2009;91(8):1985–94.
70. Freeman AL, Tornetta P 3rd, Schmidt A, et al. How much do locked screws add to the fixation of "hybrid" plate constructs in osteoporotic bone? J Orthop Trauma 2010;24(3):163–9.
71. Kofler J, Stanek C. Treatment of metacarpal and metatarsal fractures in cattle–a retrospective study (1984–1993). Wien Tierarztl Monatsschr 1995;82(3):75–89.
72. Denny HR, Sridhar B, Weaver BM, et al. The management of bovine fractures: a review of 59 cases. Vet Rec 1988;123(11):289–95.
73. Rakestraw PC. Fractures of the humerus. Vet Clin North Am Food Anim Pract 1996;12(1):153–68.
74. Nunamaker DM. Methods of internal fixation. Textbook of small animal orthopaedics. 1985. Available at: http://cal.vet.upenn.edu/projects/saortho/chapter_16/16mast.htm. Accessed April 6, 2013.
75. Rao K, Rao S. Rush pins for tibial fractures in bovines. Indian Vet J 1973;50:702–13.
76. Nichols S, Anderson DE, Miesner MD, et al. Femoral diaphysis fractures in cattle: 26 cases (1994–2005). Aust Vet J 2010;88(1–2):39–44.
77. Rodrigues LB, Las Casas EB, Lopes DS, et al. A finite element model to simulate femoral fractures in calves: testing different polymers for intramedullary interlocking nails. Vet Surg 2012;41(7):838–44.
78. Spadeto O, Faleiros RR, Alves GE, et al. Failures in the use of polyacetal and polyamide in the form of intramedullary interlocking nail for immobilization of induced femoral fracture in young cattle. Cienc Rural 2010;40(4):907–12.
79. Rakestraw PC, Nixon AJ, Kaderly RE, et al. Cranial approach to the humerus for repair of fractures in horses and cattle. Vet Surg 1991;20(1):1–8.
80. Kumar R, Prasad B, Kohli RN, et al. Repair of femoral and humeral fractures in adult cattle. Mod Vet Pract 1980;61(6):535–7.
81. Hague BA, Watkins JP, Hooper RN, et al. Tension band plating of an olecranon fracture in a bull. J Am Vet Med Assoc 1997;211(6):757–8.
82. Schneider R, Milne D, Gabel A, et al. Multidirectional in vivo strain analysis of the equine radius and tibia during dynamic loading with and without a cast. Am J Vet Res 1982;43(9):1541–50.
83. Radcliffe R, Lopez M, Turner T, et al. An in vitro biomechanical comparison of interlocking nail constructs and double plating for fixation of diaphyseal femur fractures in immature horses. Vet Surg 2001;30:179–90.

84. Hamilton G, Turner A, Ferguson J, et al. Slipped capital femoral epiphysis in calves. J Am Vet Med Assoc 1978;172(11):1318–22.
85. Kumar VR, Singh G. Use of Kuntscher nail in spiral fracture of humerus in a buffalo heifer. A case report. Indian Vet J 1976;53:64–5.
86. Coates J. Some orthopedic procedures in the young bovine. Can Vet J 1982; 23(6):205–6.
87. Dingwall JS, Duncan DB, Horney FD. Compression plating in large animal orthopedics. J Am Vet Med Assoc 1971;158(10):1651–7.
88. Winstanley EW. Fractures of the fore-leg caused by traction at calving. Irish Vet J 1973;27:218–21.
89. Steiner A, Iselin U, Auer J, et al. Physeal fractures of the metacarpus and metatarsus in cattle. Vet Comp Orthop Traumatol 1993;6:131–7.
90. Vachon A, DeBowes RM. Internal fixation of a proximal metatarsal fracture in a calf. J Am Vet Med Assoc 1987;191(11):1465–7.
91. Brown CM, Dicken JR. Intramedullary pinning of femoral fracture in a calf–a photo essay. Vet Med Small Anim Clin 1975;70(4):456–7.
92. Ames N. Comparison of methods for femoral fracture repair in young calves. J Am Vet Med Assoc 1981;179(5):458–9.
93. Kirker-Head CA, Fackelman GE. Use of the cobra head bone plate for distal long bone fractures in large animals. A report of four cases. Vet Surg 1989; 18(3):227–34.

External Skeletal Fixation of Fractures in Cattle

Susan R. Vogel, DVM, MS[a], David E. Anderson, DVM, MS[b],*

KEYWORDS

- Cattle • Fracture • External fixator • Pin cast

KEY POINTS

- External skeletal fixation (ESF) is a versatile method for rigid immobilization of long bone fractures in cattle.
- Traditional ESF devices may be used in young calves for clinical management of open fractures.
- Transfixation pinning and casting is an adaptation of ESF principles to improve clinical management of selected fractures.

Cast immobilization of fractures is most often chosen in ruminants because the most common fractures encountered can be appropriately treated with this form of external coaptation and because casts offer a reasonable economic treatment. Complications of casting include one or more of the following: muscle contracture, loss of range of motion of joints because of joint capsule and ligament contracture, reduction in articular cartilage quality and health because of prolonged immobilization, cast ulcers, impingement of soft tissues and vasculature, creation of open wounds that may communicate with the fracture, malalignment of the fracture, malunion of the fracture, delayed union of the fracture, and prolonged convalescence. Depending on the type of ESF used, these complications can be prevented or minimized. When cast immobilization is not appropriate or does not provide optimal management of fractures, other modalities must be considered. Casts cannot adequately immobilize fractures proximal to the distal radial physis or the distal tibial physis. Also, soft tissue injuries and open fractures may not be managed optimally by use of casts, splints, or splint-cast combinations. ESF presents a better option for stability and healing of fractures in many cases based on fracture configuration, soft tissue injuries, or open fractures. Usually, ESF is used in purebred animals, show animals, or other cattle of high perceived economic value.

[a] Elanco Animal Health, 2500 Innovation Way, Greenfield, IN 46140, USA; [b] Large Animal Clinical Sciences, College of Veterinary Medicine, University of Tennessee, 2407 River Drive, Knoxville, TN 37996, USA
* Corresponding author.
E-mail address: David.anderson@utk.edu

Vet Clin Food Anim 30 (2014) 127–142
http://dx.doi.org/10.1016/j.cvfa.2013.12.001
0749-0720/14/$ – see front matter © 2014 Elsevier Inc. All rights reserved.

ESF refers to the stabilization of a debilitating musculoskeletal injury (typically fractures and also joint luxation or tendon rupture) using transfixation pins (or transcortical pins) and any external frame connecting the pins and spanning the region of instability. The goal of ESF is to provide a sustainable, comfortable means to return the patient to weight bearing (or function) as soon as possible after surgery, to maintain normal joint mobility, if possible, and to provide an optimal environment for osteosynthesis and wound healing. There are 3 main types of ESF used in ruminants: (1) ESF using pins, clamps, and sidebars; (2) transfixation pin casts (TPCs) in which the fiberglass casting tape replaces the function of the clamps and sidebars; and (3) hanging limb pin casts in which the pins are only placed proximal to the fracture and a full limb cast is placed including the foot.

ADVANTAGES

ESF provides early return to function of the affected limb, management of soft tissue wounds on the limb, preservation of local blood flow to the fracture site, preservation of bone stimulatory proteins that exude into the fracture site at the time of initial injury, diversity in design for comminuted fractures, ease of implant removal after clinical union of the fracture, and relatively few complications resulting from the implants. ESF can be applied to most of the long bones. Transarticular application of external fixators may be used in the presence of severe soft tissue trauma or severe comminution of the proximal or distal end of the affected bone, and for arthrodesis or ankylosis of joints.

DISADVANTAGES

Disadvantages of ESF are suboptimal fracture reduction and poor anatomic alignment, absence of interfragmentary compression, less-rigid stabilization of the affected bone compared with bone plates, increased postoperative management compared with bone plates or casting, pain associated with micromotion at the pin-bone interface, and potential failure of the implants before clinical union of the fracture. Whenever possible, transcortical pins should be inserted between muscles and through facial planes. Pins placed through major muscle groups may result in pain and reduced usage of the affected limb.

TYPES OF ESF
Transfixation Pinning and Casting (TPC)

The most important goal of ESF is to return the animal to full weight bearing within a time frame that minimizes hindrance of limb use. Transfixation pin casting utilizes ESF pins that are incorporated into fiberglass casting material. These pins typically are inserted as *full* pins, meaning that they pass through the limb and are positioned so that the pin exits both sides of the limb (**Fig. 1**). Full pins offer the most stable construct with ESF by distributing force symmetrically across the pin. Most often, 2 to 3 positive profile pins are inserted proximal to the fracture and separated by a distance equal to 6 times the diameter of the pin (eg, two 6-mm-diameter pins should be separated by 36 mm of bone).[1] Positive profile pins are pins having threads that are greater in outer diameter than the shaft, or core, diameter of the pin. Positive profile pins are recommended because of the stronger bone-implant interface between the threads and cortical bone when compared with smooth pins.[2]

One advantage of TPC is that the distance between the bone and frame (cast) is minimized. The rigidity of the frame and bending resistance of pin are determined,

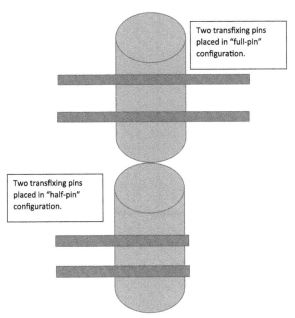

Two transfixing pins placed in "full-pin" configuration.

Two transfixing pins placed in "half-pin" configuration.

Fig. 1. Transfixation pins may be placed such that the pin exits both sides of the limb ("full pin configuration") or with the pin only exiting the insertion side of the limb ("half-pin" configuration). Full-pins contribute to a stronger construct because the external frame (side bars and clamps or fiberglass cast) is engaged on both sides. This spreads force more evenly across the near (cis) and far (trans) cortex relative to the side of pin insertion. Half-pins only engage the external frame on one side of the limb and are more prone to bending, loosening, and patient morbidity because of asymmetric force distribution.

in part, by this distance. Standard external fixation frames, composed of sidebars and clamps, require greater distance from the bone to accommodate the various pins used in the construct. Pin placement is restricted by fracture configuration and soft tissue structures. Once the TPC is constructed, biomechanical forces are transferred through the pins and to the cast. The resulting construct prevents loading of the fracture site thus preventing fracture distraction and interfragmentary movement. Possible disadvantages of this system are lack of access to soft tissues compared to traditional external fixators, greater incidence of pin loosening, pin tract infection, muscle contraction, tendon laxity, constriction of hoof growth, osteoporosis, pressure sores, and ring sequestrum formation around the pin.[3,4]

Two constructs for TPC may be used: (1) TPC with pins placed proximal and distal to the fracture site and (2) hanging limb pin cast with pins placed only proximal to the fracture site (**Fig. 2**). TPC may be used with full limb casts or using the fiberglass casting tape as a substitute for the clamps and sidebars of traditional ESF. Young calves having mid-diaphyseal fractures may benefit from placement of pins proximal and distal to the fracture followed by placement of the cast along the injured bone alone rather than as a full limb cast. This configuration allows the calf to maintain better mobility because flexion and extension of joints is not compromised. Fracture fixation using this limited TPC has been most often applied to fractures of the tibia in calves with body weight less than 100 kg. Hanging limb pin casts are more often used in adult cattle, especially for the management of tibia fractures. Pins are placed proximal to the fracture in the proximal tibia where the bone is widest, which allows placement of

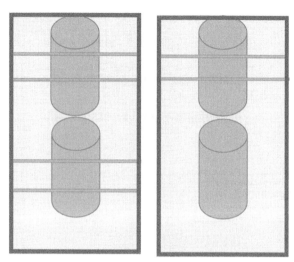

Fig. 2. Transfixation pin casts may be applied in either traditional configuration (pins proximal and distal to the fracture site, or as a hanging limb pin cast where pins are placed proximal but not distal to the fracture site. Hanging limb pin casts require a full limb cast encasing the foot so as to prevent ground reaction force loading through the fracture site.

larger and a greater number of pins. Hanging limb casts require placement of a full limb cast and inclusion of the foot within the cast. Distal pins are not necessary because weight is transferred into the cast proximal to the fracture site and transferred to the ground.

The size of the core pin diameter is crucial to the rigidity of the fixation. If the pin is too small, it will be insufficient to support the weight of the animal and may bend or break. Oversized pins may weaken the bone to a point where the integrity of the bone will become compromised and suffer pin site fracture.[5] The presence of a transcortical defect (ie, pinhole) in long bones remains the major contributing factor that reduces the strength of the bone. Defects as small as 10% of the bone diameter significantly decrease the peak torque and energy absorption under torsional loading.[6] The maximum recommended diameter of pins to be placed in a given bone is 20% to 30% of the diameter of the bone (eg, a 6-mm-diameter pin should not be used in any bone having a diameter less that 20 mm).[3,5,7–9] The geometric shape of bone is not uniform. Therefore, careful consideration must be given to the bone and to the region in which the pin is to be implanted before selecting pin diameter.

The rigidity of the TPC can be further optimized by creating divergence between the pins. Marked increases in the stability of the TPC have been determined when pins, being placed medial to lateral and perpendicular to the long axis of the bone, are placed with a 30° divergence from the frontal plane.[10] The divergence allows the pins to traverse the maximal diameter of the medullary cavity, remain engaged in cortical bone, and avoid soft tissue interference.[10]

SURGICAL TECHNIQUES FOR ESF IN FOOD ANIMALS

ESF and TPC can be applied to the affected limb of bovine patients while under general anesthesia or with a combination of sedation and nerve blockade such as a brachial plexus block for the front limbs and epidural anesthesia for the rear limbs.[11] Pins for TPC are most easily inserted with the patient in dorsal recumbency and the limb suspended vertically. This positioning facilitates fracture alignment and allows the surgeon to work without having to maintain limb position during pin placement and cast application.

Transfixation pins should be placed using strict aseptic technique, copious irrigation during drilling to minimize thermal necrosis and lubricate the drill bit, predrilling of the pinholes to a diameter slightly smaller than the diameter of the pin (0.1–0.3 mm smaller), tapping the pinhole using a transfixing pin tap for positive profile, and careful insertion of the pin through the center of the medullary cavity so that both cortices are fully engaged. If the surgeon has little experience with ESF in ruminants, we suggest placement of marker needles at the proposed site for placement of the transcortical pins. Then, radiographs are obtained and the pin sites are chosen based on the relationship of the marker needles with the fracture, fissure lines, adjacent joints, and intact cortical bone. With experience in choosing placement of pins and thorough knowledge of the limb anatomy of cattle, this step can be omitted. A l-cm incision is made through the skin at the chosen pin site. A hole is then drilled through the bone, and another incision is made for the exit site of the pin (for bilateral transcortical pins). A powered drill, pneumatic, battery, or corded, is used to drill a guide hole and insert the pins. During drilling, the drill bit should be continuously flushed with a sterile isotonic solution to help decrease thermal injury to the bone. Pins are implanted with the drill at low speed to limit heat buildup and prevent thermal necrosis of the bone surrounding the pin. Selection of drill bit and pin sizes should be done such that the pin is large enough to sustain full ambulatory weight loading by the patient (**Table 1**). A tissue protector, or pin guide, is beneficial to prevent excessive soft tissue trauma during drilling and implantation. The patient may be moved into lateral recumbency for cast preparation and application. This allows the suspension apparatus to be removed from the limb so that the foot can be enclosed within the cast. The exposed ends of the transfixing pins should be trimmed, using pin or bolt cutters, leaving sufficient length so that the pin ends can be incorporated into the fiberglass casting tape during application of the cast. The final 4 layers of the cast should cover over the pin ends and acrylic cement placed on the cast over the ends of the pins to ensure that the pin ends do not protrude through the cast.

Table 1
Guidelines for drill bit and pin diameter for creation of guide holes and pin diameter for placement in cattle

Patient Body Weight	Drill Bit Diameter	Pin Diameter	Desired Separation Between Pins	Desired Number of Pins Placed Proximal to Fracture
<150 kg	Goal: 3.0 mm Available: 2.7 mm	3.2 mm (1/8 in)	20 mm	2
150–300 kg	Goal: 4.2 mm Available: 4.0 mm	4.5 mm (3/16 in)	30 mm	2
300–500 kg	Goal: 6.1 mm Available: 6.2 mm	6.4 mm (1/4 in)	40 mm	3
>500 kg	Goal: 6.1 mm Available: 6.2 mm	6.4 mm (1/4 in)	40 mm	4

The drill bit diameter should allow for radial preloading (or compression) of bone surrounding the pin. This disparity in size should not exceed 0.3 mm so as not to propagate cracks or create cortical fractures in the surrounding bone. Limited selection of orthopedic drill bit sizes often require a size disparity of up to 0.5 mm.

Adequate padding should be placed over the entire limb with special attention paid to bony prominences, between the hooves, around the accessory digits (dew claws), and around the limb where the cast will end. TPCs can be constructed either as hanging limb pin casts or as external skeletal fixators on the injured bone. When the TPC is applied to a single bone (eg, tibia), transfixing pins are placed proximal and distal to the fracture and the fiberglass casting tape is used to span the bone and connect these pins.[12,13] The casting tape is applied similar to a cast such that a circular external fixator assembly is created. The transfixations are most often applied in a Type II external skeletal fixator construct. The fiberglass cast material should be applied without slack in the material, but it is of utmost importance not to tighten or overstretch the fiberglass material during the first few layers of application. The final layers can be applied with more tension on the material because the inner shell will protect the limb from constriction by the casting tape. The limb should remain immobile, and the fracture aligned by a dedicated assistant. Continued sedation and pain control at this point is important to ensure that the limb does not move during application. If the animal struggles or flexes its limb during cast application, the folds created in the unhardened fiberglass may cause complications such as cast sores and skin ischemia. In case this is encountered, all casting material should be removed and the application procedure started again. Each layer of the fiberglass casting material should overlap 50% of the width of the tape. Lightweight cattle should have approximately 8 layers of overlapping casting material (up and down the limb 4 times), and heavier cattle may have 12 to 20 layers of casting material depending on their weight. When the material is placed over the pins, the pins should be pushed through the material. The last few layers of the fiberglass may form a cover over the top of the pins, creating a "tent." Then, polymethylmethacrylate (PMMA) should be placed over the pin ends and cast to prevent shearing of the fiberglass. When the foot is included in the cast, PMMA should be placed over the foot to protect the end of the cast.

Distal metacarpal/metatarsal fractures are some of the most common fractures to be treated in bovine orthopedic patients.[14] When the fractures are simple and transverse in configuration, success is usually achieved with a half limb cast and pins are placed in the proximal metacarpus/metatarsus. More comminuted fractures and fractures of the proximal metacarpus/metatarsus or distal radius/tibia require a full limb cast with pins placed through the proximal radius or tibia.

JUVENILE CATTLE (<150 KG)

At birth, a calf's skeleton is mostly composed of woven bone[15]; long bones in calves have relatively thin cortices, which provide for minimal bone-implant contact. The thin cortices limit the holding power of implants and predispose implants to premature loosening.[16,17] Implant loosening can contribute to patient pain, fracture displacement, and delayed bone healing. The limited holding power of neonatal bone may increase the risk of screw pullout and failure of dynamic compression plates in young calves.[18] Transfixation pinning has been used successfully in neonates despite the limited density of cortical bone. Weight bearing results in axial loading of transfixing pins more perpendicular to their construct resulting in a "suspension" system for the limb that does not promote pin displacement or pullout.

Pins available for use in ESF include a variety of smooth, tapered, and threaded forms. Threaded pins are associated with improved longevity and torque resistance, but prospective research has demonstrated that the smallest diameter of pin suitable for the weight of the patient should be used (**Fig. 3**).[19] All pins, smooth or threaded, should be placed in the thickest portion of the bone possible so as not to compromise

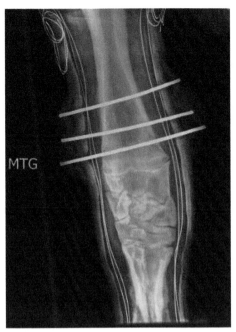

Fig. 3. Craniocaudal radiograph of TPC in a 136 Kgs calf 3 weeks after initial cast application. Three smooth pins are in the distal radius. The only pin placed in diaphyseal bone is the proximal one—note the metaphyseal location of the distal 2 pins. Fracture callus can be seen on the proximal metacarpus.

the long bone. A useful rule of thumb for selection of pin diameter is that the pin diameter should not exceed 20% of the diameter of the bone at the narrowest point (isthmus). Placement of pins through the bone results in localized weakness of the bone. Therefore, pins should not be placed close together so that this weakening is not focused to the point of causing pinhole fracture. A useful rule of thumb for pin placement is that pins should not be placed closer than 6 times the diameter of the pin (eg, two 6-mm pins should not be placed closer than 36 mm). In general, 2 pins placed proximal to the fracture are adequate for construction of a stable pin cast. Pins placed in metaphyseal bone often loosen more rapidly and may be more likely to cause patient discomfort and limb disuse.[20]

When transfixation pin casts are used, the cast must be closely monitored and changed as needed to accommodate growth and prevent cast morbidity. Diminished use of the limb during convalescence suggests that cast removal is needed. At the time of cast change, loose pins should be removed. If insufficient fracture healing requires continued ESF support, a larger pin may be placed to accommodate continued fixation. This procedure may be preferable to placement of an additional pin at a separate site because of the increased risk of pin tract fracture. The subsequent cast may be maintained until fracture healing unless healing is delayed. When fracture healing is sufficient to allow removal of the transfixation pins, removal of coaptation support should be staged to allow accommodation of the healing bone to increased weight bearing. After removal of the pin cast, a splint may be placed on the limb for 2 to 3 weeks, followed by use of a limb bandage for an additional 1 to 2 weeks, and finally pen confinement alone for 2 to 3 weeks. At this time, the calf should be sufficiently healed to return to normal management practices.

WEANED AND ADULT CATTLE (>150 KG)

Adult orthopedic patients present the challenges of greater fracture comminution, more severe soft tissue damage, and prolonged healing times. In addition, the markedly increased body weight makes it difficult to achieve adequate fracture stability and stress concentration at the bone-pin interface. A more guarded prognosis should be given to owners, and the likelihood of success decreases with increasing patient size. In adult cattle, large diameter pins (6.4 mm) that are centrally threaded are recommended. In adult cattle, 3 to 4 pins may be needed to resist loading forces and create a stable pin cast. Cast changes can be less frequent in adults than in calves. In adults, the pin cast may be maintained for 6 to 8 weeks, at which time pin removal is usually required because of loosening. Placement of a second cast may be advisable for 4 to 6 weeks to provide support during the final phases of bone callus maturation and healing of the pinhole defects. Catastrophic complications are more likely to occur in adult cattle, but careful clinical management can result in successful outcomes.[19]

COMPLICATIONS

Changes at the bone-pin interface can be difficult to detect radiographically because of the presence of cast material. In the authors' experience, patient comfort is correlated with presence of complications at the time of cast removal. When cast sores are present, they may be detected on radiographs by careful assessment of the skin-cast junction. A well-formed cast with no cast disease has a fine radiolucent line visible between the skin surface and the fiberglass casting material. When cast sores are present, there is loss of this fine line at the site of ulceration. With prolonged use of hanging limb pin casts, osteoporosis can be expected in the bones distal to the pins. Splinting the limb for about 2 weeks followed by use of a heavily padded bandage for an additional 2 weeks allows the animal to progressively gain strength in the affected limb and helps to protect the bones from fracture through the pinholes after pin removal.

Despite surgeons' best efforts and research to maximize the strength and stability of ESF, and more specifically TPC, complications are frequently encountered. The most commonly reported complications are implant loosening, infection, implant failure, bone failure, and complications associated with cast utilization (**Fig. 4**).[5,7,12,13,21–23]

The longevity of ESF is directly related to solid bone-implant interfaces and absence of pin tract osteolysis, pin tract infection, and pain to the patient.[3,19] Thermal necrosis during drilling and pin insertion causes bone resorption at the bone-implant interface and results in premature loosening.[24] Clinical techniques to avoid complications associated with pin insertion include predrilling guide holes for the pins using slightly smaller drill bits to decrease thermal damage to surrounding bone but maintain tight compression around the pin circumference (eg, use a 6.2-mm drill bit to create a guide hole for a 6.4-mm pin). This size discrepancy, termed radial preload, should not exceed 0.2 mm to avoid causing intracortical fractures during placement of the pins. Some positive profile pins have taps specifically designed to ease insertion of threaded pins. These methods of insertion increase the stability of the pins within the bone cortices and avoid the creation of microfractures.[4] Adequate padding between the limb and the cast provides protection of bony prominences and is crucial for avoiding pressure sores.[25]

Pin loosening is the most common complication seen with TPC and is usually associated with infection, instability, and pain.[26] Aseptic pin loosening can also occur as a result of the implantation technique or in osteopenic bone.[27] Loose pins are at

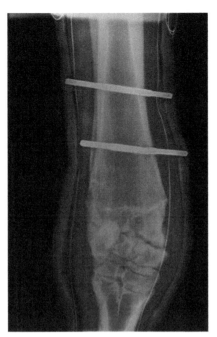

Fig. 4. TPC in an adult cow with 2 centrally threaded pins in the distal radius. Implant failure occurred with the distal pin. Note the lucency in the medullary cavity where the pin fracture occurred.

a greater risk for pin tract infection.[5] Implant loosening and infection create a vicious cycle and often occur before clinical fracture union.[22] Pin tract infection permits implant loosening by contributing to osteolysis and necrosis and can result in bone failure.[22] Clinical signs of peri-implant infection are lameness, redness, drainage, and local pain. Pin tract infection and pin tract osteolysis are not synonymous but are often present together and contribute to the development and propagation of the other.[28] It is important to be aware of the differences between a superficial infection, pin tract infection, and osteomyelitis because their influences on prognoses are not equal. These distinctions are facilitated by radiographic imaging of the pin site.

Superficial infections usually occur as a result of soft tissue irritation by pin motion, are more commonly observed with increasing soft tissue coverage, resolve quickly with pin removal, and can be minimized by avoiding placement of pins in musculotendinous areas.[27,28] Although there can be patient discomfort with these superficial infections, the integrity of the external fixation is not compromised. Pin tract infections are localized to the area immediately surrounding the pin and do not extend into the medullary cavity. The presence of infection along the surface of the pin leads to pin loosening.[22] Pin tract infections are commonly observed at the time of pin removal 6 to 8 weeks after surgery, but these infections are typically self-limiting and do not require extensive therapy. However, if the infection is left untreated, catastrophic failure may result.[7,23] Osteomyelitis is, by definition, an infection of the bone involving the medullary cavity. Osteomyelitic bone can be extremely painful for the patient, often delays healing time, is difficult to treat, and may also contribute to catastrophic failure.[22]

Last, cast complications are a result of surface pressures under the cast. Excessive pressure underneath the cast can lead to skin ulceration or diffuse ischemia.[12,29] Skin surface pressures are expected to be greater under fiberglass casts compared to plaster casts.[30] In young, fast-growing animals, cast changes should be performed at 3- to 4-week intervals to allow normal limb growth and avoid pressure sores.[31] Adults are able to tolerate a single cast for a longer period. Adequate padding between the skin and the cast is essential.[25] Additional padding may be placed under TPCs because the transfixing pins protect the distal limb from weight bearing force and thus limit pressure at prominences within the cast.

Traditional Sidebars and Clamps

ESF was designed for the use of transfixation pins, sidebars, and clamps to stabilize fractures unsuited for external coaptation alone or for internal fixation. The sidebars typically are stainless steel, but aluminum and carbon frames are also available. Traditional ESF provides rigid immobilization of a fracture with minimal soft tissue trauma and without disrupting the blood supply via soft tissue attachments to the fracture fragments. Also, this type of ESF provides optimal access to soft tissue injuries for daily management of open fractures. The clamps connecting the pins to the sidebars are a potential *weak link* in traditional external fixators. The main limitation of traditional external fixators is the ability of the assembly to resist failure during loading. The authors have used commercially available fixator frames in animals weighing less than 150 kg and do not recommend the use of traditional sidebar-clamp assemblies for cattle weighing more than 150 kg because of the higher risk of failure of the pin-damp-sidebar unit. Diameter of sidebars must be carefully chosen for use in cattle based on body weight. Regardless of the size of the animal, damps should be examined daily for tightness, position, and evidence of fatigue.

Type II ESF

Type II external skeletal fixators are used to facilitate treatment of open and contaminated wounds surrounding the fracture site.[32] Adequate space should be left between the skin and sidebars to accommodate postoperative swelling. This distance should be limited so as not to compromise the stability of the construct. The sidebars can be made to fit any pin configuration easily by drilling appropriate holes in metal bars or by using a large endotracheal tube pressed over the pin ends and filled with PMMA (**Fig. 5**).

Acrylic Polymer Sidebars

The use of methylmethacrylate as an inexpensive, conformable sidebar has biomechanical advantages compared with the use of standard steel sidebars and clamps. Use of acrylic sidebars has advantages similar to those of traditional ESF. However, acrylic sidebars cannot be adjusted after the polymer has hardened and must be replaced if an error in configuration of the frame has occurred. Acrylics (Technovit, Jorgensen Labs, Loveland, CO, USA) harden with an exothermic reaction, and potential thermal injury to the skin and bone must be considered. Transfixation pins should be rinsed with sterile fluids during the exothermic period to help dissipate heat. An adequate supply of acrylic should be readily available at the time of surgery, and the acrylic must be poured into the tubing mold while it is relatively liquid. Pouring the acrylic in multiple layers or while it is firming up causes air pockets, layering, or cracking of the sidebar and may result in catastrophic failure. Although acrylics have good mechanical stiffness, they are brittle. Therefore, acrylic sidebars must be inspected daily to ensure that failure of the fixator does not occur. The acrylic sidebars may be removed in sections by using obstetric wire to cut the acrylic surrounding the pins.

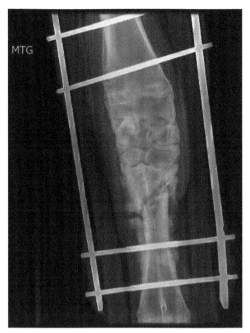

Fig. 5. Type II ESF with centrally threaded pins was used to stabilize this open, contaminated fracture. Both PMMA-filled tubes and drilled steel sidebars were used to increase the stability of the construct. ESF, external skeletal fixation; PMMA, polymethylmethacrylate.

Circular Fixators for ESF

Circular or Ilizarov fixators consist of circular frames fixed in position by threaded rods and with Kirschner wires placed under tension connected to the circular frame.[33] The wires commonly used range in diameter from 1.5 to 2 mm.[34] These wires alone are not strong enough to withstand the loads and forces placed on them by large patients. However, because the wires are tensioned, usually to 90-kg force, and multiple wires are used at each ring with at least 4 rings, the Ilizarov fixator is able to provide a stable environment for facture healing (**Fig. 6**).[35] Using at least 2 wires at each ring, and ideally oriented as close to 90° as possible, will result in the strongest construct. While most fractures can be managed with other means of fixation, the Ilizarov fixator is ideally suited for fractures with large amounts of bone loss, when there is a high degree of comminution, and for articular or periarticular fractures.[34] The authors have used circular fixators to manage MC/MT (Metacarpal or Metatarsal bones) III/IV fractures caused when calving chains caused a full cortical segment bone sequestrum and osteomyelitis. In these cases, the condyles of the metacarpus/tarsus are too small for traditional ESF but are sufficient for placement of small pins in a circular fixator assembly.

PIN-SLEEVE-CAST

The development of the pin-sleeve-cast system was reported by Brianza and colleagues[36] using an equine model. This system was designed to have 2 implants per animal, similar to TPC, but with the goal of lessening the strain at the bone-implant interface. Cyclic loading of transfixation pins concentrates strain on the outer bone

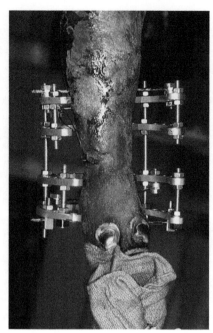

Fig. 6. A 4-ring circular fixator has been placed in this Angus calf to facilitate clinical management of an open fracture caused by crush injury by calving chains applied during a dystocia.

cortices and results in osteolysis and subsequent pin loosening. The pin-sleeve system allows some pin movement within the sleeve, but the sleeve design distributes the strain differently and more evenly to the cortices (**Fig. 7**).

A scaled-down version of the adult equine pin-sleeve system was created for use in calves and tested *ex vivo*.[37,38] This smaller, neonatal version consists of the same components: sleeve, pin, and ring. A 4-mm-diameter, 90-mm-long pin in inserted through the sleeve (27 or 30 mm long) and has contact with 2 circular support rims inside the sleeve that should be centered on each cortex once implanted. The pin is secured to the ring with an axial preload similar to the tensioning of the wires in the Ilizarov system. This system may hold promise for future use in ESF as a method to minimize pin morbidity and improve fixator longevity.

MANAGEMENT OF OPEN FRACTURES

The management of open fractures presents special challenges to the surgeon. The authors consider all fractures with a penetrating skin wound associated with the fracture to be infected because of the severity of contamination with dirt and manure typical of food animals. After induction of anesthesia, the authors clean and superficially debride the wound, prepare the limb for aseptic surgery, and copiously lavage the wound. Aerobic and anaerobic cultures of the bone and medullary cavity are obtained. This procedure decreases contamination with transient, surface bacteria and yields a more reliable indication of the true pathogen or pathogens. Empiric antibiotic therapy is initiated at the time of surgery and continued until bacterial culture and sensitivity results are obtained. Antibiotic selection for use in cattle must be made with consideration for extralabel use and potential antibiotic residues.

A   **B**

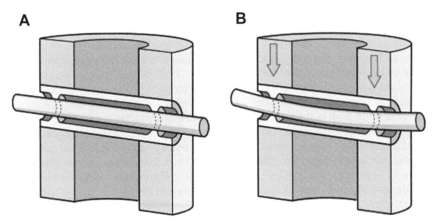

Fig. 7. (*A, B*) Drawing of the pin-sleeve system. The sleeve and bone are shown in a cutaway manner, and the ring is not illustrated but would be attached to either end of the pin. The contact points are visible, centered on the cortical bone at each end of the sleeve. (*B*) Panel shows the load an animal would place on the bone (*arrows*) and the subsequent reaction of the pin within the sleeve. Note that the sleeve has not moved or bent, only the pin has. (*From* Brianza S, Vogel S, Rothstock S, et al. Comparative biomechanical evaluation of a pin-sleeve transfixation system in cadaveric calf metacarpal bones. Vet Surg 2013;42(1):67–74; with permission.)

Empiric antibiotic therapy should be based on known osseous pathogens affecting cattle. In the authors' experience, the most common bacteria cultured from skeletal infections in cattle are *Trueperella pyogenes*, *Arcanobacterium* sp, *Actinomyces* sp, *Fusobacterium necrophorum*, *Bacteroides* spp, and coliforms. In young calves, open fracture treatment is most easily done using ESF constructed using pins and sidebars as opposed to pin casts. For open wounds that are present and have adequate drainage established from the wound, copious lavage may be performed 1 to 2 times daily depending on the degree of contamination and the severity of the infection. The wound, limb, and ESF are wrapped with clean bandage materials to prevent contamination from the environment. Sterile gauze padding is applied to the wound. The authors frequently use topical antiseptic ointments to cover the external wound and feel that the potential benefit of topical antiseptics in preventing ascending infection outweighs mild inhibitory effects on wound healing. Daily wound care is continued until a confluent granulation bed is established across the wound and covering the bone. When granulation tissue does not cover the bone, this suggests formation of a bone sequestrum. Debridement and removal of the sequestrum is indicated in these cases.

Chronic infection (osteomyelitis) of the fracture can be more difficult to resolve. Intravenous infusion of antibiotics distal to a tourniquet achieves high levels of antibiotics in the tissues, and this technique has been adapted by the authors for the treatment of chronic osseous infections in cattle. Fractures caused by calving chain injuries and those having extensive soft tissue damage often are associated with osseous sequestra. Fracture healing is slowed by the presence of the sequestrum, and sequestrectomy will usually allow fracture healing to proceed. In calves having fracture of the metacarpus or metatarsus caused by injudicious use of calving chains, full cortical sequestra can be seen and often lead to nonunion or extreme delayed union. In these calves, the authors remove the sequestrum at the earliest time possible based on radiographs or clinical findings, cleanse the wound until a healthy granulation bed is present, and then perform cancellous bone grafting from the sternum. The sternum provides the largest volume of cancellous bone for grafting. Alternatively, the proximal tibia, proximal humerus, or ileum may be used for cancellous grafts.

Infected fractures that progress to septic nonunion should be treated similarly to cortical sequestrum cases. Aerobic and anaerobic cultures and microbial susceptibility tests are repeated, and the fracture site is extensively debrided of fibrous tissue. The debridement is continued until healthy bone is exposed. A fresh, autologous cancellous bone graft is then harvested and implanted into the fracture site. In cattle having chronic nonhealing fractures, failure to ambulate and altered weight bearing caused by lameness causes medullary atrophy, which limits the volume of cancellous bone that can be harvested from the long bones. Thus, the authors use the sternum as the site of choice for cancellous bone harvest if the procedure is to be performed under general anesthesia or using methods that prevent accidental trauma to the sternum or thorax. A bone curette is used to collect the maximum quantity of cancellous bone accessible. This bone is packed into the fracture, and the skin is closed over the site, if possible.

Septic nonunion may be successfully treated by rigid immobilization and the surgical techniques described earlier. However, the economic limitations of an individual animal may be encountered before clinical union of the fracture has occurred. Amputation or euthanasia is an appropriate option for these cases.

REFERENCES

1. Hopper SA, Schneider RK, Johnson CH, et al. In vitro comparison of transfixation and standard full-limb casts for prevention of displacement of a mid-diaphyseal third metacarpal osteotomy site in horses. Am J Vet Res 2000;61:1633–5.
2. McClure SR, Hillberry BM, Fisher KE. In vitro comparison of metaphyseal and diaphyseal placement of centrally threaded, positive-profile transfixation pins in the equine third metacarpal bone. Am J Vet Res 2000;61:1304–8.
3. Anderson DE, St Jean G. External skeletal fixation in ruminants. Vet Clin North Am Food Anim Pract 1996;12:117–52.
4. Auer JA. Principles of fracture treatment. In: Auer JA, Stick JA, editors. Equine surgery. 3rd edition. St Louis (MO): Saunders; 2006. p. 1002–29.
5. Nunamaker DM, Nash RA. A tapered-sleeve transcortical pin external skeletal fixation device for use in horses: development, application, and experience. Vet Surg 2008;37:725–32.
6. Ho KW, Gilbody J, Jameson T, et al. The effect of 4 mm bicortical drill hole defect on bone strength in a pig femur model. Arch Orthop Trauma Surg 2010;130:797–802.
7. Nunamaker DM, Richardson DW, Butterweck DM, et al. A new external skeletal fixation device that allows immediate full weight bearing: application in the horse. Vet Surg 1986;15:345–55.
8. Seltzer KL, Stover SM, Taylor KT, et al. The effect of hole diameter on the torsional mechanical properties of the equine third metacarpal bone. Vet Surg 1996;25:371–5.
9. Moss DP, Tejwani NC. Biomechanics of external fixation: a review of the literature. Bull NYU Hosp Jt Dis 2007;65:294–9.
10. McClure SR, Watkins JP, Ashman RB. In vitro comparison of the effect of parallel and divergent transfixation pins on breaking strength of equine third metacarpal bones. Am J Vet Res 1994;55:1327–30.
11. Estebe JP, Le Corre P, Chevanne F, et al. Motor blockade by brachial plexus block in the sheep. Anesthesiology 2000;93:291–3.

12. St-Jean G, Clem MF, DeBowes RM. Transfixation pinning and casting of tibial fractures in calves: five cases (1985-1989). J Am Vet Med Assoc 1991;198: 139–43.
13. St-Jean G, Debowes RM. Transfixation pinning and casting of radial-ulnar fractures in calves: a review of three cases. Can Vet J 1992;33:257–62.
14. Tulleners EP. Metacarpal and metatarsal fractures in dairy cattle: 33 cases (1979-1985). J Am Vet Med Assoc 1986;189:463–8.
15. Young B, Heath J. Skeletal tissues. In: Young B, Heath J, editors. Wheater's functional histology. Edinburgh (United Kingdom): Chruchill Livingstone; 2002. p. 175–88.
16. Ames NK. Comparison of methods for femoral fracture repair in young calves. J Am Vet Med Assoc 1981;179:458–9.
17. Blikslager AT, Bowman KF, Abrams CF Jr, et al. Holding power of orthopedic screws in the large metacarpal and metatarsal bones of calves. Am J Vet Res 1994;55:415–8.
18. Trostle SS, Wilson DG, Dueland RT, et al. In vitro biomechanical comparison of solid and tubular interlocking nails in neonatal bovine femurs. Vet Surg 1995; 24:235–43.
19. Anderson D, Silviera F. Effect of pin size and pin tract osteolysis on removal torque of positively threaded transfixation pins used in external skeletal fixation in cattle: a prospective study. World Buiatrics Congress. Santiago (Chile), November 14–18, 2010.
20. Vogel S. Evaluation of a novel transcortical pin-sleeve system in a calf model. Faculte de medecine veterinaire. St-Hyacinthe (Quebec): Universite de Montreal; 2011.
21. Kaneps AJ, Schmotzer WB, Huber MJ, et al. Fracture repair with transfixation pins and fiberglass cast in llamas and small ruminants. J Am Vet Med Assoc 1989; 195:1257–61.
22. Lescun TB, McClure SR, Ward MP, et al. Evaluation of transfixation casting for treatment of third metacarpal, third metatarsal, and phalangeal fractures in horses: 37 cases (1994-2004). J Am Vet Med Assoc 2007;230:1340–9.
23. Nemeth F, Back W. The use of the walking cast to repair fractures in horses and ponies. Equine Vet J 1991;23:32–6.
24. Matthews LS, Green CA, Goldstein SA. The thermal effects of skeletal fixation-pin insertion in bone. J Bone Joint Surg Am 1984;66:1077–83.
25. Swaim SF, Vaughn DM, Spalding PJ, et al. Evaluation of the dermal effects of cast padding in coaptation casts on dogs. Am J Vet Res 1992;53:1266–72.
26. Elce YA, Southwood LL, Nutt JN, et al. Ex vivo comparison of a novel tapered-sleeve and traditional full-limb transfixation pin cast for distal radial fracture stabilization in the horse. Vet Comp Orthop Traumatol 2006;19:93–7.
27. Behrens F. General theory and principles of external fixation. Clin Orthop Relat Res 1989;(241):15–23.
28. Moroni A, Vannini F, Mosca M, et al. State of the art review: techniques to avoid pin loosening and infection in external fixation. J Orthop Trauma 2002;16:189–95.
29. Schneider RK, Ratzlaff MC, White KK, et al. Effect of three types of half-limb casts on in vitro bone strain recorded from the third metacarpal bone and proximal phalanx in equine cadaver limbs. Am J Vet Res 1998;59:1188–93.
30. Marson BM, Keenan MA. Skin surface pressures under short leg casts. J Orthop Trauma 1993;7:275–8.
31. Anderson DE, St Jean G. Management of fractures in field settings. Vet Clin North Am Food Anim Pract 2008;24:567–82, viii.

32. Singh GR, Aithal HP, Saxena RK, et al. In vitro biomechanical properties of linear, circular, and hybrid external skeletal fixation devices for use in large ruminants. Vet Surg 2007;36:80–7.
33. Marcellin-Little DJ. External skeletal fixation. In: Slatter D, editor. Textbook of small animal surgery. Philadelphia: Saunders; 2003. p. 1818–26.
34. Calhoun JH, Li F, Ledbetter BR, et al. Biomechanics of the Ilizarov fixator for fracture fixation. Clin Orthop Relat Res 1992;(280):15–22.
35. Kummer FJ. Biomechanics of the Ilizarov external fixator. Clin Orthop Relat Res 1992;(280):11–4.
36. Brianza S, Brighenti V, Boure L, et al. In vitro mechanical evaluation of a novel pin-sleeve system for external fixation of distal limb fractures in horses: a proof of concept study. Vet Surg 2010;39:601–8.
37. Brianza S, Vogel S, Rothstock S, et al. In vitro evaluation of the torsional strength reduction of neonate calf metatarsal bones with bicortical defects resulting from the removal of external fixation implants. Vet Surg 2013;42:75–8.
38. Brianza S, Vogel S, Rothstock S, et al. Comparative biomechanical evaluation of a pin-sleeve transfixation system in cadaveric calf metacarpal bones. Vet Surg 2013;42:67–74.

Limb Amputation and Prosthesis

André Desrochers, DMV, MS[a],*, Guy St-Jean, DMV, MS[b],
David E. Anderson, DVM, MS[c]

KEYWORDS

- Limb amputation • Cattle • Osteomyelitis • Lameness • Surgery • Orthopedics
- Prostheses

KEY POINTS

- Limb amputation is a drastic treatment in cases of untreatable musculoskeletal trauma or infection. Saving the limb should always be the primary goal. If this is not possible, limb amputation can be performed.
- Proximal limb disarticulation for amputation is preferred if a prosthesis is not considered.
- Distal amputations are needed to accommodate exoskeletal prosthesis.
- Prostheses are expected to provide better weight bearing and comfort to the animal and are strongly recommended if the best possible care is requested for the animal and animal welfare is important to the owner.
- It is critical to understand that the owner must be committed to daily care of the stump and well-being of the animal.
- The surgery can be successful in young and adult animals regardless of the limb affected. Amputation should always be considered as an alternative to euthanasia.

Limb amputation is an appropriate alternative to euthanasia when catastrophic injury to a limb either prevents successful restoration of the limb or the costs associated with treatment precludes this option. Although limb amputation is done as a last resort to save the life of the patient, digit amputation has been performed successfully in cattle of various ages and production types.[1–6] The procedure is simple with rapid resolution of pain and a quick return to production. Cattle having had digit amputation done can be productive; however, they only live an average of 20 months after digit amputation.[5,7] Shortened life expectancy often is associated with breakdown of the remaining digit and persistent lameness. Limb amputation is not as frequently performed as digit amputation because of the complexity of the procedure, economic consideration, prolonged aftercare, and unpredictable outcome. Clinical concerns after limb amputation include breakdown injuries to the contralateral limb, persistent lameness,

[a] Department of Clinical Sciences, Faculty of Veterinary Medicine, Université de Montréal, 3200 Sicotte, St-Hyacinthe, Quebec J2S 7C6, Canada; [b] School of Veterinary Medicine, Ross University, PO Box 334, Basseterre, St-Kitts, West Indies; [c] Large Animal Clinical Sciences, College of Veterinary Medicine, University of Tennessee, 2407 River Drive, Knoxville, TN 37996-4545, USA
* Corresponding author.
E-mail address: andre.desrochers@umontreal.ca

Vet Clin Food Anim 30 (2014) 143–155
http://dx.doi.org/10.1016/j.cvfa.2013.11.005
0749-0720/14/$ – see front matter © 2014 Elsevier Inc. All rights reserved.

recumbency, poor return to production, and poor quality of life. Construction of a custom-fitted prosthesis for the amputated limb offers the opportunity to prevent these untoward outcomes. Increasingly, valuable cattle and animal welfare concerns have resulted in limb amputation and construction of a prosthesis being performed more frequently when requested by owners.

REASON FOR LIMB AMPUTATION

Open, comminuted fracture of long bones and osteomyelitis are the most common reason for amputation (**Fig. 1**).[8–15] In cattle, these injuries are usually secondary to accidents on the farm or caused by damage from obstetric chains (**Fig. 2**).[8–18] Other indications for amputation include loss of vascular supply to the limb; clostridial infections; severe laceration of muscle, tendon and nerves; and chronic septic arthritis (**Fig. 3**).[16,19–21] Less common reasons have been reported, including a cow that was hit by a car and suffered an open comminuted tibial fracture.[18] Another animal had a severe infected laceration at the level of the left scapula with maggot infestation of the wound.[19] In a calf that was reported to suffer from chronic septic arthritis of the stifle, limb amputation was done because of fistula formation 1 month after treatment and nonfunctional ankylosis of the joint.[21]

DECISION MAKING FOR LIMB AMPUTATION

Initially, treatment should be attempted to preserve the limb unless there is evidence of irreversible distal limb ischemia or gangrene. In the case of fracture, bone fragments are reduced and immobilized; for lacerations, tissue debridement is done. The patient is most often treated with systemic and local antibiotics, daily wound care, frequent reevaluation, and pain management. Calves suffering fracture of the metacarpal bones caused by obstetric chain injury often have unnoticed vascular injury on presentation. Initially, the fractured limb is immobilized but some calves will develop full cortical sequestra, ischemic necrosis, or gangrene.[14,17] If available, infrared thermography or nuclear scintigraphy can be performed to assess vascular supply.[22] Positive contrast intravenous radiography can also be used to evaluate distal limb vascular injuries (**Fig. 4**). When extensive vascular damage is present, amputation is considered immediately.[18] Limb amputation has a dramatic impact on the quality of life and productive use of cattle. The owner must be committed to proper management of the stump postoperatively, including helping the animal to stand for the first few days

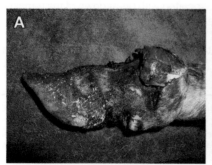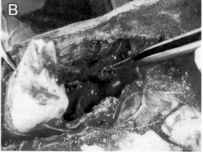

Fig. 1. (*A*) An open metacarpal physeal fracture type III on a heifer. The proximal fragment is protruding from the large skin laceration and heavily contaminated. (*B*) A 22-month-old pregnant heifer suffering from an open fracture type IIIc. The Adson forceps grab a transected thrombosed digital artery.

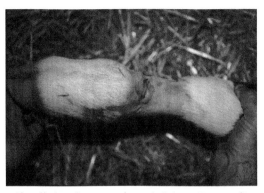

Fig. 2. A newborn calf suffering from an obstetric injury. He was diagnosed with a distal diaphyseal fracture of the metacarpi. The distal limb is swollen and there are skin marks from the obstetric chains.

and limiting the movement of the animal. After limb amputation, cattle usually require confinement to paddock or pen because they cannot easily navigate pasture terrain.

Economic constraints may limit attempts to salvage the limb. In cattle with severe and complex injuries to the limbs, the rehabilitation period is sometimes prolonged and persistent pain may be present during the convalescent period. Before making the decision to either attempt to salvage the limb or amputate it, the severity of the injury must be evaluated objectively. The following factors are considered: severity of the fracture, contamination or infection at the fracture site, integrity of the vascular and nerve supply to the limb, options for repair of the fracture, and treatment costs. The Gustilo classification of open fracture is a basic scoring system frequently used in the decision process (**Table 1**).[23] This classification system is based on soft tissue damage, severity of the fracture, blood supply, and contamination. Amputation must always be considered for Gustilo score III injuries. Other scoring systems developed by human orthopedic surgeons for lower extremity injury severity scoring include Mangled Extremity Score, Predictive Salvage Index, and Hannover Fracture Scale.[24–28] The Mangled Extremity Severity Score is well established and is based on the following criteria: limb ischemia, patient age, state of shock, and injury

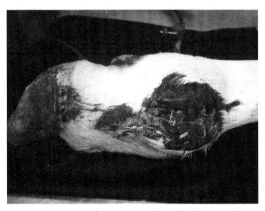

Fig. 3. A 20-month-old Holstein heifer presented with chronic laceration involving the fetlock joint. The distal limb is ischemic (blackened skin edges) and there is purulent material coming out of the joint.

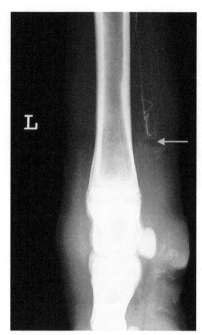

Fig. 4. Frostbite on a 5-month-old Holstein heifer. Angiographic study of the palmar digital region was obtained by injecting contrast material in the median artery. The arrow shows an interruption compatible with arterial thrombosis.

mechanism.[29,30] None of those scoring systems are infallible and they are not adapted to cattle at this time.

Criteria considered in cattle patients include the limb affected, condition of the opposite limb, intended use of the animal, treatment cost, and owner commitment. In a report of five calves that had limb amputation, calves with hind limb amputation recovered better than calves that had the front limb amputated.[31] The investigator

Table 1 Gustilo open-fracture classification	
Grade	**Description**
I	Skin lesion <1 cm, clean, simple bone fracture with minimal comminution
II	Skin lesion >1 cm, limited soft-tissue damage, minimal crushing, moderate comminution
III	Extensive skin damage with muscle and neurovascular involvement, high-speed crush injury, highly comminuted fracture, extensive contamination of the wound bed, open injury with farm contamination
IIIa	Extensive laceration of soft tissues with bone fragments covered Secondary to high-speed traumas with severe comminution
IIIb	Extensive soft-tissue lesions with periosteal stripping and contamination Severe comminution from high-speed traumas
IIIc	Exposed fracture with arterial damage that requires repair

Data from Gustilo RB, Anderson JT. Prevention of infection in the treatment of one thousand and twenty-five open fractures of long bones: retrospective and prospective analyses. J Bone Joint Surg Am 1976;58(4):453–8.

hypothesized that the pelvic limb is more stable because the hip is connected to the body through the sacroiliac joint whereas the thoracic limb is attached by a muscular belt.[31] However, another study found that hind limb amputation caused more discomfort.[32] Heavy and aged animals seemed to be less comfortable but no specific data were mentioned.[32] The contralateral limb cannot endure constant stress and is prone to injuries resulting from mechanical overload of the muscles, tendon, and ligaments. After amputation, the animal's posture will change to accommodate the altered center of gravity resulting in loss of symmetry. This compensation may contribute to long-term complications.

AMPUTATION SITE

Limb amputation may be done either through the diaphysis or by disarticulation. Disarticulation is readily performed and may be associated with less bleeding because the bone marrow is not exposed and vessels are ligated. In an experimental study, cows with amputation done by joint disarticulation healed faster, were more ambulatory, and could bear more weight on the stump.[33,34] Disarticulation has been reported at each of the high motion joints of the limbs: fetlock,[34,35] carpus,[15,17,20,34] elbow,[34] tarsus,[34] and stifle.[34] Amputation through the diaphysis has been reported through the distal third of the tibia,[16] proximal radius-ulna,[10,14] midfemur,[31] midhumerus,[31] distal femur,[18,21] proximal metatarsi,[11] and distal metacarpus.[15] Although rarely done, complete removal of the thoracic limb has been reported.[19]

The authors recommend limb amputation by joint disarticulation when possible because the joint surface provides a wider surface for weight bearing if a prosthesis is chosen. Most prostheses suitable for use in cattle significantly diminish mobility of the joints because of the rigid construct used.[36] When performing a limb amputation, the surgeon should always keep as much soft tissue as possible to cover the exposed bone or joint. This may be difficult to achieve in large animals when amputation is performed below the carpus or the tarsus because only digital flexor or extensor tendons are available to cover the distal end of the bone. Soft tissue coverage helps to prevent damage to the end of the stump and may improve patient comfort.

The location of the incisions for creation of the skin flap must be carefully planned. Skin flap proportions for limb disarticulation have been described as a "fish mouth" because of the shape of the incisions.[34] The intersection of the incisions creates the angle of the fish mouth and marks the location where the bone will be cut (**Fig. 5**). Flaps can be equal or unequal depending on whether the caudal or cranial muscle mass is different and where the sutures are expected to be.[34] Generally, the length of each flap is equal to three-fourths of the diameter of the limb at the level of the amputation. The surgeon should preserve excess skin if possible so that the skin can be trimmed as needed after the amputation. When possible, muscle and fascia should be harvested with the skin to improve chances for healing and provide additional padding between the bone and the skin at the end of the stump. Ideally, the suture line should not cross over or be centered on the distal aspect of the stump unless there is enough muscle to completely cover the exposed end of the bone. The suture line should be placed in a manner that minimizes tension. Disarticulation done at the level of the radiocarpal joint, for example, should have the suture line for the skin flap coursing along the caudal aspect of the distal radius stump.

SURGICAL TECHNIQUE

Although limb amputation can be performed while the patient sedated and after perineural anesthesia, amputation is preferably done with the patient under general

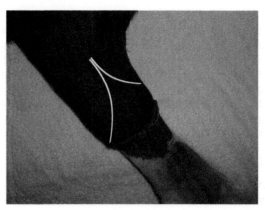

Fig. 5. A 2-month-old Holstein heifer caught herself in a rope and sustained vascular injury. There is a defined landmark between normal and abnormal skin. The yellow, curved lines are the planned fish-mouth incision to achieve amputation.

anesthesia. Some patients are poor anesthetic candidates because of shock, hemorrhage, and infection. Distal limb amputation can be done relatively quickly and these cases are more amenable to regional and epidural anesthesia. Forelimb anesthesia can be accomplished by brachial block anesthesia, which can be used for amputations at the level of the carpus (carpal disarticulation or metacarpal amputation). For the pelvic limb, epidural anesthesia can be used for amputation distal to the stifle. These patients often require assistance to stand during recovery after surgery. Distal limb amputation, especially at or distal to the level of the fetlock, can be done either by intravenous regional anesthesia distal to a tourniquet or by local infiltration of the anesthetic in a ring block fashion or as a perineural four-point block.[14,34] In all cases and whenever possible, a tourniquet should be used to aid in control of hemorrhage during the amputation. When vascularization is compromised and poorly delineated, the tourniquet may be released during the procedure to better discern the margins of nonviable tissue. In many of these cases, a more proximal amputation might be necessary to ensure proper healing of the stump. Before surgery, the segment of the limb to be amputated is wrapped with a plastic bag or other impervious barrier and the proximal portion of the limb is clipped and prepared aseptically. The skin incision is performed as planned with the appropriate flap size to cover the stump (**Fig. 6**A). Larger flaps can eventually be trimmed. All necrotic and infected tissues are resected. Removal of a more proximal section of the bone might be necessary to allow further debridement or skin closure (**Fig. 7**). If the amputation site is near the joint and skin salvage is not sufficient to close the incision, the surgical wound may be managed open and allowed to heal by second intention. Intraoperative hemorrhage is more abundant if the amputation is done through the diaphysis. Care should be taken to assess hemorrhage from the marrow cavity. Appendicular vessels and nerves are sharply cut and ligated. It is recommended to transect nerves as far proximally as possible to minimize the risk of painful neuroma formation and to prevent inadvertent contact or pressure with the ground or the prosthesis.[36]

Before closing the various tissue layers, the tourniquet may be released to allow evaluation of adequacy of hemostasis. Hemorrhage from the marrow cavity after transaction of the diaphysis may be controlled by careful suturing of a flap of muscle over the extremity of the bone. Some articular surfaces are irregular and have sharp ridges. These prominences may need to be removed with a rongeur to create a

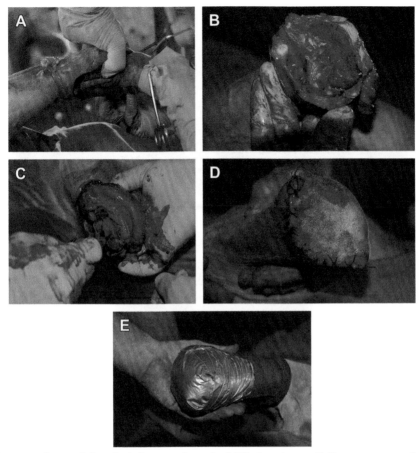

Fig. 6. Radiocarpal disarticulation on a 3-week-old Piedmontese calf. He was unsuccessfully treated for an obstetric fracture of the distal metacarpi. (*A*) A tourniquet is placed proximal to the carpal joint. The skin is incised allowing a long cranial flap of skin to be sutured without tension at the caudal aspect of the joint. (*B*) The distal radius surface is smoothed with rongeur. (*C*) The joint surface is covered with the joint capsule and tendons. (*D*) The suture line is caudal and proximal to the distal aspect of the radius. (*E*) The stump is heavily bandaged to protect the incision and provide comfort to the animal if he attempts to stand.

smooth surface before covering it with the soft tissue flap (see **Fig. 6**B, C). The soft tissues should cover the stump uniformly so as not to create imbalance while covering the distal end. The skin suture line must be located away from the maximum pressure points on the stump (see **Fig. 6**D). The skin is sutured in a routine fashion. The stump is covered by a thick pressure bandage to control swelling and prevent trauma to the suture line when the animal stands (see **Fig. 6**E).

POSTOPERATIVE TREATMENT

Following limb amputation, rapid clinical improvement in the patient is expected. In some cases, the authors have seen cattle that were anorexic and recumbent before surgery start to eat normally and stand alone the day after surgery. Analgesics are

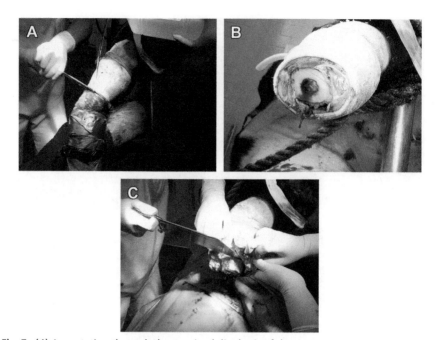

Fig. 7. (*A*) Amputation through the proximal diaphysis of the metatarsi. An amputating saw is used to cut the bone just proximal to the infected fracture. Cold sterile saline is poured over the saw to prevent thermal necrosis. (*B*) The transected end revealed more necrotic and infected tissue. (*C*) Lateral and medial incisions are made to allow a more proximal amputation of the metatarsi and provide healthy skin coverage of the stump.

usually given for several days after surgery. Nonsteroidal antiinflammatory drugs are most commonly used, but narcotics are synergistic and may benefit a patient having significant postoperative discomfort. Choice of antibiotics and duration of administration are variable depending on each case, but beta-lactam drugs are most commonly used initially. The stump should be carefully managed after surgery. Postoperative swelling must be controlled to minimize the risk of incisional complication. Dehiscence, infection, and exuberant granulation tissue are all potential complications (**Fig. 8**).[14,15] Daily care is often necessary, especially if the wound is being managed open and healing by second intention. In cases identified as candidates for a prosthesis, molding of the limb for custom fitting may be delayed by stump complications. Cattle should be confined to a stall or a small paddock during the convalescent period after surgery to avoid breakdown of the opposite leg.

PROSTHESIS

A prosthesis is strongly recommended for cattle with great genetic, economic, or personal value. The prosthesis will improve weight bearing, help protect the remaining limbs from stress breakdown, and, consequently, extend the animal's life expectancy. Limb prosthesis demands intensive aftercare by the owner. The prosthesis should be removed and cleaned daily and the stump evaluated for pressure sores. Over time, the prosthesis may need adjustment to accommodate the growth of the animal or changes in muscle mass. The authors find that orthotic and prosthetic human specialists are extremely helpful in customizing prosthetics for cattle. The prosthetic

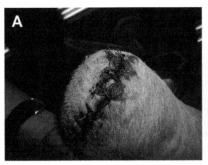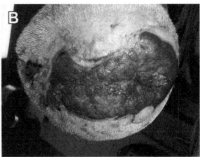

Fig. 8. (A) Ten days after a proximal amputation of the metatarsi (see **Fig. 7**), the surgical incision is healing except at its lateral aspect at the top where purulent material and blood are present. (B) The same animal 3-weeks after amputation. The incision dehisced and granulation is now covering the stump.

technician should be called before deciding where to amputate. Advances in construction technologies render the fitting to the patient and adjustment easier.[37] If the amputation is performed as an emergency procedure and prosthesis fitting is considered, it is better to keep as much of the limb as possible to create a longer stump. An experimental and clinical study demonstrated more disability with prosthesis when amputation was done proximally.[32] Revision can be made later to better fit the prosthesis. The larger the surface area of the distal extremity of the stump in contact with the prosthesis, the better will be the distribution of the weight of the animal and that will decrease the incidence of stump sores.

There are two types of prosthesis: exoskeletal and endoskeletal prosthetics.[37] An endoskeletal prosthesis has an internal framework that mimics the shape and biomechanics of bones. It is made of lightweight alloy and carbon fiber. Each part can be adjusted and replaced to the need of the patient. The exoskeletal prosthesis has an external framework made of carbon fiber or fiberglass. These prosthetics are more bulky, heavier, and can be difficult to adjust. The body mass and environment of cattle has resulted in selection of exoskeletal prostheses most often (**Fig. 9**).[10,15,17,32,35] Homemade prostheses are also usually exoskeletal with a fiberglass part that is shaped to the limb and uses a metal post as the weight-bearing part (**Fig. 10**). In a case report, a modified external fixator was fixed to the distal aspect of the tibial stump of a 2-day-old calf. A metal plate was welded at the end of four side bars as a weight-bearing surface. The prosthesis was used for a period of 4 months, at which time the calf was slaughtered for meat.[11] Some cattle will not accept or use the prosthesis. In these cattle, clinical management is better without the prosthesis.[10] These cattle should be housed in clean environments, on level ground with excellent footing, and without other livestock. This may provide sufficient comfort to allow the animal to regain productivity or quality of life.

The socket is the interface between the prosthesis and the stump. This is an extremely important part of the unit.[36,38] The socket transmits weight-bearing forces through the limb. If it is not comfortable, the animal will be reluctant to stand or walk. The socket absorbs some of the shear forces decreasing the friction between the stump and the prosthesis. If it is well-adjusted to the stump and fit tight to the prosthesis, the residual limb should be partially suspended in the prosthesis.[36] The prosthesis is removed daily to evaluate the stump, assess for pressure sores, and clean the stump and socket. If the animal is young and growing, the prosthesis must be adjustable or changed as needed.[15,17]

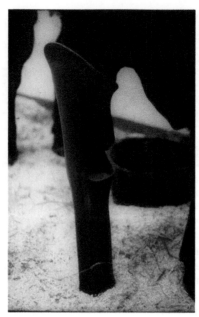

Fig. 9. A carbon fiber exoskeletal front limb prosthesis was professionally designed for this heifer. The front opening allows easy removal or the prosthesis for daily care. After prosthesis fitting, a padded carbon fiber lid is applied over the opening, securing it.

PROGNOSIS

The short-term prognosis is generally good for amputation. Commercial beef cattle will be sent to slaughter at the appropriate weight and before the breakdown of the opposite leg.[11,14] Long-term prognosis depends on the weight of the animal, management of the environment, and dedication of the owner. Cows should not be bred or allowed to be pregnant. Instead, these cows should be limited to use as embryo donors.[15] In most cases, pregnant cows that have had an amputation done are culled after calving.[16] However, there are exceptions. A heifer with a front-limb prosthesis was naturally bred and she gave birth to a normal calf.[20] A newborn female calf with

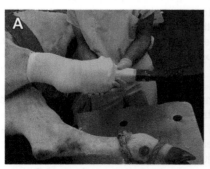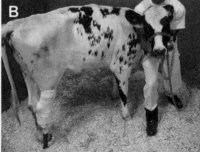

Fig. 10. Homemade hind-limb prosthesis with fiberglass cast and adjustable metal post with a rubber extremity. (*A*) The metal post was enclosed in the cast while fitted on the animal. (*B*) The animal bears full weight on the prosthetic limb. The cast was later fenestrated to allow daily removal and care.

a prosthesis was raised and calved normally but died of unknown reasons at 2.5 years old.[17] The authors were involved in cases in which the animals were kept for many years and multiple embryos were collected. In a retrospective study on 11 cattle with amputation, three mature bulls were amputated and kept in an Artificial Insemination center for 12, 27, and 32 months, postoperatively.[39] Only one of the four pregnant cows delivered a live calf. Three beef calves were raised and slaughtered between 5 and 6 months postoperatively.[39]

SUMMARY

Limb amputation is a drastic treatment in cases of untreatable musculoskeletal trauma or infection. Saving the limb should always be the primary goal. If this is not possible, limb amputation can be performed. Proximal limb disarticulation for amputation is preferred if a prosthesis is not considered. Distal amputations are needed to accommodate exoskeletal prosthesis. Prostheses are expected to provide better weight bearing and comfort to the animal and it is strongly recommended when the best possible care is requested for the animal and animal welfare is important to the owner. It is critical to understand that the owner must be committed to daily care of the stump and well-being of the animal. The surgery can be successful in young and adult animals regardless of the limb affected. Amputation should always be considered as an alternative to euthanasia.

REFERENCES

1. Bicalho RC, Cheong SH, Warnick LD, et al. The effect of digit amputation or arthrodesis surgery on culling and milk production in holstein dairy cows. J Dairy Sci 2006;89(7):2596–602.
2. Desrochers A, St Jean G. Surgical management of digit disorders in cattle. Vet Clin North Am Food Anim Pract 1996;12(1):277–98.
3. Funk KA. Late results after toe and claw amputation in cattle. Berl Munch Tierarztl Wochenschr 1977;90(8):152–6 [in German].
4. Kofler J, Feist M, Starke A, et al. Resection of the distal/proximal interphalangeal joint and digit amputation in 21 breeding bulls–indications, clinical findings and longterm outcome. Berl Munch Tierarztl Wochenschr 2007;120(3–4):156–64 [in German].
5. Pejsa TG, St Jean G, Hoffsis GF, et al. Digit amputation in cattle: 85 cases (1971–1990). J Am Vet Med Assoc 1993;202(6):981–4.
6. Starke A, Heppelmann M, Beyerbach M, et al. Septic arthritis of the distal interphalangeal joint in cattle: comparison of digital amputation and joint resection by solar approach. Vet Surg 2007;36(4):350–9.
7. Heppelmann M, Kofler J, Meyer H, et al. Advances in surgical treatment of septic arthritis of the distal interphalangeal joint in cattle: a review. Vet J 2009;182(2):162–75.
8. Aher VD, Sarkate LB, Usturge SM, et al. Amputation of thoracic limb in case of irreparable fracture of radio-ulna in cows. J Bombay Vet Coll 1991;3(1/2):61–2.
9. Aksoy O, Ozaydn I, Klc E, et al. Evaluation of fractures in calves due to forced extraction during dystocia: 27 cases (2003–2008). Kafkas Univ Vet Fak Derg 2009;15(3):339–44.
10. Casals EE. Amputation of the fore limb of a calf. Rev Vet Mil 1974;21(99/100):117.
11. Decante F. Case report: use of a prosthesis in a calf after amputation of the metatarsus. Point Veterinaire 1990;22(132):675–8.

12. Gangl M, Grulke S, Serteyn D, et al. Retrospective study of 99 cases of bone fractures in cattle treated by external coaptation or confinement. Vet Rec 2006; 158(8):264–8.
13. Gorgul OS, Seyrek-Intas D, Celimli N, et al. Evaluation of fractures in calves: 31 cases (1996–2003). Veteriner Cerrahi Dergisi 2004;10(3/4):16–20.
14. Lallemand M. Amputation of the forelimb of a calf. Point Veterinaire 2011;42(319): 44–9 [in French].
15. St Jean G. Amputation and prosthesis. Vet Clin North Am Food Anim Pract 1996; 12(1):249–61.
16. Bangel Junior JJ, Wald O, Camargo FC, et al. Amputation of a gangrenous back leg in a cow. Arq Fac Vet 1992;20:73–8.
17. Orsini JA, Warner A, Dyson S, et al. Lower-extremity amputation and application of a prosthetic device in a 1-month-old calf. Vet Surg 1985;14(4):307–9.
18. Coxon WB. Amputation of the leg of a cow. Can J Comp Med Vet Sci 1945;9(1): 14–5.
19. Rodriguez ER. Amputacion total de miembro anterior izquierdo en un vacuno. Sitio Argentino de Produccion Animal; 1975. Available at: http://www.produccion-animal.com.ar/comunicaciones/02-amputacion.pdf. Accessed 1975.
20. Morkeberg AW. Amputation through the knee of a cow. Hist Med Vet 2003;28(2): 33–7.
21. Keen FR. Amputation of the leg of a calf. J Am Vet Med Assoc 1952;120(902):307.
22. Goggin JM, Hoskinson JJ, Carpenter JW, et al. Scintigraphic assessment of distal extremity perfusion in 17 patients. Vet Radiol Ultrasound 1997;38(3):211–20.
23. Gustilo RB, Anderson JT. Prevention of infection in the treatment of one thousand and twenty-five open fractures of long bones: retrospective and prospective analyses. J Bone Joint Surg Am 1976;58(4):453–8.
24. Bosse MJ, MacKenzie EJ, Kellam JF, et al. A prospective evaluation of the clinical utility of the lower-extremity injury-severity scores. J Bone Joint Surg Am 2001; 83(1):3–14.
25. Helfet DL, Howey T, Sanders R, et al. Limb salvage versus amputation. Preliminary results of the Mangled Extremity Severity Score. Clin Orthop Relat Res 1990;(256):80–6.
26. Howe HR Jr, Poole GV Jr, Hansen KJ, et al. Salvage of lower extremities following combined orthopedic and vascular trauma. A predictive salvage index. Am Surg 1987;53(4):205–8.
27. Krettek C, Seekamp A, Kontopp H, et al. Hannover Fracture Scale '98—re-evaluation and new perspectives of an established extremity salvage score. Injury 2001;32(4):317–28.
28. Stewart DA, Coombs CJ, Graham HK. Application of lower extremity injury severity scores in children. J Child Orthop 2012;6(5):427–31.
29. Mangled extremity severity score. Available at: http://www.mdcalc.com/mangled-extremity-severity-score-mess-score/.
30. Johansen K, Daines M, Howey T, et al. Objective criteria accurately predict amputation following lower extremity trauma. J Trauma 1990;30(5):568–72 [discussion: 572–3].
31. Nguhiu M. Feasibility and prognosis of limb amputation in cattle and a goat. Bull Anim Health Prod Afr 1990;38(4):391–3.
32. Nayak S, Mohanty JN. Studies on the efficacy of prosthetic management of limb in bovine. Indian Vet J 1994;71(6):580–4.
33. Nayak S, Mohanty JN. A disability study of limb amputation in bovine by joint disarticulation and bone section. Indian J Vet Surg 1995;16(1):54–6.

34. Nayak S, Mohanty J. Joint disarticulation method for limb amputation at various levels in bovine practice. Indian Vet J 1999;76(1):42–4.
35. Prakash KK, Prakash S. Artificial limb for a heifer. Vet Rec 1990;127(25/26):623.
36. Robinson V, Sansam K, Hirst L, et al. Major lower limb amputation—what, why and how to achieve the best results. Orthop Trauma 2010;24(4):276–85.
37. Mora R, Bertani B, Pedrotti L. Amputations and prosthetic fitting. In: Mora R, editor. Nonunion of the long bones. Milan (Italy): Springer; 2006. p. 225–30.
38. Kapp SL. Transfemoral socket design and suspension options. Phys Med Rehabil Clin N Am 2000;11(3):569–83, vi.
39. Desrochers A, Gnemmi G, Nichols S, et al. A retrospective study of 11 cattle undergoing limb amputation. Presented at the 2013 American College of Veterinary Surgeons Veterinary Symposium. San Antonio (TX), October 24–26, 2013.

Diseases of the Tendons and Tendon Sheaths

Adrian Steiner, Dr med vet, MS[a],*, David E. Anderson, DVM, MS[b],
André Desrochers, DMV, MS[c]

KEYWORDS

- Cattle • Tendon • Tenosynovitis • Symptoms • Surgery • Treatment

KEY POINTS

- Contracted flexor tendon leading to flexural deformity is a common congenital defect in cattle and occurs in numerous breeds.
- Arthrogryposis is defined as a congenital syndrome of persistent joint contracture that occurs frequently in Europe as a consequence of Schmallenberg virus infection of the dam.
- Spastic paresis occurring in different breeds has a hereditary component, and affected cattle should not be used for breeding purposes.
- The most common tendon avulsion involves the deep digital flexor tendon from its insertion on the solar aspect of the third phalanx.
- Tendon disruptions may be successfully managed by tenorrhaphy and external coaptation or by external coaptation alone.
- Medical management alone is unlikely to be effective for treatment of purulent tenosynovitis because of excessive fibrin deposition within the tendon sheath.

Tendon disorders are a recognized cause of locomotor dysfunction in cattle, but the prevalence of lameness caused by tendon injury presently is unknown. Survey studies estimating the incidence of lameness in dairy herds in the United States, Canada, and the United Kingdom have not identified tendon disorders as a major cause of lameness.[1–3] However, one study indicated tendon involvement in 21% of limb lesions.[4] Another study reported that muscle and/or tendon lesions accounted for 74% of upper limb injuries in the forelimb and 7.8% in the hind limb.[5] Tendon disorders may be congenital or acquired. Relevant congenital abnormalities include:

- Hyperextension deformities
- Flexural deformities

[a] Vetsuisse-Faculty, Farm Animal Clinic, University of Bern, Bremgartenstrasse 109a, Bern 3012, Switzerland; [b] Large Animal Clinical Sciences, College of Veterinary Medicine, University of Tennessee, 2407 River Drive, Knoxville, TN 37996, USA; [c] Département des sciences cliniques, Faculté de médecine vétérinaire, Université de Montréal, 3200 Sicotte, St-Hyacinthe, Quebec J2S 7C6, Canada
* Corresponding author.
E-mail address: adrian.steiner@vetsuisse.unibe.ch

Vet Clin Food Anim 30 (2014) 157–175
http://dx.doi.org/10.1016/j.cvfa.2013.11.002
0749-0720/14/$ – see front matter © 2014 Elsevier Inc. All rights reserved.

- Arthrogryposis
- Spastic paresis

Relevant acquired tendon disorders include:

- Tendon lacerations
- Tendon avulsion
- Tendon rupture
- Septic tendinitis/tenosynovitis

CONGENITAL TENDON DISORDERS
Hyperextension Deformities

Hyperextension deformities in newborn calves generally are caused by flexor tendon laxity. This condition occurs most commonly in calves that are born prematurely or are small for their gestational age. Acquired hyperextension deformities usually result from excessive weight bearing caused by contralateral limb lameness, or occur following removal of external coaptation after a prolonged period (**Fig. 1**). Hyperextension of the tarsus can be encountered in newborn calves following forced extraction and in adults following hind limb trauma. The hyperextension of the tarsus is caused by a rupture of the peroneus tertius. The gait is abnormal but it does not appear to be painful. The affected limb may be pulled backwards by the examiner with minimal physical force. At flexion of the stifle, the tarsus remains in full extension and tension on the calcaneal tendon is reduced (**Fig. 2**).

Mild to moderate hyperextension commonly responds to limited exercise (myotactic reflex) that strengthens and tones the muscles, tendons, and ligaments. If exercise is not successful, some form of heel extension can be used to prevent hyperextension of the distal interphalangeal joint and keep the toe on the ground. The authors have used a thin wooden block glued to the hoof wall with methylmethacrylate acrylic (Technovit, Jorgensen Laboratories, Loveland, CO) to obtain heel extension. When methyl methacrylate has to be used on calves' claws, the heat from the acrylic setting must be controlled by pouring cold water otherwise the pododerma can be damaged. Rupture of the peroneus tertius is treated conservatively by stall rest for 6 to 8 weeks. The prognosis is favorable.

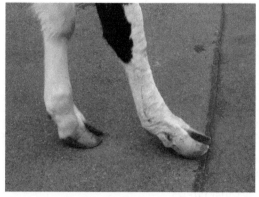

Fig. 1. Acquired hyperextension deformity following removal of external coaptation after a 7-week period.

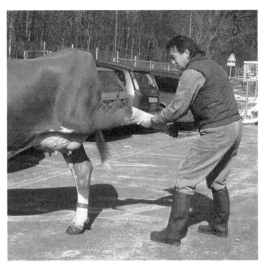

Fig. 2. Flexion of the stifle with the tarsus remaining in full extension; pay attention to the flaccid calcaneal tendon.

Flexural Deformities

Flexural limb deformities in a sagittal plane reflect an inability to achieve or maintain normal extension of the limb.[6] Flexural deformities are discussed more accurately relative to the joints affected rather than the affected tendons and ligaments, because more than one structure is often involved. Congenital contracted flexor tendon is a common defect in cattle and occurs in numerous breeds.[7] Causal origins for contracted flexor tendons include inherited factors, in utero malpositioning, and overcrowding caused by the size of the fetus relative to the dam. Contracted tendons may occur with other congenital abnormalities such as cleft palate, dwarfism, and arthrogryposis. A complete physical examination should be performed to rule out other problems before treatment is initiated for contracted tendons. Older cattle may acquire contracted tendons as a result of long-lasting reduced weight-bearing disease of the limb (for example, fracture, radial nerve paralysis, or physitis).

Most contracted tendons in calves are observed within the first day after birth. If there is reason to suspect a joint lesion as well as a tendinous lesion, radiographic examination may be useful before a prognosis is made and therapy is undertaken. Flexural deformities are generally found around the carpus or fetlock. Flexural deformities are classified as mild (if the calves are able to walk on their feet but the heels do not contact the ground), moderate (if the dorsal aspect of the claw breaks over a vertical plane perpendicular to the ground), or severe (if the affected animals are forced to walk on the dorsal aspect of the pastern, fetlock, or carpus). Nutrient or colostrum intake is often not sufficient, because the calves are unable to walk. Colostrum should be administered orally or plasma administered intravenously if the calf has difficulty walking. Also, unless adequate bedding is used or unless preventive measures are taken, rapid abrasion of the skin can occur from repeated trauma. Successful treatment of flexural deformities depends on the site and severity of the deformity and on the appropriate use of medical, physical, and possible surgical therapy. Treatment of congenital flexural deformities should be initiated soon after recognition of the problem, with the severity of the condition dictating how treatment should proceed. As the animal gets older, the contracted tissues become less responsive.

Mild to moderate flexural deformities usually respond to physical therapy with manual stretching of the tendons during exercise. The authors commonly construct an extended toe shoe, using methyl methacrylate acrylic or urethane glue and a thin wooden block, to increase the tension on the contracted tendons during walking (**Fig. 3**). Moderate cases are treated by using a bandage, splint, cast, or regular passive stretching exercise and by providing analgesia using a nonsteroidal antiinflammatory drug. Nonsteroidal antiinflammatory drugs provide analgesia to the calf and are useful to decrease the pain associated with the stretching of the contracted soft tissue that is caused by weight bearing, passive stretching exercise, splints, or casts. A single dose of oxytetracycline administered intravenously at 44 mg/kg was effective for obtaining a short-term (96 hours), moderate decrease in the metacarpophalangeal joint angle of a newborn foal.[8] The mechanism by which oxytetracycline exerts its effect is unknown, but it is most likely associated with a muscle relaxant effect.[8] Slow infusion of 60 mg/kg of oxytetracycline for the treatment of forelimb flexural deformities was attempted in 10 calves. Their average age at presentation was 6 days. The oxytetracycline was given once a day for 3 consecutive days. Fetlock angle was measured regularly after the administration of the oxytetracycline. Although small variation of angle was found, the animals did not improve significantly and they were still unable to stand on the fourth day.[9] However, we do not recommend the routine use of oxytetracycline at this high dose in cattle because of the risk of inducing renal failure. Lower doses of tetracycline have been used with some success early in the process of the disease. Relaxation of a calf limb can be induced by a firm limb bandage, possibly because of the supportive and protective effect on the muscles, tendons, and ligaments. Bandages should be placed over the limb, with the calf sedated and placed in lateral recumbency. The toes should be left unbandaged to support some weight and further stretch the tendons. Three layers of folded sheet cotton provide adequate padding and support for young calves. Splints can be changed daily or every other day, and the leg examined. In the forelimb, a splint extending from the foot to the elbow should be used. In a hind limb, the splint is placed from the foot to the point of the hock. The splint should be placed on the palmar/plantar aspect of the limb. The splint can be fashioned from polyvinylchloride (PVC) pipe cut into a semitubular shape and should be padded well to avoid pressure sores. Neglected monitoring of splints can be harmful to the animal by causing severe pressure sores. A cast may be necessary to provide more support, especially for calves with carpal flexural deformity. With the calf sedated and in lateral recumbency, a fiberglass cast is applied and

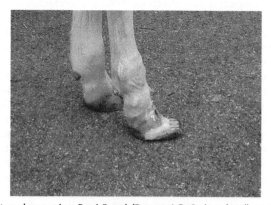

Fig. 3. Extended toe shoe, using Bovi-Bond (Provet AG, Switzerland) urethane glue and a wooden block.

allowed to harden as someone reduces the contracted limb into as normal a position as possible. The toes of the limb should be exposed, so that the calf will walk on them rather than on the cast. The cast should be removed within 1 week so that the limb can be examined. The cast can be reused as a bivalved splint if necessary. The relaxation effect of bandages, splints, and casts often provides enough improvement to allow further gradual improvement with exercise.

Most flexural limb deformities are corrected with persistent nonsurgical management. Those that do not improve may benefit from surgery, but the results in severely contracted limbs are often disappointing, and these animals are usually euthanized. In chronic cases, the joint capsule fibrosis is often severe, restricting normal movement even after a complete tenotomy of all the flexor tendons. Calves with severe flexural deformities of the fetlock may be treated by tenotomy performed in the midmetacarpal or midmetatarsal region or proximal to the carpus if the carpus is also affected by a flexural deformity.[10] With the animal anesthetized, all tendinous tissues under tension are severed through a small incision until the limb can be fully extended. Instead of a simple tenotomy, an elongation of the tendon may be achieved by a Z-tenotomy followed by a tendon suture. If the tenotomy results in some relief but complete extension of the limb is still not possible, severe trauma to the periarticular tissues may be necessary to achieve adequate extension of the affected limbs. Bandaging and splinting of the limb for 1 to 2 weeks might be required after surgery. If excessive relaxation of the limb is obtained, the limb should be placed in a cast including the foot for 3 to 4 weeks until the tendons are reunited by fibroplasia.

Arthrogryposis

Congenital arthrogryposis is defined as a syndrome of persistent joint contracture that is present at birth. Arthrogryposis may afflict 1 leg, the hind or front legs,[11] or all 4 legs, and has been reported in many breeds of cattle.[7] Arthrogryposis includes more than one causal and pathologic entity. A hereditary congenital deformity in Hereford cattle characterized by arthrogryposis, kyphosis, torticollis, scoliosis, and cleft palate has been described. Teratogens identified as causing arthrogryposis include plants and prenatal viral infections. Ingestion of lupines by pregnant cows between 40 and 70 days' gestation has caused various degrees of arthrogryposis with other associated congenital defects.[12] Lupine toxicosis is related to high alkaloid content.[7] In Europe, arthrogryposis occurs frequently after infection of the dam with the novel emerging Orthobunyavirus Schmallenberg virus (**Fig. 4**).[13] Besides arthrogryposis, the virus causes vertebral malformations, brachygnathia inferior, and malformations of the central nervous system, and it is currently responsible for severe economic losses in ruminants.[13] Cesarean section is needed in many cases because of dystocia.

Arthrogryposis should not be confused with contracted tendons, in which the joints are aligned properly and the legs are not rotated (discussed earlier). Joints of calves with contracted tendons can usually be extended with pressure or corrected surgically. In calves with arthrogryposis and crooked calf disease, the articular and osseous changes are usually permanent and become worse as the calf grows. In one retrospective study on arthrogryposis including 113 calves, 74% of the animals had only the forelimbs (carpus and fetlock) contracted; in 75% of cases, a cesarean section was needed because of dystocia.[12] Predisposing factors to arthrogryposis were male gender, posterior intrauterine presentation, and double muscling. If untreated, arthrogryposis of the carpus is usually lethal in cattle. It results in skin necrosis over the carpus, septic arthritis, and septicemia.

Surgical treatment of arthrogryposis of the forelimbs has been published and consists of desmotomy and tenotomy of contracted periarticular soft tissues.[11,12] Often,

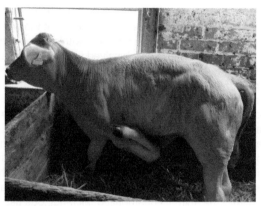

Fig. 4. Congenital arthrogryposis of the left forelimb in a 3-month-old Braunvieh calf, occurring after infection of the dam with the Schmallenberg virus.

all structures on the palmar aspect of the carpus, except blood vessels and nerves, are transected. A cast is then applied for a minimum of 6 weeks. Approximately 80% of these surgically treated animals can be kept until they reach normal slaughter weight. Because of a possible hereditary component, the authors do not recommend keeping these animals for breeding. When palmar carpal ligament transection has been performed, carpal hyperextension may occur in the postoperative period. If the palmar angulation between the metacarpus and radius is less than 100° before surgery, the prognosis is poor. In these cases, arthrodesis of the carpus may be attempted.[12]

Spastic Paresis

Spastic paresis is a progressive neuromuscular disease that occurs in dairy, beef, and crossbred cattle. Signs of spastic paresis usually appear at a few weeks to several months of age.[14] Spastic contractions of one or both gastrocnemius muscles and the superficial digital flexor (SDF) tendon lead to hyperextension of the hock. The affected leg(s) is extended caudally and is advanced in a swinging motion (**Fig. 5**). With progression of the disease, the foot often temporarily does not touch the ground when standing, and gluteal muscle atrophy occurs. Palpation of the limb shows that

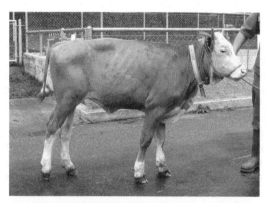

Fig. 5. Spastic paresis: spastic contractions of one or both gastrocnemius muscles and SDF tendons lead to hyperextension of the hock. The affected leg is extended caudally.

the gastrocnemius muscle is hard and rigid, but, during phases of relaxation, flexion of the hock is not painful. At first, few if any systemic effects result from the condition. However, with its progression, the animal may remain recumbent for a longer period and loses weight. Calves often must be slaughtered prematurely. No consistent pathologic lesion has been identified in the peripheral musculature or nerves or in the spinal cord or brain of animals with spastic paresis. The functional disturbance may be caused by an overactive stretch reflex present in the gastrocnemius muscles caused by overstimulation or lack of inhibition of motor neurons. Because spastic paresis is most likely inherited to some degree, affected animals should not be used as breeding stock. Surgical treatment of spastic paresis may be indicated in selected animals, mostly either to allow the cattle to reach slaughter weight or to keep an animal for sentimental value. We strongly recommend mandatory castration in males or crushing of all 4 teats with a Burdizzo clamp in females before surgical treatment of calves affected with spastic paresis. The respective breeding association should be informed.

Two surgical techniques have been described:

- Tibial neurectomy
- Transection of a portion of the gastrocnemius and superficial flexor tendons[15,16]

Partial or complete tibial neurectomy is aesthetically more pleasing. The procedure can be performed under sedation and epidural anesthesia or under general anesthesia with the animal placed in lateral recumbency with the affected limb positioned uppermost. The tibial nerve is accessed via a lateral incision through the biceps femoris muscle. It is located caudal to the peroneal nerve. The tibial nerve is isolated, and its different branches are stimulated electrically to evaluate the corresponding muscle contraction. A segment 3 cm long is excised from each of the 2 nerve branches innervating the gastrocnemius. The surgical incision is sutured in a routine fashion. Only 1 leg should be operated on at a time to assess the efficacy of the procedure. Partial tibial neurectomy has resulted in good to excellent results in 131 of 138 (95%) calves.[15]

Transection of a portion of the gastrocnemius and SDF tendons is performed after sedation, with the animal placed in lateral recumbency and with the affected limb positioned uppermost.[16] The leg is surgically prepared from the midmetatarsus to the stifle and 2% lidocaine is locally infiltrated over a l0-cm length proximal to the calcaneus and over the cranial border of the lateral aspect of the calcaneal tendon. A 5-cm skin incision is performed over the cranial border and lateral aspect of the gastrocnemius tendinous portion. The 2 tendons of insertion of the gastrocnemius muscle (lateral and medial head of the gastrocnemius muscle) and half of the SDF tendon are transected for a length of 2 cm, approximately 6 cm proximal to the point of the hock. The subcutis is closed with a simple continuous pattern, followed by a layer of simple interrupted skin sutures of nonabsorbable monofilament material. A bandage is applied over the surgical site for 5 days, and the skin sutures are removed after 10 days. The immediate effect of surgery is that the hock becomes profoundly flexed and the metatarsus becomes nearly parallel to the ground. Fibrous unions generally develop between the tendon ends, and limb posture returns in 4 to 6 weeks. Spasticity often returns slowly over several months. The results often do not allow the calf to return to a level of productive performance expected by the owner.

ACQUIRED TENDON DISORDERS

Dairy breeds, feedlot cattle, and cattle maintained in confinement housing are commonly affected, and the incidence of lameness in dairy herds ranges widely.

Lesions in dairy cattle occur most frequently during the early lactational period and in first-lactation heifers, and may occur more frequently during the spring and summer. However, based on these studies, lameness caused by tendon injury is uncommon in cattle. Therefore, information regarding acquired tendon disorders in ruminants is limited. Injuries observed in cattle include traumatic tendon disruptions (laceration, avulsion, and rupture) and septic tendinitis/tenosynovitis.

Tendon Laceration

Tendon laceration is an uncommon cause of lameness in cattle and occurs most commonly when the cow falls onto or kicks a sharp object (**Fig. 6**). The rear limbs are affected most commonly.[17] An open wound with contamination or infection is typically present at the site of tendon rupture. Management practices may be associated with the higher incidence of tendon lacerations among dairy breeds. Adult dairy cattle are maintained in a high-concentration environment and are often moved on concrete flooring. Concrete flooring requires frequent cleaning, which is often done using a tractor with a blade attachment. Therefore, dairy cattle are exposed to potential hazards on the farm. Feedlot cattle are also housed in concentrated environments with frequent exposure to farm machinery. However, feedlot cattle may be infrequently presented for treatment because of their lower perceived individual economic value.

Lacerations occur most commonly in a single hind limb at the level of the metatarsus. Ultrasound examination of the involved tissues may be limited because of the presence of an open wound and emphysema of the peritendinous tissues.[18] Radiographs (survey, contrast studies) may be useful to determine whether a joint or tendon sheath is involved and to evaluate for the presence of a foreign body.

Tendon Avulsion

In our experience, the most common tendon avulsion of cattle is avulsion of the deep digital flexor (DDF) tendon from its insertion on the solar aspect of the third phalanx

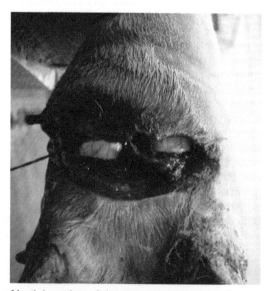

Fig. 6. Laceration of both branches of the SDF and deep digital flexor tendons proximal to the dewclaws after kicking a sharp object.

(discussed later). We have observed avulsion of the calcaneal tendon from its insertion on the calcaneus secondary to septic apophysitis in calves. Furthermore, we have diagnosed several animals affected with avulsion of the gastrocnemius muscle from its origin on the distal caudal femur (**Fig. 7**). Traumatic tendon avulsion affecting the peroneus tertius muscle has occurred in calves immediately after removal of a full-limb cast. We have seen traumatic avulsion of the tendon of insertion of the extensor carpi radialis (ECR) muscle in a calf after manual extraction for treatment of dystocia.

Management should be directed toward support of the limb and treatment of the inciting disease. Supportive treatment may include stall rest and antiinflammatory medication. A full-limb cast was used to treat a calf with avulsion of the tendon of insertion of the ECR muscle. The cast was removed after 21 days, and stall rest continued for 14 days. The calf made a full recovery, without any complications. Avulsion of the gastrocnemius muscle may be treated using a Thomas splint to stabilize the limb, but a poor prognosis for return to productive soundness should be given for complete avulsion. Stall rest for 8 to 12 weeks is recommended for partial gastrocnemius muscle avulsion, and a guarded to fair prognosis is given to the owner. Rupture of the peroneus tertius is treated conservatively by stall rest for 6 to 8 weeks. The prognosis is favorable.

Tendon Rupture

Spontaneous tendon rupture is most commonly associated with breeding accidents, bull fights, or postparturient neuropathy and usually involves the gastrocnemius muscle-tendon unit. Spontaneous rupture of the gastrocnemius muscle usually occurs at the junction of the muscle fibers and tendon.[17,19] Rupture of the gastrocnemius tendon adjacent to the insertion on the tuber calcaneus may be caused by direct trauma.

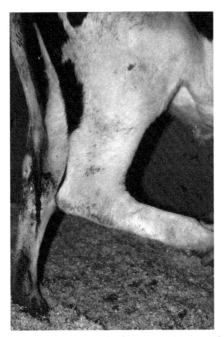

Fig. 7. Avulsion of the gastrocnemius muscle from its origin on the distal caudal femur, which allows passive flexion of the tarsus while the stifle remains in extension.

Treatment of Tendon Disruption

Flexor tendon lacerations can be managed successfully in cattle by tenorrhaphy and external coaptation or by external coaptation alone and supportive therapy such as stall rest, use of a wooden or rubber block on the healthy digit, and corrective farriery.[20] Economic costs associated with treatment and prolonged convalescence should be discussed with the owner before attempting therapy. Also, the owner's expectation for long-term productivity should include the likelihood of persistent lameness.

The location of the lesion, individual tendon involvement, and concurrent injuries are important factors for treatment selection. Stall confinement may be adequate for incomplete lacerations and partial disruption of the gastrocnemius muscle or tendon (**Fig. 8**). Application of a wooden block is useful when disruption of the branches of the DDF tendons (III or IV) to a single digit is present. A full-limb or half-limb cast may be indicated for injuries disrupting the flexor tendons to both digits of the same limb. Stall rest, use of a wooden block, and external coaptation of the limb result in healing of the tendon by second intention (fibroplasia) and scar tissue formation. Flexor tendon laceration located distal to the hock may be treated with application of a cast including the foot and extending to the level of the hock but not spanning the hock.[21,22] The fetlock may be flexed during casting or the solar surface of both digits positioned on a wooden wedge to release tension from the flexor tendons and allow closer apposition of the tendon ends. As an alternative, the limb may be cast in a normal, standing position. We recommend that the cast be maintained for 3 to 4 weeks longer than when a flexed fetlock or a wedge cast is used. The fetlock must be lightly padded on the dorsal and palmar/plantar aspects to protect the limb from pressure-induced perforating cast sores. Laceration of the calcaneal tendon may be treated with

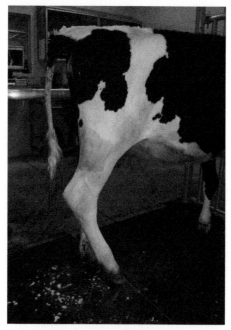

Fig. 8. Partial disruption of gastrocnemius muscle/tendon on a 16-month-old Holstein heifer. The calcaneum is slightly dropped while the stifle is in extension.

application of a cast including the foot and extending to the proximal tibia (level of the tibial crest). The portion of the cast spanning the hock must be thicker than the remainder to prevent breakage of the cast at this point. Reinforcing splints may provide a stronger construct, and if used should be placed on the cranial aspect of the limb. Thomas splints may be used to stabilize gastrocnemius muscle-tendon disruption, but in our experience the results have been poor. We prefer to use a full-limb cast when the disruption is close to the calcaneus.

Suture repair (tenorrhaphy) of transected tendons in addition to external coaptation achieves a more mature scar, resulting in a stronger and more rapidly healing scar-tendon unit than does healing by second intention. Biomechanical tests of the various methods of tenorrhaphy in SDF tendons of fresh equine cadavers have resulted in the recommendation that triple-interlocking loop or 3-loop pulley suture patterns be used.[23] Recent research revealed that the 6-strand Savage pattern was superior to the 3-loop pulley pattern concerning strength and resistance to suture pull-through (**Fig. 9**).[24]

The bodies of the tendons in the metacarpal and metatarsal regions are wide and thin and present a challenge for anchorage of tendon sutures. Nylon, polydioxanone, and polyglyconate are the most common suture materials used for tendon repair. However, no suture material or suture pattern currently in use can provide adequate breaking strength to allow ambulation without external coaptation. Cast immobilization has been advocated for a minimum of 6 to 8 weeks based on biomechanical studies of tendon healing and on clinical observations. Supportive farriery also has been recommended after cast removal. At present, the authors recommend external coaptation be maintained for a minimum of 60 days after complete transection of flexor tendons. During and after cast removal, a wedge block is used to elevate the heel. After cast removal, the angle of the wedge should be reduced in several steps

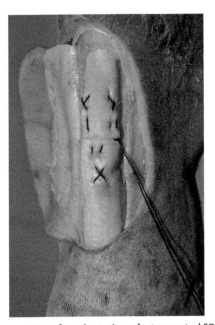

Fig. 9. The 6-strand Savage pattern for adaptation of a transected SDF tendon at the level of midmetatarsus III/IV shown on a cadaveric bovine hind foot.

and stall confinement continued for 4 to 6 weeks. Heel elevation after cast removal is not required when a standing conformation cast has been used.

The prognosis for tendon rupture in cattle is considered good for injuries involving the SDF tendon alone. In our experience, the prognosis for survival and for long-term productivity of cattle with traumatic rupture of both digital flexor tendons (SDF and DDF) is fair. Ultrasound examination of the healing tendon may provide valuable information regarding treatment and prognosis. Treatment of gastrocnemius tendon rupture has only been recommended for young, lightweight cattle. With complete disruption of the calcaneal tendon or gastrocnemius muscle, we provide a grave prognosis for cattle weighing more than 500 kg, and a poor prognosis for cattle weighing less than 500 kg. However, the prognosis for production soundness after disruption of the extensor tendons is considered excellent.

Septic Tendinitis

Septic tendinitis is most commonly associated with extension of digital sepsis, subsolar abscess, or sole ulcer (pododermatitis circumscripta, Rusterholz ulcer) to involve the DDF tendon.[25–27] Avulsion of the DDF from its insertion on the flexor tuberosity of the third phalanx may result, if sufficient necrosis of the tendon or underlying bone occurs. Surgical debridement, lavage, and daily wound management are indicated for deep sole ulcer, subsolar abscess, and septic pedal osteitis. A facilitated ankylosis of the distal interphalangeal joint is favored to stabilize the foot.[28] Affected cattle should be confined to a small pen or a stall for 6 to 8 weeks. The prognosis for unilateral DDF tendon avulsion is good if the cause of infection is treated.

Septic tendinitis also may occur when degloving injuries involve the flexor or extensor tendons of the distal limbs. Degloving wounds are often associated with injury from wire fencing, farm machinery, metal sidings on buildings, trailer accidents, and dog attacks. Treatment includes thorough surgical debridement, lavage, daily wound management, and systemic antibiotic and antiinflammatory medication. If DDF tendon involvement is confined to a single digit, a wooden or rubber block (claw block) may be applied to the solar surface of the healthy digit to improve comfort and ambulation. We recommend that these animals be maintained in a restricted environment (stall or small pen) during convalescence (6–8 weeks). Prognosis for septic tendinitis is good for superficial wounds. Deep wounds causing extensive tissue necrosis or sepsis of adjacent synovial cavities (joints, tendon sheaths) warrant a more guarded prognosis (discussed later).

Tenosynovitis (Tenovaginitis)

Based on research reported for horses, the tendon sheath is different in structure compared with that of diarthrodial joints. The synovial lining cells of the tendon sheath are fibroblastic in appearance and are composed of a single synovial cell type (diarthrodial joints have 2 distinct cell types).[29] Also, the tendon sheath contains abundant blood vessels but sparse nerve fibers. Synovial fluid produced by the tendon sheath has a lower concentration of hyaluronic acid and a lower mucinous precipitate quality than that of diarthrodial joint fluid. However, the cellular constituents and protein concentrations in tendon sheath fluid and joint fluid are similar. Cellular and protein changes in response to trauma and sepsis are also similar.

Pathologic lesions occur most commonly in the common digital flexor tendon sheath (CDFTS). The CDFTS originates from a point 6 to 8 cm proximal to the fetlock and extends distally to a point immediately distal to the coronary band. The tendon sheath is confined on its palmar/plantar surface by the palmar/plantar annular ligament of the fetlock, the palmar/plantar digital annular ligament (distal to the dewclaw), and the distal interdigital ligaments (proximal to the heel bulbs). Inflammation of the CDFTS should be suspected when focal swelling of the palmar/plantar aspect of the pastern is observed concurrent with focal swelling extending some centimeters proximally from the level of the dewclaws (**Fig. 10**).

Inflammation of synovial structures may be caused by trauma, injection of irritant chemicals, immune-mediated synovitis, or sepsis. Inflammation and distension of the tendon sheath result in pain. Adhesions between the tendon and tendon sheath may result from sustained trauma or inflammation. Restrictive adhesions may cause recurrent pain and lead to decreased productive soundness. Two forms of tenosynovitis have been recognized in cattle: aseptic (traumatic, secondary synovitis, idiopathic) and septic. The authors have successfully treated various cattle affected with aseptic tenosynovitis using nonsteroidal antiinflammatory drugs, hydrotherapy (30 minutes, 2–3 times per day for 10–14 days), tendon sheath drainage and lavage (1 L of 0.9% saline or lactated Ringers solution, once), pressure bandages (changed every 2 days for 7–10 days), and/or intrathecal administration of sodium hyaluronate (20 mg, once).[30]

Septic Tenosynovitis

Septic tenosynovitis is most frequently diagnosed in the CDFTS but also occurs in the tendon sheath of the ECR muscle. Sepsis of the tendon sheath typically occurs as a result of extension of local sepsis (such as with sole ulcer, a septic distal interphalangeal joint, a septic distal sesamoid bursa or podotrochleosis, or a heel bulb abscess) or by direct inoculation (via penetrating wounds, foreign bodies, or iatrogenic trauma from farm implements such as a pitchfork or front-end loader).[25] Septic tenosynovitis caused by hematogenous translocation of bacteria (septicemia) is rare. Clinical signs

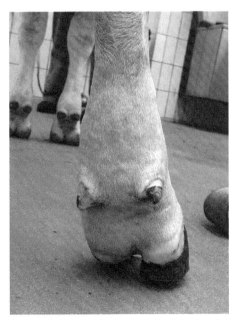

Fig. 10. Septic tenosynovitis of the CDFTS characterized by focal swelling of the plantar aspect of the pastern, extending some centimeters proximally from the level of the dewclaws.

include lameness (moderate to non–weight bearing), recumbency, decreased milk production, and decreased feed intake. When standing, affected cattle may be reluctant to walk or may walk with the limb abducted or adducted to shift weight to the unaffected digit and with a shortened second phase of the stride. Effusion of the tendon sheath results in swelling proximal to the dewclaws. Swelling in the pastern region is limited by the annular ligament of the fetlock, the digital annular ligament, and the proximal interdigital ligament. The lateral hind limb tendon sheath is the most frequently affected. Diagnosis of septic tenosynovitis may include:

- Orthopedic examination
- Ultrasonographic examination
- Synovial fluid collection for cytologic evaluation, culture, and total protein analysis

Each digital branch of the SDF and DDF tendon has its own tendon sheath, and the two sheaths rarely communicate near their proximal extent.[26,31] Treatment of septic tenosynovitis should include management of the inciting disease and of the infected tendon sheath. Medical management alone (systemic antibiotics, hydrotherapy, protective bandages) is unlikely to be effective because of the severity of the inciting disease and the excessive fibrin deposition within the tendon sheath. Antibiotics cannot effectively penetrate fibrin foci to achieve therapeutic concentrations.[32,33] Effective treatment options of septic tenosynovitis include:

- Arthroscopic lavage
- Surgical implantation of an active lavage/drainage system
- Tenovaginotomy with surgical debridement and passive ventral drainage
- Digit amputation

Selection of the most appropriate treatment option depends on economic constraints and on the severity of the septic process, ranging from the least invasive technique (lavage) adequate for treatment of serofibrinous tenosynovitis to the most invasive technique (tenovaginotomy and debridement with ventral drainage) in chronic cases with severe septic involvement of the tendons. Amputation may be classified as a salvage procedure. Before any type of surgery (except amputation) is initiated, a wooden block is applied to the healthy digit to improve comfort and ambulation during the convalescent period.

Tenovaginoscopic lavage, combining through-and-through and distension-irrigation lavage, was described for successful treatment of septic serofibrinous tenosynovitis with minor tendon involvement in 4 adult cattle (**Fig. 11**).[31] With the animal in lateral recumbency and the affected limb uppermost, a 1-cm skin incision was made 4 to 5 cm proximal to the dewclaws in the midline of the respective CDFTS. The sleeve with a blunt trocar was introduced into the proximal pouch of the CDFTS, just proximal to the palmar/plantar annular ligament, and advanced along its length in a distal direction, plantar or palmar to the SDF tendon. The arthroscope was then introduced into the sleeve, and the CDFTS examined and thoroughly flushed, using 3 to 6 L of physiologic Ringer solution. At the end of the procedure, 12×10^6 IU of sodium benzylpenicillin and 10 mL of 2% lidocaine were injected into the CDFTS. Aftercare included 30,000 IU/kg sodium benzylpenicillin every 8 hours intravenously through an indwelling catheter in the jugular vein for 7 days, whereas 4 mg/kg ketoprofen was administered orally once a day for 3 to 5 days. Recommendations for further care after discharge from the clinic were daily intramuscular administration of benzylpenicillin procaine (30,000 IU/kg) until day 10 after surgery, removal of the skin sutures on day 11, removal of the wooden block on day 30, and stall confinement until day 60

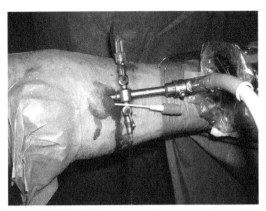

Fig. 11. Position of the arthroscope for tenosynovioscopy of the CDFTS.

after surgery.[31] In cases of fibrinous tenosynovitis with minor tendon involvement, removal of fibrin clots may be achieved with a Ferris-Smith forceps under arthroscopic control (**Fig. 12**).

Surgical implantation of an active lavage/drainage system represents an alternative to tenovaginoscopic lavage for septic tenosynovitis without necrotic tendinitis in cattle, using a multifenestrated silicone rubber drain (Snyder Hemovac, Zimmer, Dover, OH). This procedure is best performed with the animal sedated and restrained in lateral recumbency on a tilt table. Intravenous regional anesthesia (lidocaine 2%, 20 mL) is infused distal to a tourniquet before surgery. A 14-gauge needle is inserted into the tendon sheath proximally and distally to guide optimal placement of the stab incisions. Limited debridement is then performed through a stab incision placed into the proximal aspect of the tendon sheath and a second stab incision placed into the distal tendon sheath. A large, curved forceps or clamp (Rochester-Carmalt forceps) is inserted from proximal to distal within the CDFTS. The instrument is used

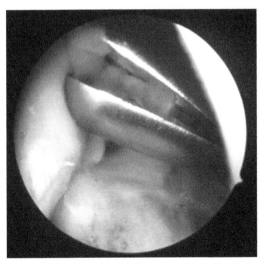

Fig. 12. Removal of fibrin clots from the CDFTS, using Ferris-Smith forceps under arthroscopic control.

to grasp the proximal tubing of the drain, and the drain is pulled through the tendon sheath. The excess fenestrated portion of the drain is discarded. Drainage and lavage are performed by high-pressure infusion of sterile, isotonic electrolyte solutions into the drain. We use a 60-mL syringe and 3-way stopcock to achieve high-pressure lavage. The distal end of the drain is sutured closed to occlude the lumen and force the fluids to exit the drain into the tendon sheath. The drain is sutured to the skin proximally and maintained under a sterile bandage between flushing. High-pressure lavage is performed once daily for 5 to 7 days, using 1 to 2 L of saline or lactated Ringer solution. Crystalline antibiotic solutions may be instilled into the drain and tendon sheath after each lavage and when the drain is removed. Many veterinarians add antiseptic chemicals (such as povidone iodine or chlorhexidine) to lavage fluids. However, research has shown that povidone iodine (concentration>0.2%) and chlorhexidine (concentration>0.05%) induce significant synovitis and may exacerbate intrathecal disease.[34,35] It is optimal for the drain to be cultured at the time of removal and the results compared with initial microbial cultures. Systemic antibiotics and antiinflammatory medication are administered concurrently. A possible complication with this technique is ascending infection of the tendon sheath through or along the drain. In our experience, a fair to favorable prognosis for long-term productive soundness may be given with this technique.

If purulent tenosynovitis is present, tenosynoviotomy with surgical debridement and passive ventral drainage is indicated. Surgical exploration provides optimal access for thorough debridement of the tendon sheath and tendons. Exploration is performed by incising the sheath beginning at its origin proximal to the accessory digits and extending in a curvilinear fashion distally between the dewclaws to the coronary band. Thorough debridement and lavage of the tendons and the sheath are performed. If the tendons are necrotic, affected aspects are rigorously resected (**Fig. 13**).[36,37] Thereafter, an indwelling Penrose drain exiting distally is introduced to facilitate drainage after surgery, and the proximal three-fourths of the sheath and the skin are sutured. The Penrose drain is removed at 3 to 5 days after surgery, and a bandage is maintained until suture removal at day 11 (**Fig. 14**). Antibiotic and antiinflammatory medications should be administered for at least 10 days after surgery. Dehiscence of the surgical wound is a potential complication because of the high motion occurring in the palmar/plantar aspect of the fetlock. In our experience, the prognosis of this procedure is fair to favorable.

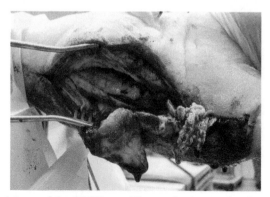

Fig. 13. Tenosynoviotomy of the CDFTS, providing optimal access for thorough debridement and rigorous resection of necrotic tissues.

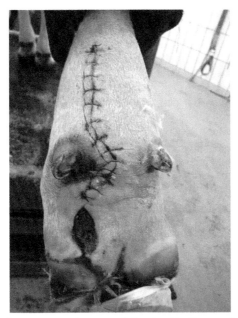

Fig. 14. Seven days after tenosynoviotomy of the CDFTS. The proximal four-fifths of the sheath and the skin were sutured. Drainage is maintained through the opening in the distal aspect of the wound.

Digit amputation proximal to the middle phalanx provides ventral drainage of purulent material and fibrin from the tendon sheath. Immediate relief from pain and swelling may be noted after surgery. Antibiotics should be administered for 7 to 10 days after surgery, but may be omitted if early salvage is performed.

REFERENCES

1. Choquette-Levy L, Baril J, Levy M, et al. A study of foot disease of dairy cattle in Quebec. Can Vet J 1985;26(9):278–81.
2. Wells SJ, Trent AM, Marsh WE, et al. Prevalence and severity of lameness in lactating dairy cows in a sample of Minnesota and Wisconsin herds. J Am Vet Med Assoc 1993;202(1):78–82.
3. Whitaker DA, Kelly JM, Smith EJ. Incidence of lameness in dairy cows. Vet Rec 1983;113(3):60–2.
4. Russell AM, Rowlands GJ, Shaw SR, et al. Survey of lameness in British dairy cattle. Vet Rec 1982;111(8):155–60.
5. Arkins S. Lameness in dairy cows. Ir Vet J 1981;35:135–40.
6. Tulleners EP. Management of bovine orthopedic problems. Part II: coxofemoral luxation, soft tissue problems, sepsis, and miscellaneous skull problems. Comp Cont Educ Pract 1986;8:S117–23.
7. Leipold HW, Hirarga T, Dennis SM. Congenital defects of the bovine musculoskeletal system and joints. Vet Clin North Am Food Anim Pract 1993;9:93–104.
8. Madison JB, Garber JL, Rice B, et al. Effect of oxytetracycline on metacarpophalangeal and distal interphalangeal joint angles in newborn foals. J Am Vet Med Assoc 1994;204(2):246–9.

9. Metzner M, Baumgart I, Klee W. Effect of infusion of 60 mg/kg oxytetracycline on forelimb flexor tendon contracture in calves. Vet Rec 2007;160(5):166–7.
10. Weaver AD, St Jean G, Steiner A. Contracted flexor tendons. In: Weaver AD, St Jean G, Steiner A, editors. Bovine surgery and lameness, vol. 1, 2nd edition. Oxford (IA): Blackwell Publishing; 2005. p. 240–2.
11. Verschooten F, DeMoor A, Desmet P, et al. Surgical treatment of congenital arthrogryposis of the carpal joint, associated with contraction of the flexor tendons in calves. Vet Rec 1969;85:140–2.
12. Van Huffel X, DeMoor A. Congenital multiple arthrogryposis of the forelimb in calves. Comp Cont Educ Pract 1987;9:F333–9.
13. Herder V, Wohlsein P, Peters M, et al. Salient lesions in domestic ruminants infected with the emerging so-called Schmallenberg virus in Germany. Vet Pathol 2012;49(4):588–91.
14. Leipold HW, Huston K, Guffy MM, et al. Spastic paresis in beef shorthorn cattle. J Am Vet Med Assoc 1967;151(5):598–601.
15. Vlaminck L, De Moor A, Martens A, et al. Partial tibial neurectomy in 113 Belgian blue calves with spastic paresis. Vet Rec 2000;147(1):16–9.
16. Weaver AD, St Jean G, Steiner A. Spastic paresis. In: Weaver AD, St Jean G, Steiner A, editors. Bovine surgery and lameness, vol. 1, 2nd edition. Oxford (IA): Blackwell Publishing; 2005. p. 246–8.
17. Weaver AD. Muscles. In: Greenough P, editor. Lameness in cattle, vol. 1, 3rd edition. Philadelphia, London, Toronto, Montreal (Canada), Sydney (Australia), Tokyo: WB Saunders; 1997. p. 194–9.
18. Miles KG. Basic principles and clinical applications of diagnostic ultrasonography. Comp Cont Educ Pract 1989;11:609–22.
19. Wheat JD, Asbury AC. Rupture of the gastrocnemius muscle in a cow–A case report. J Am Vet Med Assoc 1958;132:331–2.
20. Anderson DE, St-Jean G, Morin DE, et al. Traumatic flexor tendon injuries in 27 cattle. Vet Surg 1996;25(4):320–6.
21. Wilson DG, Vanderby R Jr. An evaluation of fiberglass cast application techniques. Vet Surg 1995;24(2):118–21.
22. Wilson DG, Vanderby R Jr. An evaluation of six synthetic casting materials: strength of cylinders in bending. Vet Surg 1995;24(1):55–9.
23. Easley KJ, Stashak TS, Smith FW, et al. Mechanical properties of four suture patterns for transected equine tendon repair. Vet Surg 1990;19(2):102–6.
24. Everett E, Barrett JG, Morelli J, et al. Biomechanical testing of a novel suture pattern for repair of equine tendon lacerations. Vet Surg 2012;41(2):278–85.
25. Greenough PR. Observations on some of the diseases of the bovine foot, Part II. Vet Rec 1962;74:53–63.
26. Stanek C. Septic tenosynovitis of the digital flexor tendon sheath. In: Greenough P, editor. Lameness in cattle, vol. 1, 3rd edition. Philadelphia, London, Toronto, Montreal (Canada), Sydney (Australia), Tokyo: WB Saunders; 1997. p. 188–90.
27. Weaver AD, St Jean G, Steiner A. Deep digital sepsis. In: Weaver AD, St Jean G, Steiner A, editors. Bovine surgery and lameness, vol. 1, 2nd edition. Oxford (IA): Blackwell Publishing; 2005. p. 219–20.
28. Starke A, Heppelmann M, Beyerbach M, et al. Septic arthritis of the distal interphalangeal joint in cattle: comparison of digital amputation and joint resection by solar approach. Vet Surg 2007;36(4):350–9.
29. Hago BE, Plummer JM, Vaughan LC. Equine synovial tendon sheaths and bursae: an histological and scanning electron microscopical study. Equine Vet J 1990;22(4):264–72.

30. Gaughan EM, Nixon AJ, Krook LP, et al. Effects of sodium hyaluronate on tendon healing and adhesion formation in horses. Am J Vet Res 1991;52(5):764–73.
31. Bertagnoli A, Raber M, Morandi N, et al. Tenovaginoscopic approach to the common digital flexor tendon sheath of adult cattle: technique, normal findings and preliminary results in four clinical cases. Vet J 2012;191(1):121–7.
32. Barza M, Samuelson T, Weinstein L. Penetration of antibiotics into fibrin loci in vivo. II. Comparison of nine antibiotics: effect of dose and degree of protein binding. J Infect Dis 1974;129(1):66–72.
33. Barza M, Weinstein L. Penetration of antibiotics into fibrin loci in vivo. I. Comparison of penetration of ampicillin into fibrin clots, abscesses, and "interstitial fluid". J Infect Dis 1974;129(1):59–65.
34. Smith JA, Williams RJ, Knight AP. Drug therapy for arthritis in food-producing animals. Comp Cont Educ Pract 1989;11:87–94.
35. Wilson DG, Cooley AJ, MacWilliams PS, et al. Effects of 0.05% chlorhexidine lavage on the tarsocrural joints of horses. Vet Surg 1994;23(6):442–7.
36. Nuss K, Hänichen T. Fibrino-purulent flexor tendinitis in infected tenosynovitis of the digital flexor tendon sheath in cattle. Tierarztl Prax 1995;23:565–9.
37. Weaver AD, St Jean G, Steiner A. Resection of the deep and superficial flexor tendons and sheaths. In: Weaver AD, St Jean G, Steiner A, editors. Bovine surgery and lameness, vol. 1, 2nd edition. Oxford (IA): Blackwell Publishing; 2005. p. 226–7.

Clinical Management of Septic Arthritis in Cattle

André Desrochers, DMV, MS*, David Francoz, DMV, DES, MSc

KEYWORDS

- Cattle • Septic arthritis • Surgery • Joint disease • Diagnostic

KEY POINTS

- Synovial fluid, ultrasound, and radiographic imaging are common diagnostic tools for septic arthritis.
- Mycoplasma septic arthritis is suspected in calves with clinical signs of otitis and pneumonia.
- Commonly affected joints are carpus, stifle, and tarsus.
- Treatment strategy must include long-term antibiotics, anti-inflammatories, and joint lavage.
- Knowledge of communication and boundaries for commonly affected joints is essential to perform joint lavage and arthrotomy.

Lameness in cattle originates from the digits. The second most common cause of lameness is from the joint; 47.0% to 72.2% of all lameness other from the foot is located to the joint and ligament.[1,2] The most common lesions affecting the joint are of traumatic origin, developmental (osteochondrosis), and septic. Few data are available on the importance of septic arthritis (SA) in cattle. In Israel, arthritis accounts for 13.8% of lameness cases.[3] In American feedlots, swollen joints are linked to 12% of lameness. The most common joints infected are front fetlock, hock, and elbow.[4] A Canadian survey in feedlot calves from Saskatchewan showed that 1.3% became chronic; 39% of these calves had a diagnosis of polyarthritis.[5] In Sweden, the incidence rate of arthritis in dairy calves was reported to be 0.002 cases per calf-months at risk.[6] In a study in veal calves in Belgium, the incidence rate of SA was 0.11 cases per 1000 calf days at risk.[7]

Although not as common as claw diseases, the consequences of SA are dramatic if left untreated, with potential irreversible joint function. It is a painful disease demanding a rapid medical decision. It also can be the first sign of a contagious disease like *Histophilus somni*[8,9] or *Mycoplasma bovis*.[10–13]

Faculty of Veterinary Medicine, Department of Clinical Sciences, Université de Montréal, 3200 Sicotte, St-Hyacinthe, Quebec J2S 7C6, Canada
* Corresponding author.
E-mail address: andre.desrochers@umontreal.ca

Vet Clin Food Anim 30 (2014) 177–203
http://dx.doi.org/10.1016/j.cvfa.2013.11.006
0749-0720/14/$ – see front matter © 2014 Elsevier Inc. All rights reserved.

PATHOPHYSIOLOGY

Bacterial arthritis is the most common form of SA in cattle.[14] There is anecdotal report of virus infection.[15] Bacterial arthritis is certainly the most damaging joint pathology. The origin of the bacterial infection is from direct trauma or contamination, adjacent infection, or hematogenous seeding. The distal joints like the interphalangeal joints and the fetlock are mostly affected by direct trauma. Iatrogenic infection following intra-articular (IA) injection is also possible, but rare in cattle compared with horses.[16] Infection adjacent to a joint is another cause of septic joint. A solar or bulbar abscess can expend and contaminate the distal interphalangeal joint.[17,18] Finally, the systemic or remote infection has to be considered when a calf is diagnosed with SA, especially if more than one joint is affected and no wound can be seen. The umbilicus is a very common route of infection. Inadequate hygiene and disinfection of the umbilicus after birth and passive immunity transfer failure are the most important factors contributing to umbilical infection. Other frequent newborn infections have to be considered if the umbilicus is normal at the physical or ultrasound examination: pneumonia, diarrhea, and septicemia. Because passive immunity transfer failure is the most important risk factor for all these diseases, it should also be considered Systemic origin rather than local trauma will increase the probability of more than one joint being infected.[19] In adult endocarditis, Lyme disease, pneumonia, or mastitis can be the source of SA.[10,20,21]

Even if the synovial membrane has a relative effectiveness on the control of the bacteria, multiple villosities support the establishment and the attachment of microorganisms. Bacteria will take action on the cartilage, the synovial membrane, and fluid but the most perverse effects are of immunologic origin. First, microorganisms are destroyed by neutrophils and their enzymes: elastase, cathepsin, gelatinase, and the collagenase. These enzymes destroy not only the bacteria but also the cartilage and its components. Moreover, the neutrophils and the inflamed tissues release free radicals, which have the same harmful effects on articulation. The inflammation will increase the permeability of the capillaries and let other mediators arrive at the site of infection (kinine, factor of coagulation, cascade of the complement, fibrinolytic system). These mediators will stimulate the synoviocytes and the chondrocytes. The chondrocytes will release mediators as the MMP (matrix metalloproteinase), which will decrease the production of proteoglycan. The reduction in production and the degradation of the proteoglycans deteriorate the physical properties of the cartilage, thus decreasing its potential of compression. The cartilage is therefore more fragile. The presence of fibrin on the cartilage and the synovial membrane decreases the nutritive effectiveness of the synovial fluid and the diffusion of antibiotics used in the treatment of SA. If left untreated, this fibrin will form a pannus covering all surfaces of the joint cavity.

PATHOGEN

Numerous bacteria have been isolated from infected joints in cattle. To our knowledge, only a few studies are available on the prevalence of the different pathogens isolated for septic joints. In our hospital, we have performed a retrospective study of joint bacterial culture in 172 cases of SA (between 1980 and 2000).[14] No bacterium was cultured in 40% of cases (n = 69), 1 bacterium in 47% (n = 80), 2 bacteria in 9% (n = 16), and more than 3 in 4% (n = 7). The proportion among the different bacteria cultured is presented in **Table 1**. *Truepurella pyogenes* was by far the most frequent bacterium cultured. Because their specific culture was not requested for all cases, the importance of anaerobic bacteria and *Mycoplasma* spp is probably

Table 1
Proportion of the different bacteria cultured and their repartition according to the age in a retrospective study of 172 cases of septic arthritis

	Cattle Younger than 6 mo of Age (n = 71)	Cattle Older than 6 mo of Age (n = 65)	Total (n = 136)
Truepurella pyogenes	35 (25)	48 (31)	41 (56)
Streptococci	20 (14)	8 (5)	14 (19)
Enterobacteriaceae	14 (10)	11 (7)	12 (17)
Staphylococci	6 (4)	17 (11)	11 (15)
Pasteurellaceae	8 (6)	0 (0)	4 (6)
Pseudomonas	1 (1)	1 (1)	1 (2)
Anaerobacteriaceae[a]	8 (6)	14 (9)	11 (15)
Mycoplasma[a]	7 (5)	1 (1)	4 (6)

Numbers in parentheses are those with a positive culture.
[a] Anaerobic and *Mycoplasma*-specific cultures were not performed on all cases.
Data from Francoz D, Desrochers A, Fecteau G, et al. A retrospective study of joint bacterial culture in 172 cases of septic arthritis in cattle. Paper presented at: 20th ACVIM forum, Dallas, May 29 - June 1, 2002.

underestimated in this retrospective study. Actually in our hospital, we believe that *Mycoplasma* spp is one of the most commonly isolated bacteria in calves. Other bacterial pathogens have been anecdotally associated with cases of SA in calves. They include *Lactococcus lactis*,[22] *Chlamydophila* spp,[23] *Salmonella typhimurium* DT 104,[24] *Erysipelothrix insidiosa*,[25] *Erysipelothrix rhusopathiae*,[26] and *Streptococcus dysgalactiae*.[27]

Borrelia burgdorferi, the agent of Lyme disease or borreliosis, is associated with swollen joints and lameness in different species. In cattle, the clinical presentation of borreliosis is unclear; only a few data on natural *B burgdorferi* associated infection are available.[28] However, lameness and swollen joints are common clinical signs.[28,29] Swollen joint and arthritis are also clinical signs reported with brucellosis in cattle.[28]

As mentioned previously, *Mycoplasma*-associated SA is probably underestimated, and to date no data are available on the prevalence in North America. In one study from Iran, *Mycoplasma* spp was isolated in 46.3% of the positive cultures of synovial fluid sampled at abattoir on cases of SA.[30] Among all *Mycoplasma* species, *Mycoplasma bovis* is probably the most important species involved in joint diseases. Clinical cases of *M bovis*–induced arthritis tend to be sporadic and are typically considered as a sequel of respiratory disease or mastitis within a herd or animal. Nevertheless, outbreaks of *M bovis* infections have been reported in calves,[31,32] and dairy cows[33–35] with arthritis as the primary and/or predominant clinical manifestation. A specific syndrome, chronic pneumonia and polyarthritis syndrome, is described in weaned beef calves and in beef cattle, which appears 3 to 4 weeks after entering the feedlot.[11,36] Clinical signs of *M bovis* arthritis are typically those of SA, but involvement of tendon sheaths with periarticular soft tissue swelling is also frequently observed.[33,35,37] Any joint may be affected, and multiple joints can be involved. Poor response to treatment is a common feature of *M bovis* arthritis.[34,35,37–39]

CLINICAL PRESENTATION

Typical clinical signs of SA include acute non–weight-bearing lameness, joint swelling, and pain and heat on joint palpation and manipulation. The animal may also have fever and decreased appetite. One or multiple joints may be affected at the same time. Polyarthritis is commonly associated with blood dissemination of bacteria from a primary site of infections and is more common in calves. The most commonly affected joints are carpus, tarsus, stifle, and fetlock.[40–42] Carpal and stifle joints were the most frequently affected joints in young animals, whereas fetlock and tarsal joints were more frequently involved in adults.[14]

Most lameness is obvious by observing the animal's stance (**Fig. 1**). Attention should first be paid to the posture of the animal, including the back, shoulders, pelvis, and major limb joints. With the animal standing, the general stance is observed first, then attention is drawn toward the limbs from the digit to the proximal limb. Compare one region to the opposite side and determine if obvious swelling, wounds, shifting of weight, and foot posture, such as toe touching or favored weight bearing on the medial or lateral claw, are present. In long-standing diseases with severe lameness, the heels are taller and the wall longer on the affected digit compared with that of the healthy claw. A dropped fetlock (eg, hyperextension of the fetlock joint) may be noticed on the sound limb because of excessive load on the flexor tendons and suspensory ligament.

In young animals, angular limb deformities secondary to uneven weight bearing occur rapidly with chronic lameness. The affected limb will have flexural deformities from chronic pain and muscular atrophy secondary to disuse. The contralateral limb is supporting more weight and its axial positioning will change to keep the animal in balance. Depending of the chronicity and the severity of the lameness, this posture change may deform the limb. Attention should be paid to differentiate this muscular atrophy from the one caused by nerve injury. Neurogenic muscle atrophy occurs very rapidly (7–10 days) and is severe. The animal will still attempt to bear weight but will fail because of weakness. Chronic lameness of the front limb will usually bring atrophy of the triceps, biceps, and scapular muscles. The consequence of this atrophy is more a prominent shoulder and the animal may be falsely diagnosed with shoulder joint diseases. Similarly, atrophy of gluteal muscles makes the greater trochanter prominent, which may be misdiagnosed as a coxofemoral joint luxation.

Once the affected limb or limbs are identified, palpation and localization of the swelling is the second step. Knowledge of the joint boundaries and communication

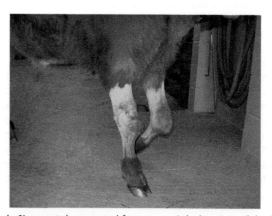

Fig. 1. A young male Simmental presented for non–weight bearing of the left thoracic limb. The left carpus is swollen and the animal keeps it in flexion. The dorsal aspect of the right carpus is swollen as well, but is more limited around the bursae and tendon sheath of the extensors. Although painful, it is less than that of a septic joint.

is important while evaluating a joint (**Fig. 2**). SA is generally painful to pressure. The joint is distended and joint instability may be palpable. One must pay attention not to confound this laxity with that observed in cases of ligament or tendon injury and joint luxation. Joint distension may not be obvious for proximal joints, such as the hip and the shoulder. Joint palpation also may help the veterinary practitioner to identify if the infection is secondary to a direct trauma or to an extension from a periarticular infection (**Fig. 3**). In young animals, all the other joints must be palpated and any distension must be considered as septic until proven otherwise.

When SA is likely to be the consequence of blood dissemination of infection, it is important to identify the primary source of infection to be able to institute appropriate treatment. Such cases may be suspected (1) when proximal joints are implicated (stifle, hip, shoulder), (2) in cases of polyarthritis, or (3) when direct trauma or infected area near the joint is not found during joint manipulation. As mentioned previously, the primary source of infection may be the umbilicus, the respiratory tract, the digestive tract, or the mammary gland. A complete workup must be achieved to rule out potential involvement of these systems.

DIFFERENTIAL DIAGNOSIS

Differential diagnoses for non–weight-bearing lameness should always include sole abscess, fracture, major joint luxation (eg, tarsus), critical weight-bearing ligament, or tendon injury (eg, gastrocnemius muscle), critical nerve injury (eg, radial nerve, femoral nerve, and sciatic nerve), SA, and septic tenosynovitis. An abnormal deviation of the limb is usually related to a fracture or joint luxation. The stance and position of the limb is abnormal with nerve damage, tendon rupture, or a severe ligament injury.

The differential diagnosis of swollen joint in calves should include SA, ligament injury, osteochondrosis, articular fracture, and idiopathic arthritis. Septic arthritis should remain high on the list of possible diagnosis for swollen joint in calves. Animals with periarticular swelling (bursitis or hygroma) can be sound to mildly lame. If lameness is obvious, an articular involvement must be considered. Soft, indolent swelling over a joint is typical of osteochondrosis or a bursitis. Animals affected with osteochondrosis will usually have a moderate lameness but weigh bearing is always present. Osteoarthritis clinical signs are extremely variable as far as degree of lameness. Generally it affects older animals and the lameness is moderate but with

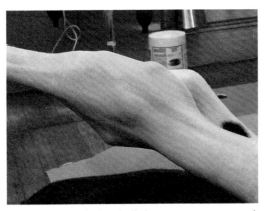

Fig. 2. This tarsus is severely distended and all the compartments can be identified.

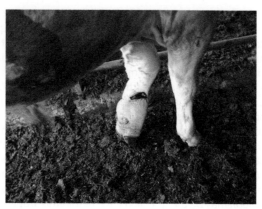

Fig. 3. This Charolais bull has a deep infected laceration on the medio-palmar aspect of the left thoracic limb. Without appropriate examination, it is impossible to determine if the sheath of the flexor tendons and the fetlock joint are affected.

a slow chronic progression. Animals affected with osteochondrosis might have bilateral lesions. Animals with ligament injury will react to joint movement or direct pressure on the affected ligament (collateral ligaments). Any fractures involving the joint are very painful. However, some animals with a slipped capital physis of the femur might be able to bear weight.

DIAGNOSTIC
Arthrocentesis

Arthrocentesis and subsequent cytologic and bacteriologic analyses of the synovial fluid are the complementary tests of choice for the diagnosis and the management of SA. It is simple and cost-effective. Sterile technique is mandatory to avoid contamination or worst, an iatrogenic infection.[16,43] Most of the joints can be done blindly, just with basic knowledge of the anatomy.[44,45] However, the coxofemoral joint is better performed under ultrasound guidance.

Arthrocentesis can be easily performed on a standing or lying sedated animal. The joint must always be surgically prepared. Recently, the necessity of hair clipping before arthrocentesis has been questioned in horses based on nonsignificant bacterial reduction compared with clipped skin or by observation of tissue or hair debris.[46] However, small-gauge needles were used (20 G and 22 G) to perform arthrocentesis.[46] The use of a disposable spinal needle with the stylet inserted with an angle into the joint decreases joint contamination with debris as well.[46] Those findings should be considered if the suspicion of a septic joint is rather low. Otherwise, if SA is highly probable, larger-diameter needles are suitable because of their high cellular and protein content and the difficulty aspirating the thick synovial fluid. An 18-G or 20-G 1.5-inch is then insert in specific sites related to joint anatomy, boundaries and communication (**Table 2**).

Unsuccessful aspiration is rather rare but possible. It can be caused by inadequate technique, low volume of fluid, or needle obstruction with fibrin or plica of synovial membrane or fat pads (stifle). If the synovial fluid is purulent, thick, or contains a lot of fibrin, a 14-G needle can be used but only if SA is highly suspected based on ultrasound or radiographic images. The synovial fluid is collected by passive flow or by using a 10-mL needle. The synovial fluid should be placed in a purple tube for cytologic analysis and in a sterile tube for bacteriologic culture. The synovial fluid is collected in a red-top tube for glucose and enzyme dosage if appropriate. The joint is then left unbandaged unless necessary large needles have been used. If only a small volume can be collected, the priority should be bacteriology. The samples are refrigerated if immediate shipping or analysis is not possible. It is reported that delayed analysis can influence cell counts, which can be important to differentiate some suppurative arthritis from inflamed joints.[47]

Bacteriologic Culture

Ideally, routine, specific anaerobic and mycoplasma cultures must be requested in all cases of SA. Samples should be submitted as soon as possible and should be transported refrigerated when a delay between sampling and culture is suspected. Contacting the bacteriology laboratory is strongly recommended to confirm the ideal shipping procedure and to specify the culture of bacteria, such as *Mycoplasma* spp or *H somni*, that require specific media. The success rate of bacterial culture is reported to be approximately 60% in cattle.[14] Blood culture bottles have been reported to increase recovery of bacteria in synovial fluid.[48] It has the advantage of promoting growth of fastidious bacteria, bacteria with low load, and minimizing the impact of previous antimicrobial treatment. Some of these systems have the advantage of allowing growth of anaerobic and aerobic bacteria. However, most of blood culture bottles contain sodium polyanethol sulfonate, which inhibits *Mycoplasma* growth.[49] Once isolated, performing antimicrobial drug susceptibility testing may be useful for case management. However, one must remember that actually no cutoff points are available for the determination of antimicrobial susceptibilities in synovial fluid and that antimicrobial susceptibility is not routinely performed in most laboratories for anaerobic bacteria or bacteria, such as *Mycoplasma* spp or *T pyogenes*.

Polymerase chain reaction (PCR) is a very interesting alternative to culture.[50] It could provide results more rapidly than culture and is expected to be more sensitive. However, PCR has some limitations that must be taken into account. First, most PCRs are made for the detection of a specific pathogen, and consequently may be of limited value when looking for nonspecific bacteria. PCR by definition detects only DNA and it is difficult to determine if viable bacteria are still present in the joint. Additionally, it is not possible to determine the antimicrobial susceptibility using PCR. Finally, it is important to keep in mind that all PCRs are not similar and that PCR inhibitors are present in synovial fluid. Consequently, the choice of the PCR and DNA technique extraction are crucial points when analyzing synovial fluids.[51]

Cytologic Examination

Macroscopic examination of the fluid is often diagnostic (increased turbidity, decrease viscosity, fibrin) (**Fig. 4**). If macroscopic changes are subtle, the sample should be submitted for cellular count and differential. Nuclear cell count greater than 25,000 cells/μL, polymorphonuclear (PMN) cell count greater than 20,000 cells/μL, or more than 80% PMN cells and total proteins greater than 4.5 g/dL is compatible with an SA.[52] Microorganisms are not always seen on cytology.

Other Markers

Numerous biomarkers have been studied in other species for their potential use as a help for the diagnosis of SA as well as for the establishment of prognosis. Only a few data are available in cattle. Older studies have been performed on the evaluation of different enzymes, such as Alkaline Phosphatase (ALP) and more recently studies were done on MMPs.[53–55] On the other hand, measurements of glucose or lactate dehydrogenase (LDH) appear of more limited value.[56] To be of value in cattle, these

Table 2
Common sites for arthrocentesis in cattle

Articulation	Compartments	Arthrocentesis Site	Difficulty	Communication in Compound Joints
Scapulohumeral		Between the cranial portion of the major tubercle and the tendon portion of the infraspinatus with a spinal needle aiming caudomedially. A needle can be inserted caudally to the joint by distending first the joint and inserting a spinal needle where bulging is apparent.	++	There is a bursa underneath the infraspinatus tendon. If it cannot be localized with ultrasound, the needle should be inserted 1 cm more proximally and slightly directed ventrally to avoid it.
Elbow		Cranial to the colateral ligament If distended, cranial lateral to the lateral humeral epicondyle In the angle formed by the lateral epicondyle of the humerus and the olecranon with the needle in a craniodistal direction	+	
Carpus	a. Antebrachiocarpal	Lateral and medial to extensor carpi radialis (a-b)	a. 0	Antebrachiocarpal and midcarpal: 13%
	b. Midcarpal	Lateral and medial to common digital extensor (a-b-c)	b. 0	Mid-carpal and carpometacarpal: 100%
	c. Carpometacarpal	Medial to lateral digital extensor (c)	c. +	
Fetlock	a. Lateral	In flexion, needle inserted dorsally with an angle of 45° in a distal direction	+	Lateral and medial: 100%
	b. Medial	Between the proximal sesamoid and metatarsus or metacarpus	0	
		If distended, proximal to the proximal sesamoid bones and just adjacent to the metatarsus or metacarpus	0	

Joint	Approach	Difficulty	Communication
P2-P3	Immediately proximal to the coronary band with and angle of 60° in a distal direction	++	
Coxofemoral joint	Cranial to the greater trochanter of the femur and the spinal needle is kept horizontal in a caudomedial direction	+++	
Tarsus	a. Tarsocrural	Proximal, dorsal and lateral or medial to the digital extensors (a-b)	a. 0	Tarsocrural and proximal intertarsal: 100%
	b. Proximal intertarsal	Lateral and medial plantar pouch for joint lavage and arthrotomy	b. 0	
	c. Distal intertarsal	Rarely performed	c. ++++	Distal intertarsal and tarsometatarsal 30%
	d. Tarsometatarsal		d. +++	
Stifle	a. Lateral femorotibial	a. Cranial or caudal to the collateral ligament	a. +	Lateral femorotibial and femoropatellar: 60%
	b. Medial femorotibial	b. Cranial or caudal to the collateral ligament	b. +	No direct communication between the lateral and medial femoropatellar joints
	c. Femoropatellar	c. Between the medial and middle patellar ligaments with a spinal needle aiming under the patella	c. ++	Medial femorotibial and femoropatellar: 100%

Difficulty level: 0 being easy to perform and +++: being extremely difficult.

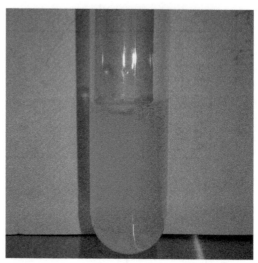

Fig. 4. A septic synovial fluid. It is opaque, cloudy, and yellow.

biomarkers need to be cheap and performed cowside, easily, and rapidly. Recently in horses, D-dimer, serum amyloid A, myeloperoxidase, and neutrophil viability have been evaluated in this way.[57–60] In human medicine, a systematic review concludes that synovial fluid lactate concentration is a promising tool based on its diagnosis accuracy but additional studies are needed for its implication in the management of SA.[50,56] Synovial fluid lactate concentration also has to be reported to be useful in horses and more particularly in the acute phase of the disease and it can be easily evaluated horseside by using a portable clinical analyzer.[61–63] Unfortunately, none of these biomarkers have been studied in cattle. The need for a biomarker for the diagnosis of SA is probably more limited in cattle than in humans or horses. Contrary to other species, SA is by far the most frequent joint disease and cytologic evaluation is frequently sufficient for confirmation of diagnosis. However, they could be useful when bacterial culture is negative and/or cytologic changes are equivocal and could play a role as prognosis markers.

Radiographic Images

When interpreting the radiographic views, the clinician has to remember that the lesions seen are 10 to 14 days later than the actual process. The cartilage is not visible on radiographs. In the acute condition, we will observe swelling of soft tissue with the presence of gas in certain cases and increased articular space (**Fig. 5**). Chronic lesions are more visible: subchondral bone lysis, decreased joint space by articular destruction, osteomyelitis, periosteal reaction, and bony proliferation (**Fig. 6**). These lesions can be focal or multicentric. With chronic SA, severe bone neoformation is more frequently observed in adults than in calves, where bone lysis is more typical.

Ultrasound Images

Soft tissues are better evaluated with ultrasound examination. In acute SA, the synovial fluid will increase in volume and echogenic (gray) material (fibrin) could be seen floating in the joint. Cartilage is anechogenic (black) because of its high content of water but the subchondral bone is hyperechogenic (white) and lysis or defect will change its contour. In our clinics, we have been using ultrasound to determine the presence

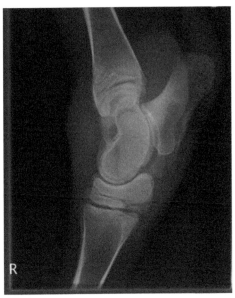

Fig. 5. Lateral radiographic view of a tarsus of a young calf. There is soft tissue swelling but no obvious bone lesions are observed.

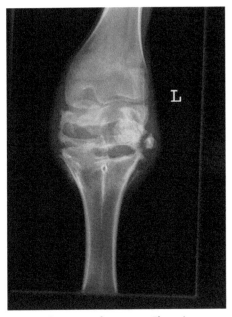

Fig. 6. Cranio-caudal radiographic view of a carpus. There is severe subchondral bone lysis of the cuboidal bones and the proximo-lateral aspect of the metacarpus. There is bone proliferation especially surrounding the middle carpal and carpometacarpal joints.

and location of fibrin in the joint (**Fig. 7**). These findings will help the clinician decide which treatment should be applied to a particular animal.

TREATMENT

There are 3 important parts to the treatment: decreasing bacterial load, controlling the inflammatory process, and pain management. Clinically, it means to give antibiotics, anti-inflammatories, and joint lavage. Depending on the bacteria, joint affected, and chronicity of the disease, case management will vary. Bone lesions identified on radiographic views also will influence the treatment protocol. Osteomyelitis associated with SA will be managed differently with the possibility of local debridement and longer administration of antibiotics.

Antimicrobial Therapy

Selection of the antimicrobial

Choice of an antimicrobial should always be based on culture and sensitivity. However, it takes days to obtain a result and delaying the treatment can be harmful for the patient. Animals with a diagnosis of SA are started on empiric therapy. Because of the wide diversity of bacteria that may be involved, large-spectrum antimicrobials are frequently used in first intent. However, the choice of the antimicrobial drugs may be guided by the suspected cause of the septic joint. In adult animals, the selected antimicrobial drug should be effective against *T. pyogenes* (such as one in the β-lactam family). In young animals, an antimicrobial drug effective against gram-positive and gram-negative bacteria, as well as *Mycoplasma*, should be favored. Antimicrobials effective against *Mycoplasma* should be used in calves, and in animals with associated clinical signs of pneumonia, otitis, or mastitis. The antimicrobial treatment regimen should then be reassessed and changed based on bacterial culture and

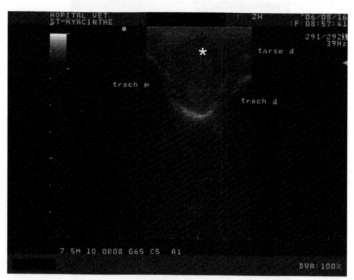

Fig. 7. Dorsolateral longitudinal ultrasound view of the tarsus. A 7.5-MHz linear probe was used. The probe is centered over the talus showing the proximal trochlea (troch p) and the distal trochlea (troch d). The asterisk indicates the synovial cavity. It is filled with an echogenic material that is compatible with highly cellular synovial fluid. An arthrotomy might be indicated.

sensitivity results when available. Other nonmedical factors, like homologation, breed, production type, behavior, facilities, and value of the animal are always considered when establishing a treatment. To our knowledge, none of the antimicrobials in North America are homologated for specific treatment of SA in cattle. Extra-label antibiotics of already approved antimicrobial have to be used. Antimicrobial diffusion is usually adequate in inflamed joints. In cases of SA, 3 main factors could influence the diffusion and efficacy of the drugs within the joint and are generally taken into account. First, the IA pH becomes acid. Second, numerous tissue debris will be present in the joint, and, finally, even if an inflamed membrane is generally considered as more permeable, that could affect exchanges between blood and the joint. However, our choices are often driven by bacterial sensitivity, economic reason, and withdrawal time or country regulation.

No studies are available on the efficacy of specific antimicrobial treatments in cases of naturally acquired SA. Trimethoprim sulfadiazine (TMS), cefapirin, penicillin, and oxytetracycline have demonstrated good IA diffusion in cases of SA in calves following systemic administration.[64–66] Joint diffusion of ampicillin trihydrate has been shown to decrease in cases of infection but concentration remains effective.[67] Marbofloxacin has been successfully used to treat calves with acquired SA.[68] In an experimental model of SA in calves with *Escherichia coli*, intravenous (IV) ceftiofur was administered for 21 days.[69] At day 8 post infection, all cultures were negative.

Administration route

Antimicrobials may be administered by the systemic, locoregional, or IA route. The systemic route is by far the most frequently used. In humans it is now recommended to give the antimicrobial drugs IV for the first days followed by oral administration.[70,71] Because an early and aggressive antimicrobial treatment is mandatory for optimizing the prognosis, the recommendation in bovine medicine is to begin IV and then to use the intramuscular (IM) or subcutaneous route. Because of the long duration of the treatment, in our clinic we favor implementation of a long-term polyurethane IV catheter and to administer the antimicrobials IV for the whole duration of treatment. Limitations of the systemic route are the use of high-dose antibiotic and associated costs and potential toxicity, as well as the constraint of daily administration. In chronic cases in which fibrin and infected bone are present, regional antibiotics are often used to increase local therapeutic level.[19,72–74]

The main goal of locoregional or IA administration of antimicrobial drugs is to achieve high IA antimicrobial drug concentration with lower doses (and lower costs) and less risk of toxicity, or when tissue perfusion is compromised. Locoregional antimicrobial drug perfusion may be an alternative for the distal joints. Administration of 500 mg ceftiofur HCl, 250 mg cefazolin, or 1000 mg tetracycline hydrochloride has been demonstrated to reach effective IA concentrations in normal joints.[75–77] Limitations of this technique are that multiple injections may be difficult and in some cases surrounding tissues are also infected and IV administration cannot be performed safely. In our clinic, we put in place a locoregional catheter to administer the antimicrobials locally for several days in selected animals like chronic, unresponsive severely swollen distal limbs.

Even if frequently used, IA injection of antimicrobials is controversial. Development of chemical synovitis or bacterial colonization of the joint may be an issue. The excellent diffusion of most of antimicrobial drugs into an infected joint makes the justification of repetitive IA administration limited. There are actually no data on the risk versus benefit of this procedure in cattle. In one study in India, there was no advantage of administration of IA gentamycin in addition to IM administration versus IM administration alone for the treatment of SA in calves.[78] On the other hand, studies in horses have demonstrated that IA concentrations of gentamycin were greatly increased when administered IA in comparison with only systemic administration.[79] Additionally, lincomycin, penicillin, kanamycin, gentamycin, and doxycycline do not induce chemical synovitis when administered IA.[80,81] Although still controversial, the authors of this paper or we give IA antibiotics but only after a confirmed diagnosis of septic joint (macroscopic examination of the fluid or cytology) and at the end of a joint lavage. One alternative to repetitive IA injection is a system of drug delivery into the joint for slow release of the antimicrobial drugs.[82] To date, 2 different systems have been described and used in cattle: gentamicin-impregnated polymethyl methacrylate beads[83] and gentamicin-impregnated collagen sponges.[41,82,84,85] Not all the antimicrobial drugs are compatible with these systems.[82] Moreover, gentamicin is not approved for cattle in North America and neither is the use of slow-releasing devices, making their use problematic.

Duration of treatment

Duration of antibiotic treatment in cases of SA remains empiric in cattle, and it is still controversial in humans where control studies are difficult to do.[86–88] It is usually recommended to last at least 3 to 4 weeks after clinical improvement. Bacteria involved in the diseases, and response to treatment, should be taken into consideration before deciding treatment duration.[69] If the bone is not infected, there is a trend to shorten the duration of antibiotic administration in humans.[86–88] A randomized clinical trial has shown that the combination of less than 2 weeks of antimicrobial drugs with one joint aspiration is sufficient for the treatment of SA in children.[88] However, most of those short-term protocols are based on frequent administration of time-dependent antibiotics, such as β-lactams, and higher dosages, which are not always practical in cattle.[88,89] In an experimental SA in calves treated with IV antibiotics, PCR identification of a known bacterium was negative after 8 days. However, the PMN counts were still higher than normal, indicating that inflammation was still present.[69]

Anti-inflammatory Drugs

Anti-inflammatory drugs are useful for pain management and control of the inflammatory process. As mentioned previously, the inflammatory response is as much, if not more, deleterious by itself for the joint than the presence of bacteria alone. Until recently, nonsteroidal anti-inflammatory drugs (NSAIDs) were the only anti-inflammatory drugs recommended for the treatment of SA. One must be aware of potential negative secondary effects of administration of NSAIDs, particularly when prolonged treatment may be necessary. NSAIDs have gastrointestinal and renal toxicity. They must be used with caution in cattle with decreased appetite or those that are dehydrated. Additionally, renal function must be followed cautiously when NSAIDs are combined with drugs with renal toxicity (eg, gentamicin). Nowadays, specific cylooxygenase-2 inhibitors are available in cattle, and their use may potentially decrease these risks of toxicity. To our knowledge, there are no published studies on the efficacy of NSAIDs in cattle for the control of inflammation with SA. However, flunixine meglumine was reported to be effective in controlling pain in dairy steers with induced synovitis.[90] The analgesic effect of meloxicam also was demonstrated in cows with resection of the distal interphalangeal joint.[91] In horses, meloxicam, diclofenac, ketoprofen, and phenylbutazone have been reported to significantly decrease PGE2 IA concentration in cases of induced synovitis or osteoarthritis.[92–94] However, phenylbutazone had a stronger effect on lameness and joint swelling in comparison with ketoprofen.[92] Despite these apparent advantages, phenylbutazone cannot be recommended anymore in North America in dairy cattle for legal consideration. Finally, cost, risk of toxicity, and facilities must be taken in consideration when selecting an NSAID.

Despite their strong anti-inflammatory properties, systemic or IA administration of corticosteroids is controversial because of their immunosuppressive properties and risk of deleterious effect on clearance of bacteria. In horses, corticosteroids also are reported to have negative effects on cartilage. Studies with induced SA have demonstrated a protective effect on cartilage of a combination of IA administration of corticosteroids with a systemic antimicrobial.[95,96] In human medicine, 2 randomized clinical trials are available for the evaluation of short-term dexamethasone therapy (4 days orally) associated with systemic antimicrobial therapy in the treatment of SA in children.[97,98] In both studies, the dexamethasone groups had shorter duration of clinical signs. No short-term or long-term negative effects were observed. In horses and cattle, IA administration of corticosteroids has already been used with positive outcome when administered after the period of joint lavage and when no bacteria were cultured in cases of idiopathic gonitis of after repeated joint lavage for SA.[99,100]

Sodium iodide 20% IV is occasionally used to treat chronic nonresponding SA at recommended dosage of 15mL/45kg. Although its exact mechanism of action is unknown, it seems particularly effective when inflammation is chronic and granulomatous (*T. pyogenes*).

Joint Lavage

Joint lavage allows the evacuation of fibrin, microorganisms, and the inflammation by-products that are detrimental for the joint. The metalloproteinases and other enzymes are still present even in the absence of bacteria. Antibiotic efficiency also is improved with the removal of excessive purulent material. In chronic suppurative arthritis, a pannus (fibrovascular tissue) is often present and decreases normal fluid exchange between the synovial membrane and the joint cavity. Depending on the thickness, strength, and area affected, joint lavage might not be enough to dislodge it. Arthrotomy or arthroscopy is indicated to debride the pannus.

Although use of 0.1% of povidone iodine solution has been suggested to treat SA in horses, we usually recommend the use of a large volume of isotonic and iso-osmolar solution to avoid detrimental effect on the synoviocytes and chondrocytes.[101]

Techniques

There are 4 techniques of lavage: tidal lavage, through and through, arthroscopy, and arthrotomy. The less invasive, the better it is for the patient. However, there are some criteria that can help the clinician to choose the appropriate technique at the first place: acute or chronic, quantity of fibrin, number of joints infected, and their location. Acute SA without fibrin can be easily lavaged with needles without invasive technique. Studies in children have shown no advantage to using the arthroscopy over simple needle drainage in acute SA.[102] Unfortunately, chronic presentation is more common in cattle with a history of failed medical treatment. *T pyogenes* is a bacterium that stimulates fibrin production, making lavage with needle difficult in chronic SA. Arthroscopy or arthrotomy is then favored to achieve better joint lavage.

Surgical preparation of the site is essential, whichever technique is chosen. If there is a wound or laceration over the joint, the needle should be inserted away from it to avoid cross-contaminating the joint with a different microorganism (**Fig. 8**). The sedation, analgesia, and anesthesia will differ significantly among them and is discussed separately. The size of the needle is usually 18 to 16 G for a calf and up to 14 G for a cow. If fibrin is plugging the needles, then a larger needle is used. The authors have used

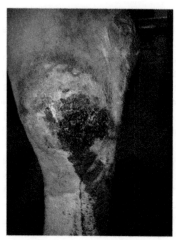

Fig. 8. An adult dairy cow with an infected skin wound on the lateral aspect of the tarsus. There is pus coming out of the open wound. There is mild swelling of the joint as well. Ultrasound of the surrounding joint allows the clinician to select a secure area where cellulitis is not present before performing the arthrocentesis.

5-mm trocar and cannula arthroscopic units to perform through-and-through lavage. However, arthrotomy or arthroscopy must be considered if there is constant obstruction of the needle with fibrin. The volume of fluid to be used is variable according to the volume of the joint and the amount of purulent materiel. Subjectively, we stop the lavage when the liquid becomes clear. Large joints, such as the tarsus or the stifle, in adult cattle would benefit from 2 to 4 L of fluids whereas 100 mL might be enough for an acute SA of the coxofemoral joint on a calf. The lavage is repeated if necessary the next 2 consecutive days depending of the chronicity of the arthritis and response to treatment. A fibrinous joint would benefit from a second and third lavage, whereas only one might be enough on an acutely septic joint.

Tidal irrigation

Tidal irrigation was developed for the treatment of osteoarthritis in humans.[103] It is the less invasive irrigation technique because only one needle is needed. The principle is to distend the joint and aspirate its contents through the same needle, creating a tidal effect (wave). It is usually used in smaller joints without large cul-de-sacs and communications with other adjacent joints. Otherwise, it would be difficult to achieve appropriate irrigation through only one needle. The distension-irrigation cycle is repeated until the liquid is clear without fibrin.

This procedure can be performed under sedation, systemic analgesia, and local infiltration of lidocaine. The joint cavity is infiltrated with lidocaine after joint decompression as well and before the distension with the lavage solution. An 18-G to 14-G needle is inserted in the joint. A syringe is filled with a sterile solution and the joint distended. The fluid is discarded and the procedure repeated. A 3-way valve can be used to improve the efficiency of the procedure by making the instillation from one port and exiting fluid from another port easier. The fluid from the same syringe can be re-instilled a few times to distend the joint and create turbulence to dislodge the fibrin. Tidal irrigation is often used with joints where inserting a second needle is difficult or ineffective, such as the coxofemoral joint.

Through-and-through lavage

At least 2 needles are needed with the through-and-through lavage technique. Some joints with cul-de-sac and complex boundaries benefit from more needles, rendering the lavage more efficient. The needles have to be far from each other to improve irrigation (**Fig. 9**). The analgesic protocol is similar to the one described previously. If the animal suffers from polyarthritis, sedation might have to be repeated. A sterile drip set attached to a 1-L fluid bag is plugged into the ingress needle to distend the joint until joint distention is achieved. Then an egress needle is inserted until the fluid is coming out under pressure. The liter bag is squeezed to increase pressure or place into a pressurized fluid bag with a pressure up to 300 mm Hg. The fluid is stopped and the needle reinserted or redirected at any time the fluid is not coming out easily.

Arthrotomy

Arthrotomy is performed if the medical treatment failed or the joint is filled with fibrin or pus and through-and-through lavage is impossible. Sites of arthrotomy are similar to the sites of arthrocentesis (see **Table 2**). This is a painful procedure, and the animal must be deeply sedated to prevent further cartilage damage while incising and inserting instruments in the joint cavity. The arthrotomy sites are infiltrated with lidocaine as well as each joint compartment to be invaded. Synovial bursa and tendon sheaths are located and carefully avoided when entering the joint. A stab incision through the joint is first performed followed by the insertion of a hemostat or any blunt instrument to confirm IA location (**Fig. 10**). The incision is then lengthened to fully access the joint compartment. More than one incision per joint is necessary to access the entire cavity and improve the debridement. Atraumatic forceps are inserted into the joint and fibrin is removed from all accessible compartments (**Fig. 11**). As discussed earlier, some joints have cul-de-sacs that are difficult to reach, limiting debridement by conventional access. The antebrachiocarpal joints have a pouch between the first row and the accessory bone.[45,104] They can be carefully accessed by the medial aspect of the accessory bone under ultrasound guidance. A plantar approach of the fetlock has been described in cases with concurrent septic tenosynovitis.[105] The caudomedial and caudolateral pouches of the tarsus are often filled with fibrin and must be accessed (see **Fig. 11B**). A caudolateral approach of the stifle was described to

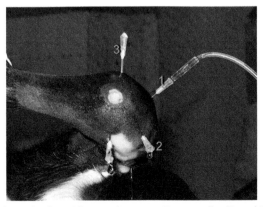

Fig. 9. A young Holstein heifer with a septic carpus. Two needles (1 and 2) are inserted into the middle carpal joint. The needles 3 and 4 are in the carpometacarpal joint far from the wound.

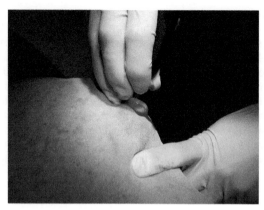

Fig. 10. A stab incision is performed into the stifle joint. Purulent material is coming out of the incision already.

access osteolytic lesions of the femorotibial joint.[106] After fibrin has been removed from all the compartments, lavage is done to remove loose debris.

Postoperatively, the incisions are covered with a bandage or stents, and additional lavage is performed the following days if necessary (**Fig. 12**). After 24 to 48 hours, the incision is often closed and reopening is necessary to access the joint cavity. Joint lavage is performed until synovial fluid is clear and the fibrin removed from the cavity is negligible. A clean bandage must cover the incisions for at least 5 days postoperatively or until no apparent fluid is coming out. Synovial fistula is rather rare in cattle according to the authors.

Arthrodesis

Arthrodesis is the final solution when no treatments were efficient or because of the chronicity of the disease, joint function will never be restored. Decision making for arthrodesis is indicated when capsule fibrosis is extensive and joint motion cannot be restored or there is radiographic evidence of extensive irreversible osteomyelitis lesions. Articulations of the distal limb are easily arthrodesed (fetlock, proximal and distal interphalangeal joints). Joint resection, facilitated ankylosis of the distal interphalangeal joint is commonly performed and is highly successful.[107–110] It has been extensively described and will not be covered in this article. Severe carpal infection

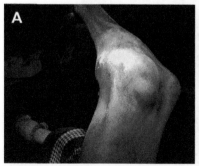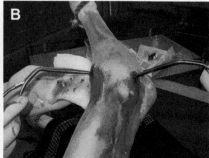

Fig. 11. (*A*) A septic right tarsus chronically infected. There is a severe distension of the lateral compartment. (*B*) Two Magill forceps are used to remove the fibrin and other debris from the joint cavity.

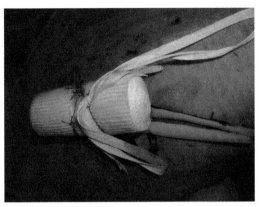

Fig. 12. A stent is covering an arthrotomy incision of the stifle. It can be easily removed to access the joint and lavage it for the next 2 days if necessary.

also has been treated with arthrodesis. For a high-motion joint, the clinician will have to take in consideration the facilities (stall or small pasture), value, and purpose of the animal before proposing surgery to the owner. Fetlock arthrodesis was successfully used in 4 adult cattle diagnosed with SA.[111] The joint was approached through 4 incisions (dorsolateral, dorsomedial, lateral, and medial abaxial).[111]

Carpus arthrodesis in calves has been described.[112–114] To our knowledge, there is no successful report of stifle, hip, elbow, and shoulder arthrodesis in cattle. At this point, if one of those joints is affected, amputation might be considered to save the animal's life.

General anesthesia is highly recommended because this is an invasive surgery and a second surgery site is often necessary to harvest cancellous bone graft. The surgery also can be performed under deep sedation and brachial block. A long transverse incision dorsal to the flexed carpus is centered over the affected joint. If the 3 carpal joints are severely affected and cuboidal resection is considered, the incision is centered over the middle carpal joint. The tendons are transected and the joint capsule is invaded. The cartilage is removed with a curette or an electric burr. The decision to remove carpal bones is made during surgery and is based on preoperative radiographic images of the joint and intraoperative evaluation of the cartilage and bones (**Fig. 13**A, B). If a cuboidal bone has to be resected, the complete row is removed.[112] Rows of carpal bones are sharply removed by transecting the intercarpal ligaments. The caudal aspect is carefully dissected because the major vessels and nerves are situated outside the capsule. The joint is lavaged and excessive skin removed if a row of carpal bones is resected. Cancellous bone graft is placed and the dorsal aspect of the joint reconstructed layer by layer. The authors have used antibiotics impregnated with plaster of Paris beads to fill the space in the carpus and increase local antibiotic concentration (**Fig. 14**). The joint is immobilized in a cast or a pin cast for up to 6 weeks.[112] The cast must be changed in between to evaluate the incision and also if it is a young, growing animal.

Prognosis

The prognosis should always be guarded unless the onset is acute and there are no bone lesions on the radiographic images. Many factors will influence the prognosis:

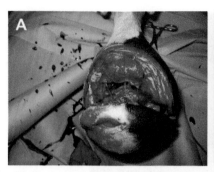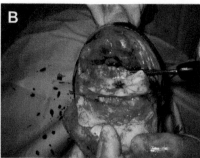

Fig. 13. A young Holstein calf with a chronic septic arthritis of the carpus undergoing an arthrodesis. (*A*) A long transverse dorsal incision from lateral to medial gives appropriate exposure to debride the joint and remove the cartilage or rows of cuboidal bones as needed. (*B*) The proximal row of carpal bones (*asterisk*) is dissected out and is ready to be resected.

age, joint affected, microorganism isolated, time of presentation, number of joints involved, concomitant diseases, and value of the animal. If more than 2 joints are infected, it is the authors' opinion that the prognosis is poor. Nuss[115] reported that of the 17 cattle treated for SA of the shoulder and hip, 10 survived more than 6.5 months (median). Two of them were lame and had to be euthanized later. Conservative (systemic and IA antibiotics) and surgical treatment (arthrotomy and debridement) have been compared in a retrospective study of 81 cattle.[116] Of the 42 cattle treated surgically, 29 recovered, whereas of the 39 treated conservatively, 13 recovered.[116] The least favorable prognosis in both treatment groups was associated with the tarsus, and postoperative ankylosis of the carpus was frequent.[116]

Joint lavage in 20 calves with SA showed that 80% of 20 calves responded positively to the treatment requiring 2 or more flushes.[40] In this study, animals with septic tarsus had a better prognosis compared with the other joints involved. Arthroscopic lavage and implantation of gentamicin-impregnated collagen sponges were successful in 12 of 14 animals treated.[41] Seventeen adult cattle of 20 returned to production

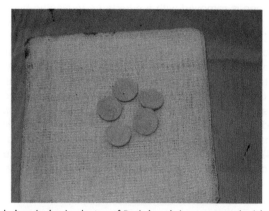

Fig. 14. Homemade hemispheric plaster of Paris beads impregnated with ceftiofur (Excenel, Zoetis canada, canada). They will be placed in the carpal joint after extensive flushing, just before articular capsule closure.

after being treated with joint lavage and antibiotics.[42] In this study, cattle with septic tarsi had less chance of recovery.

Pain-free arthrodesis of the carpus permitting full weight bearing was obtained in 69% of the 72 cattle treated.[112] When breaking down the results related to type of arthrodesis, the surgery was successful in 87% without carpal bone resection, 72% with 1 row resected, and 35% of fusions in which a radio-metacarpal arthrodesis was performed.[112]

REFERENCES

1. Russell AM, Rowlands GJ, Shaw SR, et al. Survey of lameness in British dairy cattle. Vet Rec 1982;111(8):155–60.
2. McLennan MW. Incidence of lameness requiring veterinary treatment in dairy cattle in Queensland. Aust Vet J 1988;65(5):144–7.
3. Bargai U, Levin D. Lameness in the Israeli dairy herd—a national survey of incidence, types, distribution and estimated cost (first report). Isr J Vet Med 1993; 48(2):88–91.
4. Griffin D, Perino L, Hudson D. Feedlot lameness. Historical materials from University of Nebraska-Lincoln extension 1993. paper 196. Available at http:// digitalcommons.unl.edu/cgi/viewcontent.cgi?article=1195&context=exte.
5. Pollock CM, Campbell JR, Janzen ED. Descriptive epidemiology of chronic disease of calves in a Western Canadian feedlot. Paper presented at: 33rd meeting the American Association Bovine Practitioners, Rapid City (SD), September 20-23, 2000.
6. Svensson C, Lundborg K, Emanuelson U, et al. Morbidity in Swedish dairy calves from birth to 90 days of age and individual calf-level risk factors for infectious diseases. Prev Vet Med 2003;58:179–97.
7. Pardon B, De Bleecker K, Hostens M, et al. Longitudinal study on morbidity and mortality in white veal calves in Belgium. BMC Vet Res 2012;8:26.
8. Donkersgoed JV, Janzen ED, Harland RJ. Epidemiological features of calf mortality due to hemophilosis in a large feedlot. Can Vet J 1990;31(12): 821–5.
9. Pritchard DG, Shreeve J, Bradley R. Experimental infection of calves with a British strain of *Haemophilus somnus*. Res Vet Sci 1979;26(1):7–11.
10. Maunsell FP, Woolums AR, Francoz D, et al. *Mycoplasma bovis* infections in cattle. J Vet Intern Med 2011;25(4):772–83.
11. Gagea MI, Bateman KG, Shanahan RA, et al. Naturally occurring *Mycoplasma bovis*-associated pneumonia and polyarthritis in feedlot beef calves. J Vet Diagn Invest 2006;18(1):29–40.
12. Hewicker-Trautwein M, Feldmann M, Kehler W, et al. Outbreak of pneumonia and arthritis in beef calves associated with *Mycoplasma bovis* and *Mycoplasma californicum*. Vet Rec 2002;151(23):699–703.
13. Hughes KL, Edwards MJ, Hartley WJ, et al. Polyarthritis in calves caused by *Mycoplasma* sp. Vet Rec 1966;78(8):276–81.
14. Francoz D, Desrochers A, Fecteau G, et al. A retrospective study of joint bacterial culture in 172 cases of septic arthritis in cattle. Paper presented at: 20th ACVIM forum, Dallas, May 29 - June 1, 2002.
15. Cavirani S, Foni E, Cabassi CS, et al. Bovid herpesvirus 4 from tarsal synovitis of the cow. Bologna (Italy): Societa Italiana di Buiatria; 1994.
16. Lapointe JM, Laverty S, Lavoie JP. Septic arthritis in 15 standardbred racehorses after intra-articular injection. Equine Vet J 1992;24(6):430–4.

17. Heppelmann M, Kofler J, Meyer H, et al. Advances in surgical treatment of septic arthritis of the distal interphalangeal joint in cattle: a review. Vet J 2009; 182(2):162–75.
18. Kostlin RG, Nuss K. Treatment of septic pedal arthritis in cattle by resection—results. Tierarztl Prax 1988;16(2):123–31 [in German].
19. Desrochers A. Septic arthritis. In: Fubini SL, Ducharme NG, editors. Farm animal surgery. (MO): Saunders; 2004. p. 494–7.
20. Power HT, Rebhun WC. Bacterial endocarditis in adult dairy cattle. J Am Vet Med Assoc 1983;182(8):806–8.
21. Rothwell JT, Christie BM, Williams C, et al. Suspected Lyme disease in a cow. Aust Vet J 1989;66(9):296–8.
22. Wichtel ME, Fenwick SG, Hunter J, et al. Septicaemia and septic arthritis in a neonatal calf caused by *Lactococcus lactis.* Vet Rec 2003;153(1):22–3.
23. Twomey DF, Griffiths PC, Hignett BC, et al. Suspected chlamydial polyarthritis in a calf in the UK. London: British Veterinary Association; 2003.
24. Blake N, Scott PR, Munroe GA. Septic physitis, arthritis and osteomyelitis probably caused by *Salmonella typhimurium* DT104 in beef suckler calves. Cattle Pract 1997;5(4):345–6.
25. Biancardi P. Septic arthritis caused by *Erysipelothrix insidiosa* in a calf. Obiettivi e Documenti Veterinari 1992;13(11):61–2.
26. Dreyfuss DJ, Stephens PR. *Erysipelothrix rhusiopathiae*-induced septic arthritis in a calf. J Am Vet Med Assoc 1990;197(10):1361–2.
27. Ryan DP, Rothwell JT, Hornitzky MA. *Streptococcus dysgalactiae* infection in calves. Aust Vet J 1991;68(6):210.
28. Boulouis HJ, Maillard R, Haddad N. Lyme borreliosis in cattle. XXIV World Buiatrics Congress. Nice (France), October 15-19, 2006. p. 527–31.
29. Burgess EC. *Borrelia burgdorferi* infection in Wisconsin horses and cows. Ann N Y Acad Sci 1988;539:235–43.
30. Khazrainia P, Gharagooslu MJ, Nazifi S, et al. Microbiological and clinicopathological studies on bovine arthritis in Iran. J Facul Vet Med 2006;61(1):33–8 University of Tehran.
31. Butler JA, Sickles SA, Johanns CJ, et al. Pasteurization of discard mycoplasma mastitic milk used to feed calves: thermal effects on various mycoplasma. J Dairy Sci 2000;83(10):2285–8.
32. Stipkovits L, Rady M, Glavits R. Mycoplasmal arthritis and meningitis in calves. Acta Vet Hung 1993;41(1–2):73–88.
33. Henderson JP, Ball HJ. Polyarthritis due to *Mycoplasma bovis* infection in adult dairy cattle in Northern Ireland. Vet Rec 1999;145(13):374–6.
34. Houlihan MG, Veenstra B, Christian MK, et al. Mastitis and arthritis in two dairy herds caused by *Mycoplasma bovis.* Vet Rec 2007;160(4):126–7.
35. Wilson DJ, Skirpstunas RT, Trujillo JD, et al. Unusual history and initial clinical signs of *Mycoplasma bovis* mastitis and arthritis in first-lactation cows in a closed commercial dairy herd. J Am Vet Med Assoc 2007;230(10): 1519–23.
36. Langford EV. *Mycoplasma agalactiae* subsp. *bovis* in pneumonia and arthritis of the bovine. Can J Comp Med 1977;41(1):89–94.
37. Adegboye DS, Halbur PG, Nutsch RG, et al. *Mycoplasma bovis*-associated pneumonia and arthritis complicated with pyogranulomatous tenosynovitis in calves. J Am Vet Med Assoc 1996;209(3):647–9.
38. Brice N, Finlay D, Bryson DG, et al. Isolation of *Mycoplasma bovis* from cattle in Northern Ireland, 1993 to 1998. Vet Rec 2000;146(22):643–4.

39. Byrne WJ, McCormack R, Brice N, et al. Isolation of *Mycoplasma bovis* from bovine clinical samples in the Republic of Ireland. Vet Rec 2001;148(11):331–3.
40. Jackson PG, Strachan WD, Tucker AW, et al. Treatment of septic arthritis in calves by joint lavage: a study of 20 cases. Ir Vet J 1999;52(10):563–9.
41. Steiner A, Hirsbrunner G, Miserez R, et al. Arthroscopic lavage and implantation of gentamicin-impregnated collagen sponges for treatment of chronic septic arthritis in cattle. Vet Comp Orthop Traumatol 1999;12(2):64–9.
42. Meier C. Procedure in purulent arthritis of adult cattle and clinical experience with joint lavage. Prakt Tierarzt 1997;78(10):893–906 [in German].
43. Schneider RK, Bramlage LR, Moore RM, et al. A retrospective study of 192 horses affected with septic arthritis/tenosynovitis. Equine Vet J 1992;24(6):436–42.
44. Nuss K, Hecht S, Maierl J, et al. Arthrocentesis in cattle. Part 2: pelvic limb. Tierarztl Prax Ausg G Grosstiere Nutztiere 2002;30(5):301–7.
45. Nuss K, Hecht S, Maierl J, et al. Arthrocentesis in cattle. Part 1: thoracic limb. Tierarztl Prax Ausg G Grosstiere Nutztiere 2002;30(4):226–32.
46. Wahl K, Adams SB, Moore GE. Contamination of joints with tissue debris and hair after arthrocentesis: the effect of needle insertion angle, spinal needle gauge, and insertion of spinal needles with and without a stylet. Vet Surg 2012;41(3):391–8.
47. Kerolus G, Clayburne G, Schumacher HR Jr. Is it mandatory to examine synovial fluids promptly after arthrocentesis? Arthritis Rheum 1989;32(3):271–8.
48. von Essen R. Culture of joint specimens in bacterial arthritis. Impact of blood culture bottle utilization. Scand J Rheumatol 1997;26(4):293–300.
49. Smaron MF, Boonlayangoor S, Zierdt CH. Detection of Mycoplasma hominis septicemia by radiometric blood culture. J Clin Microbiol 1985;21(3):298–301.
50. Carpenter CR, Schuur JD, Everett WW, et al. Evidence-based diagnostics: adult septic arthritis. Acad Emerg Med 2011;18(8):781–96.
51. Schneeweiss W, Stanek C, Wagner M, et al. Inhibitor-free DNA for real-time PCR analysis of synovial fluid from horses, cattle and pigs. Vet Microbiol 2007; 121(1/2):189–93.
52. Rohde C, Anderson DE, Desrochers A, et al. Synovial fluid analysis in cattle: a review of 130 cases. Vet Surg 2000;29(4):341–6.
53. Arican M, Coughlan AR, Clegg D, et al. Matrix metalloproteinases 2 and 9 activity in bovine synovial fluids. J Vet Med A Physiol Pathol Clin Med 2000;47(8):449–56.
54. Francoz D, Desrochers A, Simard N, et al. Relative expression of matrix metalloproteinase-2 and -9 in synovial fluid from healthy calves and calves with experimentally induced septic arthritis. Am J Vet Res 2008;69(8):1022–8.
55. Van Pelt RW, Langham RF. Synovial fluid changes produced by infectious arthritis in cattle. Am J Vet Res 1968;29(3):507–16.
56. Margaretten ME, Kohlwes J, Moore D, et al. Does this adult patient have septic arthritis? JAMA 2007;297(13):1478–88.
57. Ribera T, Monreal L, Armengou L, et al. Synovial fluid D-dimer concentration in foals with septic joint disease. J Vet Intern Med 2011;25(5):1113–7.
58. Jacobsen S, Niewold TA, Halling-Thomsen M, et al. Serum amyloid A isoforms in serum and synovial fluid in horses with lipopolysaccharide-induced arthritis. Vet Immunol Immunopathol 2006;110(3–4):325–30.
59. Wauters J, Pille F, Martens A, et al. Equine myeloperoxidase: a novel biomarker in synovial fluid for the diagnosis of infection. Equine Vet J 2013;45(3):278–83.
60. Wauters J, Martens A, Pille F, et al. Viability and cell death of synovial fluid neutrophils as diagnostic biomarkers in equine infectious joint disease: a pilot study. Res Vet Sci 2012;92(1):132–7.

61. Tennent-Brown BS. Interpreting lactate measurement in critically ill horses: diagnosis, treatment, and prognosis. Compend Contin Educ Vet 2012;34(1):E2.

62. Tulamo RM, Bramlage LR, Gabel AA. Sequential clinical and synovial fluid changes associated with acute infectious arthritis in the horse. Equine Vet J 1989;21(5):325–31.

63. Dechant JE, Symm WA, Nieto JE. Comparison of pH, lactate, and glucose analysis of equine synovial fluid using a portable clinical analyzer with a bench-top blood gas analyzer. Vet Surg 2011;40(7):811–6.

64. Shoaf SE, Schwark WS, Guard CL, et al. Pharmacokinetics of trimethoprim/sulfadiazine in neonatal calves: influence of synovitis. J Vet Pharmacol Ther 1986; 9(4):446–54.

65. Guard CL, Byman KW, Schwark WS. Effect of experimental synovitis on disposition of penicillin and oxytetracycline in neonatal calves. Cornell Vet 1989;79(2): 161–71.

66. Brown MP, Gronwall RR, Pattio N, et al. Pharmacokinetics and synovial fluid concentrations of cephapirin in calves with suppurative arthritis. Am J Vet Res 1991; 52(9):1438–40.

67. Brown MP, Mayo MB, Gronwall RR. Serum and synovial fluid concentrations of ampicillin trihydrate in calves with suppurative arthritis. Cornell Vet 1991;81(2): 137–43.

68. Grandemange E, Gunst S, Woehrle F, et al. Field evaluation of the efficacy of MarbocylReg. 2% in the treatment of infectious arthritis in calves. Ir Vet J 2002;55(5):237–40.

69. Francoz D, Desrochers A, Fecteau G, et al. Synovial fluid changes in induced infectious arthritis in calves. J Vet Intern Med 2005;19(3):336–43.

70. Paakkonen M, Peltola H. Simplifying the treatment of acute bacterial bone and joint infections in children. Expert Rev Anti Infect Ther 2011;9(12): 1125–31.

71. Rutz E, Spoerri M. Septic arthritis of the paediatric hip—A review of current diagnostic approaches and therapeutic concepts. Acta Orthop Belg 2013;79(2): 123–34.

72. Paakkonen M, Peltola H. Bone and joint infections. Pediatr Clin North Am 2013; 60(2):425–36.

73. Desrochers A. Medical and surgical therapies in the pathology of the hock and fetlock joint of beef cattle: International Congress SIVAR, Cremona, Italy, 6-7 May 2011. Available at: http://cabdirect.org/abstracts/20123328420.html; jsessionid=2139268F80A9E8D8CCCF1B537638EAF5.

74. Trostle SS, Hendrickson DA, Stone WC, et al. Use of antimicrobial-impregnated polymethyl methacrylate beads for treatment of chronic, refractory septic arthritis and osteomyelitis of the digit in a bull. J Am Vet Med Assoc 1996; 208(3):404–7.

75. Gagnon H, Ferguson JG, Papich MG, et al. Single-dose pharmacokinetics of cefazolin in bovine synovial fluid after intravenous regional injection. J Vet Pharmacol Ther 1994;17(1):31–7.

76. Navarre CB, Zhang L, Sunkara G, et al. Ceftiofur distribution in plasma and joint fluid following regional limb injection in cattle. J Vet Pharmacol Ther 1999;22(1): 13–9.

77. Rodrigues CA, Hussni CA, Nascimento ES, et al. Pharmacokinetics of tetracycline in plasma, synovial fluid and milk using single intravenous and single intravenous regional doses in dairy cattle with papillomatous digital dermatitis. J Vet Pharmacol Ther 2010;33(4):363–70.

78. Moulvi BA, Chandna IS, Rishi T, et al. Efficacy of intramuscular along with intra-articular gentamicin in the treatment of infectious arthritis in calves. Indian J Vet Surg 2002;23(2):111.

79. Lloyd KC, Stover SM, Pascoe JR, et al. Synovial fluid pH, cytologic characteristics, and gentamicin concentration after intra-articular administration of the drug in an experimental model of infectious arthritis in horses. Am J Vet Res 1990; 51(9):1363–9.

80. Haerdi-Landerer MC, Suter MM, Steiner A. Intra-articular administration of doxycycline in calves. Am J Vet Res 2007;68(12):1324–31.

81. Trent AM, Plumb D. Treatment of infectious arthritis and osteomyelitis. Vet Clin North Am Food Anim Pract 1991;7(3):747–78.

82. Haerdi-Landerer MC, Habermacher J, Wenger B, et al. Slow release antibiotics for treatment of septic arthritis in large animals. Vet J 2010;184(1): 14–20.

83. Butson RJ, Schramme MC, Garlick MH, et al. Treatment of intrasynovial infection with gentamicin-impregnated polymethylmethacrylate beads. Vet Rec 1996; 138(19):460–4.

84. Hirsbrunner G, Steiner A. Treatment of infectious arthritis of the radiocarpal joint of cattle with gentamicin-impregnated collagen sponges. Vet Rec 1998;142(15): 399–402.

85. Zulauf M, Jordan P, Steiner A. Fenestration of the abaxial hoof wall and implantation of gentamicin-impregnated collagen sponges for the treatment of septic arthritis of the distal interphalangeal joint in cattle. Vet Rec 2001;149(17): 516–8.

86. Paakkonen M, Kallio MJ, Kallio PE, et al. Shortened hospital stay for childhood bone and joint infections: analysis of 265 prospectively collected culture-positive cases in 1983-2005. Scand J Infect Dis 2012;44(9):683–8.

87. Paakkonen M, Peltola H. How short is long enough for treatment of bone and joint infection? Adv Exp Med Biol 2011;719:39–46.

88. Peltola H, Paakkonen M, Kallio P, et al. Prospective, randomized trial of 10 days versus 30 days of antimicrobial treatment, including a short-term course of parenteral therapy, for childhood septic arthritis. Clin Infect Dis 2009;48(9): 1201–10.

89. Paakkonen M, Peltola H. Treatment of acute septic arthritis. Pediatr Infect Dis J 2013;32(6):684–5.

90. Schulz KL, Anderson DE, Coetzee JF, et al. Effect of flunixin meglumine on the amelioration of lameness in dairy steers with amphotericin B-induced transient synovitis-arthritis. Am J Vet Res 2011;72(11):1431–8.

91. Offinger J, Herdtweck S, Rizk A, et al. Postoperative analgesic efficacy of meloxicam in lame dairy cows undergoing resection of the distal interphalangeal joint. J Dairy Sci 2013;96(2):866–76.

92. Owens JG, Kamerling SG, Stanton SR, et al. Effects of pretreatment with ketoprofen and phenylbutazone on experimentally induced synovitis in horses. Am J Vet Res 1996;57(6):866–74.

93. Lynn RC, Hepler DI, Kelch WJ, et al. Double-blinded placebo-controlled clinical field trial to evaluate the safety and efficacy of topically applied 1% diclofenac liposomal cream for the relief of lameness in horses. Vet Ther 2004;5(2): 128–38.

94. de Grauw JC, van de Lest CH, Brama PA, et al. In vivo effects of meloxicam on inflammatory mediators, MMP activity and cartilage biomarkers in equine joints with acute synovitis. Equine Vet J 2009;41(7):693–9.

95. Sakiniene E, Bremell T, Tarkowski A. Addition of corticosteroids to antibiotic treatment ameliorates the course of experimental *Staphylococcus aureus* arthritis. Arthritis Rheum 1996;39(9):1596–605.

96. Wysenbeek AJ, Volchek J, Amit M, et al. Treatment of staphylococcal septic arthritis in rabbits by systemic antibiotics and intra-articular corticosteroids. Ann Rheum Dis 1998;57(11):687–90.

97. Odio CM, Ramirez T, Arias G, et al. Double blind, randomized, placebo-controlled study of dexamethasone therapy for hematogenous septic arthritis in children. Pediatr Infect Dis J 2003;22(10):883–8.

98. Harel L, Prais D, Bar-On E, et al. Dexamethasone therapy for septic arthritis in children: results of a randomized double-blind placebo-controlled study. J Pediatr Orthop 2011;31(2):211–5.

99. Madison JB, Tulleners EP, Ducharme NG, et al. Idiopathic gonitis in heifers: 34 cases (1976-1986). J Am Vet Med Assoc 1989;194(2):273–7.

100. Meijer MC, van Weeren PR, Rijkenhuizen AB. Clinical experiences of treating septic arthritis in the equine by repeated joint lavage: a series of 39 cases. J Vet Med A Physiol Pathol Clin Med 2000;47(6):351–65.

101. Bertone AL, McIlwraith CW, Jones RL, et al. Povidone-iodine lavage treatment of experimentally induced equine infectious arthritis. Am J Vet Res 1987;48(4):712–5.

102. Ayral X. Arthroscopy and joint lavage. Best Pract Res Clin Rheumatol 2005;19(3):401–15.

103. Bradley JD, Heilman DK, Katz BP, et al. Tidal irrigation as treatment for knee osteoarthritis: a sham-controlled, randomized, double-blinded evaluation. Arthritis Rheum 2002;46(1):100–8.

104. Desrochers A, St-Jean G, Cash WC, et al. Characterization of anatomic communications among the antebrachiocarpal, middle carpal, and carpometacarpal joints in cattle, using intra-articular latex, positive-contrast arthrography, and fluoroscopy. Am J Vet Res 1997;58(1):7–10.

105. Kofler J, Martinek B. New surgical approach to the plantar fetlock joint through the digital flexor tendon sheath wall and suspensory ligament apparatus in cases of concurrent septic synovitis in two cattle. Vet J 2005;169(3):370–5.

106. Heppelmann M, Staszyk C, Rehage J, et al. Arthrotomy for the treatment of chronic purulent septic gonitis with subchondral osteolysis in two calves. N Z Vet J 2012;60(5):310–4.

107. Bicalho RC, Cheong SH, Guard CL. Field technique for the resection of the distal interphalangeal joint and proximal resection of the deep digital flexor tendon in cows. Vet Rec 2007;160(13):435–9.

108. Desrochers A, St-Jean G, Anderson DE. Use of facilitated ankylosis in the treatment of septic arthritis of the distal interphalangeal joint in cattle: 12 cases (1987-1992). J Am Vet Med Assoc 1995;206(12):1923–7.

109. Nuss K. Surgery of the bovine digits—current techniques and perspectives. Prakt Tierarzt 2004;85(8):586–93.

110. Starke A, Heppelmann M, Beyerbach M, et al. Septic arthritis of the distal interphalangeal joint in cattle: comparison of digital amputation and joint resection by solar approach. Vet Surg 2007;36(4):350–9.

111. Starke A, Kehler W, Rehage J. Arthrotomy and arthrodesis in the treatment of complicated arthritis of the fetlock joint in adult cattle. Vet Rec 2006;159(23):772–7.

112. Van Huffel X, Steenhaut M, Imschoot J, et al. Carpal joint arthrodesis as a treatment for chronic septic carpitis in calves and cattle. Vet Surg 1989;18(4):304–11.

113. Riley CB, Farrow CS. Partial carpal arthrodesis in a calf with chronic infectious arthritis of the carpus and osteomyelitis of the carpal and metacarpal bones. Can Vet J 1998;39(7):438–41.
114. Pistani JR, Miscione H, Redondo A, et al. Clinical use of Ilizarov's compression technique in the treatment of a septic pseudoarthrosis in a calf. Vet Comp Orthop Traumatol 1997;10(1):12–5.
115. Nuss K. Septic arthritis of the shoulder and hip joint in cattle: diagnosis and therapy. Schweiz Arch Tierheilkd 2003;145(10):455–63 [in German].
116. Verschooten F, De Moor A, Steenhaut M, et al. Surgical and conservative treatment of infectious arthritis in cattle. J Am Vet Med Assoc 1974;165(3):271–5.

Noninfectious Joint Disease in Cattle

Sylvain Nichols, DMV, MS[a],*, Hélène Lardé, Dr Med Vet, DES[b]

KEYWORDS

- Cattle • Osteochondrosis • Degenerative joint disease • Osteoarthritis • Surgery

KEY POINTS

- Osteochondrosis causes variable degrees of joint effusion and lameness. Arthroscopic debridement of the lesions provides the best long-term outcome.
- Articular fracture or joint instability following collateral ligament rupture causes severe joint effusion and lameness. Internal fixation combined with external coaptation is the treatment of choice.
- Degenerative joint disease in young animals has a guarded prognosis. Arthroscopy combined with medical therapy may slow down the disease process.
- Degenerative joint disease involving the distal interphalangeal joint has a good prognosis following joint resection.

INTRODUCTION

Noninfectious joint diseases are uncommonly diagnosed in cattle.[1] Typical clinical signs include joint effusion and various degree of lameness. Joint trauma can be diagnosed in cattle of all ages. However, osteochondrosis and degenerative joint disease (DJD) are usually recognized in young cattle.[1–9] This article discusses all the aforementioned disorders with regard to the causes, clinical and diagnostic features, treatments, and prognosis.

OSTEOCHONDROSIS

Osteochondrosis is a complex arthropathy that is rarely identified in cattle. The atlanto-occipital and the femoropatellar joints are the most commonly affected joints in feedlot cattle.[2]

Osteochondrosis usually refers to either osteochondritis dissecans (OCD) or subchondral bone cysts. However, these qualifications have been challenged. Because

a Department of Clinical Sciences, Faculty of Veterinary Medicine, Université de Montréal, 3200 Rue Sicotte, St-Hyacinthe, Quebec J2S 2M2, Canada; b Centre Hospitalier Universitaire Vétérinaire, Université de Montréal, 3200 Rue Sicotte, St-Hyacinthe, Quebec J2S 2M2, Canada
* Corresponding author.
E-mail address: sylvain.nichols@umontreal.ca

Vet Clin Food Anim 30 (2014) 205–223
http://dx.doi.org/10.1016/j.cvfa.2013.11.010
0749-0720/14/$ – see front matter © 2014 Elsevier Inc. All rights reserved.

there is no inflammation associated with OCD, the term osteochondritis is inappropriate and has been changed to osteochondrosis dissecans.[10] Two earlier stages of the disease have been recognized and named osteochondrosis latens and osteochondrosis manifesta.[10] Osteochondrosis latens is the first stage of the disease and is characterized by a focal area of necrotic cartilage within the epiphyseal cartilage. This lesion is only visible histologically. Osteochondrosis manifesta is the second stage of the disease, which is characterized by a focal failure of endochondral ossification caused by the necrotic cartilage. This lesion is visible macroscopically and radiographically and is similar to a subchondral bone cyst. Osteochondrosis dissecans is the final stage of the disease. A fissure originating from the necrotic cartilage extends to the articular cartilage, creating a cartilage flap or a loose body within the joint. This fissure is probably secondary to mild traumatic injury to the joint.

Causes and Pathophysiology

The causes and pathophysiology of osteochondrosis are complex. Studies often involve subjects with late clinical manifestations of the disease (osteochondrosis dissecans), with chronic remodeling of the joint already present. Among the many theories explaining this disorder, the one that currently answers most of the interrogations is the cartilage canal blood vessel necrosis theory.[10]

Cartilage canals are essential to nourish chondrocytes that are beyond the reach of synovial fluid nutrients. They are also essential to the formation and to the function of secondary ossification centers. Early in life, the blood supply to the canal comes from the perichondral vasculature. At some point, the blood supply shifts from the perichondral vessels to the metaphyseal vessels. At that moment, the fragile anastomoses created at the chondro-osseous junctions are more susceptible to trauma, which may damage the vessels and deprive the cartilage of its blood supply. The cartilage becomes necrotic and a lesion of osteochondrosis latens forms. Depending on the size of the lesion, it may resolve spontaneously and allow normal endochondral ossification, or it may remain and impede mineralization or vascularization. The lesion becomes radiographically visible and can be called osteochondrosis manifesta. At this stage, the lesion can still resolve, and the void created by the necrotic cartilage becomes granulation tissue and eventually bone; the same way a fracture heals. However, if the necrotic material cannot be removed or if the subchondral bone cannot heal properly, an osteochondrosis dissecans lesion appears following minor trauma to the unhealthy cartilage and subchondral bone (**Fig. 1**).

Risk Factors

For a long time, it was thought that fast-growing animals fed a high-energy diet were more likely to develop osteochondrosis.[3,6] This hypothesis was never confirmed and it is now thought that it might not be an important factor in the development of the disease. Being an intact male was also implicated.[6] Nowadays, with high-value females, males are not as overrepresented as they were in the past. In pigs and horses, osteochondrosis has a heritable component.[11,12] It was thought that the heritable component was at the level of the quality of the bone or cartilage. However, this theory does not explain why osteochondrosis is always diagnosed at the same location and rarely involves other articulations except for the contralateral joint. Therefore, the hereditable component seems to be more at the level of certain anatomic characteristics.[13] In pigs, the incidence of osteochondrosis can be decreased or increased significantly by selecting the breeding stock according to joint shape and conformation.[14]

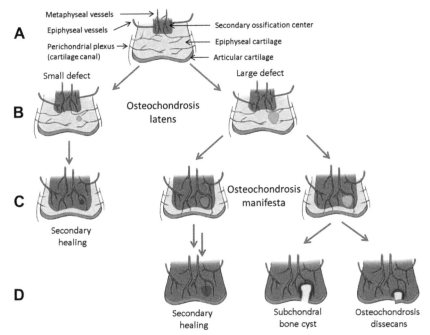

Fig. 1. Pathophysiology of osteochondrosis. (*A*) The epiphyseal cartilage is well vascularized by the perichondral vessel. (*B*) Anastomoses between the cartilage canal and the vessels of the secondary ossification center (metaphyseal vessels). Failure to anastomose may create an ischemic area within the epiphyseal cartilage. (*C*) Small defects may resolve as they are reached by the secondary ossification front. Large defects may become osteochondrosis manifesta because the ossification front fails to invade the lesion. (*D*) Osteochondrosis manifesta may be replaced my granulation tissue and healed by second intention, or it may become a subchondral bone cyst or a lesion of osteochondrosis dissecans. (*Adapted from* Ytrehus B, Carlson CS, Ekman S. Etiology and pathogenesis of osteochondrosis. Vet Pathol 2007;44:429–48. *Data from* Catherine Lardé.)

Dietary factors such as copper deficiency have been associated with osteochondrosis. Studies have shown that low copper levels in foals create lesions similar to osteochondrosis.[15–18] However, these lesions are more severe and diffuse, and affect multiple joints compared with the typical cases of osteochondrosis. It is now thought that copper deficiency is a systemic disease that is different from naturally occurring osteochondrosis.

The same observations as are seen in foals were made in a report of an outbreak of OCD-like lesions in bulls.[8] Imbalance in minerals and vitamins such as calcium; copper; and vitamins A, D, and E was implicated in this outbreak.

It was thought that an articular trauma was necessary to initiate osteochondrosis. This theory has also been challenged because osteochondrosis is often bilateral. It is improbable that a similar trauma would occur on both limbs at the same location and create similar lesions of osteochondrosis. However, minor trauma caused by daily ambulation can, in an animal with anatomic predisposition, cause damage to cartilage canals leading to osteochondrosis latens.[10] More minor trauma can make the disease progress from osteochondrosis manifesta to osteochondrosis dissecans. Therefore, traumatic events are still a factor in this disorder.

In conclusion, animals with specific joint anatomy sustaining a minor trauma at a critical moment in the period of growth and maturation of articular cartilage could develop osteochondrosis lesions. These lesions may or may not progress to osteochondrosis dissecans, the most frequent presentation of osteochondrosis. This theory takes into account the distribution of the lesions, the frequent bilateral nature of the disease (same anatomic characteristic on each leg), and the juvenile nature of the condition.

Clinical Presentation

Cattle with osteochondrosis are usually presented with variable degree of lameness and joint effusion (**Fig. 2**). The more chronic the lameness, the worse the lesions are. In some cases, the animal is presented for cosmetic reasons (joint effusion). They are usually between 1 and 2 years old and are valuable animals (show heifers and breeding bulls) with rapid growth rates.[1–9] The physical examination often reveals effusion of the contralateral limb.

Diagnostic Technique

Arthrocentesis

Using a small-gauge needle, articular fluid is obtained and submitted for cytology. The fluid flows easily from the needle, has a normal color, and may or may not have decreased viscosity. The cytology reveals mild inflammation with a mild increase in proteins.[19]

Radiography

It is recommended always to evaluate the contralateral joint radiographically. Depending on the articulation involved, 4 radiographic views (lateral, craniocaudal, and 2 obliques) might be necessary to localize the lesion. The use of computed radiography significantly improves the ability to find small subchondral bone lesions (**Fig. 3**). Poor correlation has been found between radiology and arthroscopic findings in other species.[20]

Ultrasonography

Joint cartilage can be evaluated through ultrasonography (**Fig. 4**). It is recommended to use a high-frequency linear probe to improve evaluation of superficial structures. Flexion and extension help to find irregularities of the cartilage or even of subchondral bone. The main disadvantage of ultrasonography is the impossibility of evaluating the

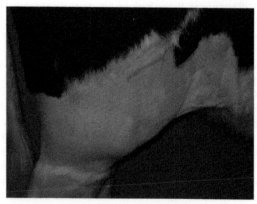

Fig. 2. Severe distension of the right stifle on this Holstein heifer.

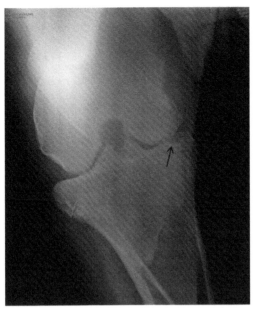

Fig. 3. A radiographic craniocaudal view of the stifle of yearling Holstein heifer is shown. Subchondral bone cyst of the medial condyle of the proximal tibia (*black arrow*).

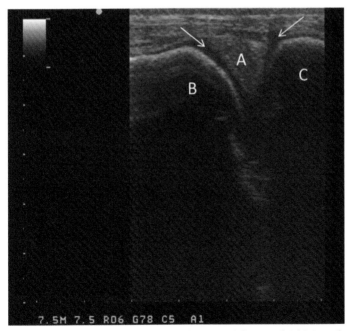

Fig. 4. Longitudinal ultrasound evaluation of the medial femorotibial joint of a yearling Holstein heifer using a 7.5-mHz linear probe. The small white arrows indicate articular cartilage. A, medial meniscus; B, medial femoral condyle; C, medial tibial condyle.

entire joint cartilage. However, because osteochondrosis lesions are rarely in the middle of the joints, ultrasound evaluation was shown to be more sensitive than radiography to detect osteochondral lesions in the horse.[21,22,23]

Computed tomography and magnetic resonance imaging

A diagnosis is usually obtained with the use of digital radiography and ultrasonography. Computed tomography (CT) and magnetic resonance imaging (MRI) have been used in horse research to help understand the pathophysiology of the disease.[24,25] In humans, MRI has been used to help decide which therapeutic plan is best for small osteochondrosis lesions.[26] Small lesions showing signs of healing (intake of contrast product), without cystic lesions or cartilage lesions on MRI, are treated conservatively. In cattle, the cost associated with the procedure and the difficulty in getting proximal joints in the tube explain why these diagnostic modalities are rarely used.

Distribution of Lesions in Cattle

In feedlot cattle, the atlanto-occipital joint is the most frequent joint involved, followed by the femoropatellar joint.[2] In bull studs, the lateral trochlear ridge of the femoropatellar joint and the distal intermediate ridge of the tibia of the tarsocrural joint, especially, are the most frequent locations of osteochondrosis.[3–6] Osteochondrosis lesions are found in other bovine joints less frequently. Osteochondrosis dissecans is the most frequent presentation of osteochondrosis. Subchondral bone cysts are less frequent and need to be differentiated from cystic lesions associated with septic arthritis (**Fig. 5**). The origin of lesions associated with septic arthritis is unclear. It is the author's belief that they are caused by bone abscesses that rupture in the joint, leading to septic arthritis.

Treatment

Conservative treatment

Conservative treatment consists of stall rest (3–6 months) and nonsteroidal antiinflammatory drugs (NSAIDs). Phenylbutazone was an ideal molecule before it became highly restricted or even prohibited in dairy milking cows in the United States. Other NSAIDs have been approved in cattle but their homologation limits their used in lame patients. The regulation differs between countries. In addition, frequent use is expensive and might not be possible in commercial animals. However, because of lack of alternatives in pain management, extralabel use of NSAIDs is common.

Molecules containing hyaluronic acid (Legend) or polysulfated glycosaminoglycan (Adequan) have been used extralabel in cattle. These molecules can be used locally or systemically. Septic arthritis is a serious potential complication of intra-articular injections; this might explain why the systemic route is used more often. Legend has been used intravenously (2 mL) once a week for 3 weeks and Adequan has been used at a dose of 1 mg/kg intramuscularly once a week for 3 weeks followed by once every 2 weeks for 3 other treatments. The beneficial effects of these molecules are difficult to evaluate. There is anecdotal evidence that it improves comfort and may slow down the progression of DJD.

Surgical treatment

Surgical debridement of an osteochondrosis lesion can be achieved through an arthrotomy incision or by arthroscopy (**Fig. 6**).[6] Arthrotomy is more invasive and therefore necessitates more postoperative care compared with arthroscopy. Also, cattle have thick joint capsules, making it difficult to access the joint without making a large incision.

Arthroscopy is the ideal surgical technique, allowing a thorough evaluation of the joint through a small incision. The surgery remains challenging in cattle because of

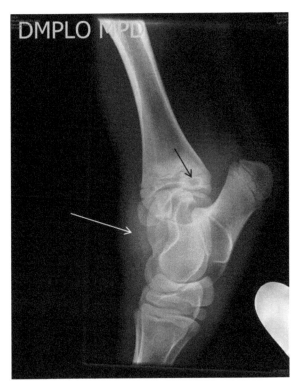

Fig. 5. A radiographic dorsomedial plantarolateral oblique view of the hock of a 2-month-old Holstein bull calf with an acute septic arthritis. The small white arrow indicates severe joint distension, and the small black arrow indicates a cystlike lesion caused by osteomyelitis of the distal tibia.

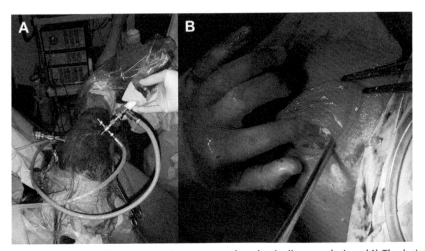

Fig. 6. Surgical approaches to removing an osteochondrosis dissecans lesion. (*A*) The lesion on the lateral trochlear ridge of the femur is removed through arthroscopy using triangulation. (*B*) The lesion on the caudal aspect of the medial femoral condyle is removed through arthrotomy.

the thick joint capsule and the proliferative synovium associated with chronic articular disease.[27–30] A motorized synovial resector is mandatory to properly view the joint structures. The surgical approach and portal placement of specific joints are discussed by Lardé and colleagues elsewhere in this issue. This article emphasizes the specific arthroscopic treatment of lesions.

Prophylactic antibiotics and an NSAID are given before the procedure. With proper joint distension and with adequate portal location, the lesion is observed. Using the triangulation principle, the lesion is treated using the techniques described later.

DEBRIDEMENT

Full-thickness cartilage is debrided all the way to healthy subchondral bone. Healthy subchondral bone is firm and reddish from the diffuse bleeding (**Fig. 7**). The edge of the cartilage lesion is left perpendicular to the exposed bone. No attempt should be made to taper the edge of the lesion. Tapering the edge only increases the size of the lesion. Debridement is performed using a bone curette and a rongeur.

CHONDROPLASTY

Partial-thickness lesions or cartilage fibrillation should be partially debrided (chondroplasty). The deep cartilage still attached to subchondral bone is stronger than the fibrocartilage that replaces a full-thickness lesion. Chondroplasty can only be achieved with a motorized synovial resector (**Fig. 8**).

FORAGE OR MICROFRACTURE

Forage has been replaced by microfracture (**Fig. 9**). Forage involves drilling small holes through the subchondral bone to reach the marrow and allowing marrow elements to enter the defect and promote cartilage healing. It is simple and inexpensive. However, it requires more instruments and it can be difficult to reach centrally located lesions. Therefore, it was replaced by microfracture. The basic principle is the same: reaching the bone marrow. A specialized instrument called a micropick, an angled tapered awl, is used. This instrument allows better control and creates a tapered hole in the shape of a crater that improves attachment of the newly formed fibrocartilage. This technique is now widely used in both human and equine arthroscopy.

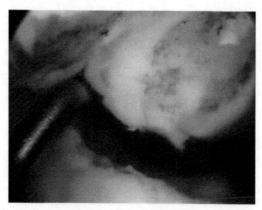

Fig. 7. Osteochondrosis dissecans lesion of the intermediate carpal bone after removal of the osteochondral fragment and debridement of the subchondral bone.

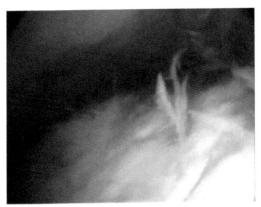

Fig. 8. Arthroscopic view of the distal radius showing severe cartilage fibrillation. These partial-thickness cartilaginous lesions are better debrided using a motorized synovial resector.

CARTILAGE REATTACHMENT

Only large, partially attached cartilage flaps with minimal fibrillation are worth being reattached. This type of lesion is uncommon in cattle. Therefore, the technique has only been described in horses. It involves drilling the subchondral bone and placing polydioxanone pins through the flap down to the bone.[31,32]

Postoperative Treatment

The joint is kept bandaged until the sutures are removed. Depending on the joint involved and the environment in which the animal is kept, antibiotics might also be given during the postoperative period. The conservative treatment described earlier is usually used in the postoperative period.

Prognosis

Conservative management seems to have a guarded prognosis. The lesions eventually lead to DJD and worsening of the lameness.[6] Arthroscopic debridement seems to improve the prognosis if the surgery is performed before radiographic evidence of DJD is observed. However, this hypothesis has never been validated in a multiple case study.

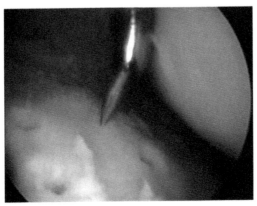

Fig. 9. Microfracture of the subchondral bone using a micropick to promote cartilage healing.

JOINT TRAUMA

Most cases of joint trauma are secondary to a deep laceration exposing the joint and frequently result in septic arthritis. Articular trauma, as seen in the horse, is uncommon in cattle. In this species, repetitive trauma to bone and cartilage can cause fracture and damage to the cartilage, causing osteoarthritis.[33,34]

In cattle, the trauma usually takes place as a single but catastrophic event. The most frequent causes of joint trauma are joint luxation, cuboidal bone fracture, avulsion fracture of tendinous or ligamentous attachments, and rupture of collateral or intra-articular ligaments. All these conditions can cause hemarthrosis and severe lameness.

Joint Luxation

The joint most frequently involved is the coxofemoral joint. It is always associated with rupture of the femoral head ligament.[35] This condition has a grave prognosis, especially in mature cattle. It is extensively discussed by Marchionatti and colleagues elsewhere in this issue.

Joint luxation of the scapulohumeral and the tibiotarsal joints has been reported.[36–38] Scapulohumeral joint luxation often necessitates lateral reinforcement to avoid reluxation. Tibiotarsal joint luxation is often difficult to reduce. However, when in place, external coaptation during the healing period is usually sufficient to prevent reluxation. Proximal intertarsal joint luxation involving the calcaneum and the central tarsal bone has been described. This luxation is in a plantarodistal orientation. General anesthesia or deep sedation combined with traction is usually sufficient to reduce the luxation. When in place, the articulation is stable. No splint or bandage is required in the postoperative period but the animal is confined in a stall for 1 to 2 months.

Cuboidal Bone Fracture

Tarsal bone fractures are more frequent than carpal bone fractures. They are secondary to a trauma, like a kick from another animal. In our experience, the talus and the calcaneum are the bones most frequently involved. The animal is painful and the joint is severely distended. Hemarthrosis is also present in acute cases. The final diagnosis is obtained by radiography (**Fig. 10**). With complex fractures, a CT scan may be of better diagnostic value. Without adequate treatment, the joint develops osteoarthritis, and ankylosis might follow. Nondisplaced fractures may heal if the joint can be adequately immobilized. However, without internal stabilization and reduction, complex or displaced fractures either fail to heal or develop an exuberant callus that fuses the joint and is likely to cause chronic pain.

Arthrodesis of the proximal joints of the hock is difficult to achieve and seems to be more problematic (chronic lameness) compared with partial or pancarpal arthrodesis. The distal trochlea of the talus in cattle is mobile and biomechanically important when the animal is either rising or lying down. Severe trauma to the carpal bone can be successfully treated with a combination of joint resection and immobilization. The surgical technique is similar to what has been described in cases of partial carpal joint resection secondary to septic arthritis in calves.[38]

Avulsion Fracture

Olecranon and calcaneal fractures are avulsion fractures that affect the mechanical function of the elbow and the tarsocrural joints (**Fig. 11**). These fractures may or may not involve the articular surface. If they do, anatomically precise reconstruction is crucial to avoid secondary osteoarthritis. Nondisplaced or minimally displaced olecranon fractures can be treated with external coaptation alone and stall rest.

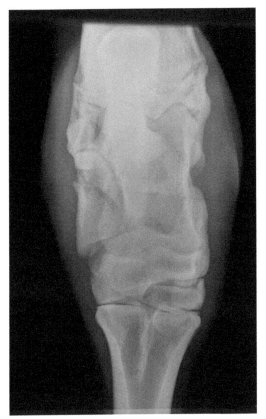

Fig. 10. A radiographic dorsopalmar view of the left hock of yearling bull with a traumatic fracture of the body of its calcaneum.

Calcaneum fractures are usually severely displaced and need to be repaired surgically (see **Fig. 11**). The tension side of the calcaneum is on the plantar surface (caudal surface for the olecranon) and is readily available to place a combination of plate, screws, and tension wires. External coaptation is important during the postoperative period following internal fixation of a calcaneal fracture.

Proximal sesamoid bone fractures are seen sporadically (**Fig. 12**). They are thought to be secondary to severe hyperextension of the fetlock joint in immature animals. In young animals, the bone is often softer than the tendons and ligaments. Therefore, trauma to the fetlock joint is more likely to cause a fracture than a tendon or ligament rupture. The fracture is often comminuted and involves multiple sesamoid bones, making it unsuitable for open reduction and internal fixation. These fractures have been treated conservatively using external coaptation. This condition has a guarded prognosis because healing by second intention of these bones results in osteoarthritis and chronic pain without subsequent fetlock arthrodesis.

Rupture of Collateral or Intra-articular Ligament

The most frequent collateral or intra-articular ligament rupture occurs in the stifle (cranial cruciate ligament and collaterals). These disorders are discussed further elsewhere in this issue.

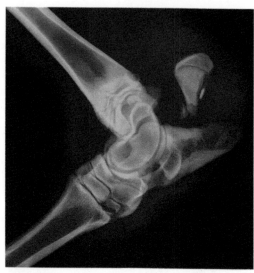

Fig. 11. A 6-month-old Holstein heifer with an avulsion fracture of the right calcaneum.

The collateral ligaments of the hock and fetlock are also at risk of rupture, causing instability of the joint and severe lameness. This condition can be treated conservatively with external coaptation alone or surgically by using a combination of bone anchors, screws, washers, and large nonabsorbent sutures (eg, nylon). Even with surgical treatment, the articulation involved must be stabilized during the early phases of the healing process.

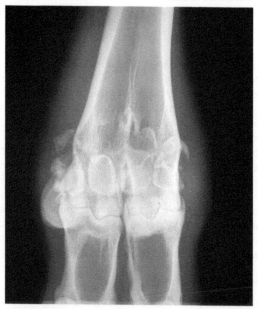

Fig. 12. A dorsopalmar view of the right fetlock of this 20-month-old Holstein heifer. A comminuted fracture of the abaxial proximal sesamoid bones is present.

It is important not to improperly diagnose a collateral ligament rupture and a subsequent fetlock luxation in case of epiphyseal fracture of the metacarpal and metatarsal bones. The displacement of the distal limb could be similar.

DJD

DJD is a term used to describe severe, progressive, nonseptic arthropathy in growing animals. It needs to be differentiated from the term osteoarthritis, which is used to describe acquired progressive arthropathy in older animals. DJD in cattle is uncommon. The exact cause of this condition is unknown but it may be associated with osteochondrosis. There are only a few reports of this condition in cattle.[3,39,40] One report involved 9 cases of DJD of the distal interphalangeal joint (DIJ) in calves.[40] The DIJ seems to be the joint that is most often involved.

Clinical Presentation

Calves with this condition are moderately lame. The lameness usually affects 1 or both forelimbs. The calves typically walk on their toes and have a shortened anterior stride to avoid putting any weight on their heels (**Fig. 13**). No joint distension is present on palpation. Hoof testers applied to the heel induce severe pain.

Diagnostic Technique

Regional anesthesia
Perineural anesthesia (4-point block) or locoregional intravenous anesthesia should improve the lameness significantly.

Arthrocentesis
Because there is no synovial effusion with this disorder and the DIJ is small, it is difficult to obtain synovial fluid for analysis. If successfully obtained, cytology results are likely to be within normal limits.

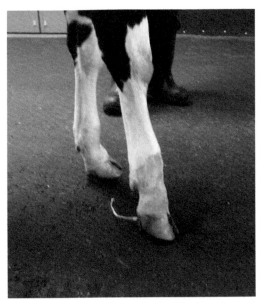

Fig. 13. Typical toe-touching lameness of an animal with distal interphalangeal (DIP) joint degenerative disease.

Radiography

Oblique views of the DIJ are ideally taken to isolate the palmar aspect of the joint and the distal sesamoid bone (**Fig. 14**). Interdigital views can be helpful as well. With this view, it is important to get the cassette high enough between the heel bulbs to get the entire articular surface and the distal sesamoid bone. Even if the lameness is unilateral, it is also important to evaluate both forelimbs and both claws on each forelimb.

On radiographs, the lesions appears aggressive and septic (see **Fig. 13**). However, the clinical presentation does not fit with a septic process (multiple joint involvement, no synovial effusion, very focal lesion always located at the palmar aspect of the joint).

CT

A CT scan, if available, is probably the best diagnostic tool in cases of DJD of the DIJ. Both forelimbs can be evaluated at the same time, and the degree of severity of the lesions can be determined with the help of three-dimensional reconstruction software. Cost of the procedure and risks associated with deep sedation are the main disadvantages of CT imaging in cattle.

Treatment

Conservative treatment

Conservative management consists of gluing a wooden block to the unaffected claw. This treatment is possible only if one claw, on the affected limb, is radiographically normal. NSAIDs should also be given, especially if both claws on the same limb are affected. Meloxicam can be used extralabel every other day for an extended period of time, apparently without any side effects on an otherwise healthy animal. It is not as potent for orthopedic pain as phenylbutazone but it is our clinical impression that it might be better than other NSAIDs that are available for use in cattle at the moment.

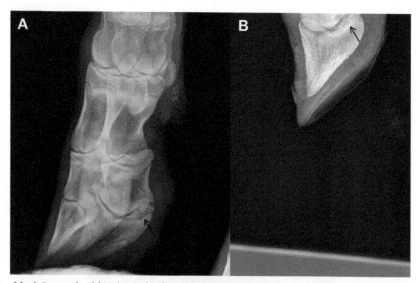

Fig. 14. A 9-month-old Holstein heifer with DIP joint degenerative disease. (*A*) Dorsomedial palmarolateral view exposing the palmar aspect of P2 and P3. (*B*) Interdigital view of the affected digit. On both radiographs, lysis and sclerosis of the subchondral bone are present on the palmar aspect of P2 and P3 (*black arrows*).

Surgical treatment

Surgical treatment of DJD involves joint resection to facilitate ankylosis of the DIJ. Ankylosis of this joint eliminates the pain associated with this condition without causing mechanical lameness or changing the angulation of the limb.

Many techniques have been described for DIJ resection.[41–45] These techniques are described elsewhere in this issue. The abaxial approach is ideal for this condition because it often has to be performed on more than one joint (**Fig. 15**). This approach is fast and does not involve incising the soft tissue of the palmar and bulbar surfaces. The main disadvantage of this approach is that it is impossible to reach the distal sesamoid bone.

The postoperative treatment is similar to the conservative management. When both claws are involved on the same limb, a short limb cast can be used to immobilize the joint. The cast is kept for 3 to 4 weeks.

Prognosis

Calves managed conservatively may reach soundness. It is thought that the joint will eventually fuse by itself. However, without joint resection, this process may take a long time and some calves with chronic pain have a decreased growth rate and may develop angular limb deformities on the unaffected limb. Joint resection speeds up ankylosis and may prevent some of these complications.[40]

Degenerative Disease in Other Joints

DJD in cattle has principally been reported in the fetlock, carpus, and tarsus.[46,47] The author has seen DJD in other joints, especially the carpus and tarsus. The lesions are

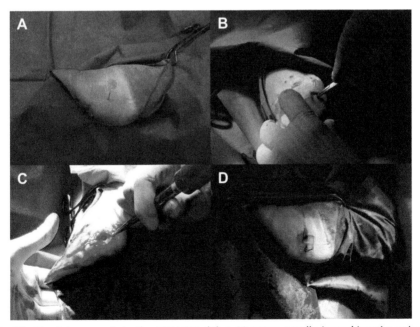

Fig. 15. Abaxial approach to the DIP joint. (*A*) A 20-gauge needle is marking the palmar aspect of the joint. (*B*) A 1 × 1 cm² piece of the abaxial hoof wall was removed to get access to the DIP joint. (*C*) A curette is used to remove the cartilage. (*D*) The piece of hoof wall that was removed is reattached to cover the surgery site.

variable and the exact origin unknown. The hard concrete floor and collecting practices were suspected in a Artificial insemination (AI) center.[46] DJD was also described in cattle with cruciate ligament injury,[48] which causes joint effusion and varying degrees of lameness. Because these are high-motion joints, joint resection or arthrodesis are not the ideal surgical options for achieving soundness without mechanical lameness. These joints have therefore been treated conservatively (discussed earlier) or surgically through arthroscopy. Arthroscopy reveals a diffusely abnormal cartilage. Wear lines, fibrillations, and cartilage erosions of varying depths are detected (see **Fig. 8**). Only full-thickness lesions are debrided down to the subchondral bone. The fibrillations are shaved with a motorized synovial resector.

Because of the extensive damage to the cartilage, arthroscopic debridement and synovial lavage provide only temporary relief of lameness. Therefore, we think that the prognosis for DJD of high-motion joints such as the carpus and tarsus is guarded at best.

OSTEOARTHRITIS

Osteoarthritis (OA) in cattle is rarely diagnosed. However, it is probably more common than we think. Because cattle are not performance animals, mild osteoarthritis might not have any recognizable clinical implication.

OA might be primary or secondary. Primary OA could have a hereditary component in its pathophysiology. Secondary OA could be the consequence of repeated trauma to the joint caused by inappropriate husbandry, nutritional imbalance, joint instability caused by a ruptured ligament or tendon, or a previous insult such as septic arthritis.

The goal of the treatment is to decrease pain (NSAID), to protect the joint from further damage (improve husbandry), and to improve the quality of synovial fluid (hyaluronic acid [Legend] or polysulfated glycosaminoglycan [Adequan]). In low-motion joints where resection or arthrodesis is possible, those surgeries might be the best treatment to alleviate pain.

In cases refractory to the aforementioned treatments, corticosteroids can be injected intra-articularly. Triamcinolone acetonide (Vetalog, 6 mg/joint) and methylprednisolone (Depo-Medrol, 40 mg/joint) can be used extralabel. The authors have always worried about the possibility of causing septic arthritis with intra-articular corticosteroid injections. Strict aseptic technique must be used. Use of these drugs in cattle has yielded mixed results.

SUMMARY

It is important to recognize noninfectious joint disease in cattle. Ultrasonography and radiography help obtain a precise diagnosis, elaborate the best treatment plan (which frequently involves performing an arthroscopy), and determine the prognosis. Long-term prognosis of DJD is poor except when it involves joints where an arthrodesis or a facilitated ankylosis can be performed.

ACKNOWLEDGMENTS

The authors thank Dr Marketa Kopal for her support and her help in the preparation of this article.

REFERENCES

1. Tryon KA, Farrow CS. Osteochondrosis in cattle. Vet Clin North Am Food Anim Pract 1999;15(2):265–74.

2. Jensen R, Park RD, Lauerman LH, et al. Osteochondrosis in feedlot cattle. Vet Pathol 1981;18:529–35.
3. Weisbrode SE, Monke DR, Dodaro ST, et al. Osteochondrosis, degenerative joint disease, and vertebral osteophytosis in middle-aged bulls. J Am Vet Med Assoc 1982;181(7):700–5.
4. Baxter GM, Hay WP, Selcer BA. Osteochondritis dissecans of the medial trochlear ridge of the talus in a calf. J Am Vet Med Assoc 1991;198(4):669–71.
5. Wegener KM, Heje NI. Dyschondroplasia (osteochondrosis) in articular-epiphyseal cartilage complexes of three calves from 24 to 103 days of age. Vet Pathol 1992;29:562–3.
6. Trostle SS, Nicoll RG, Forrest LJ, et al. Clinical and radiographic findings, treatment, and outcome in cattle with osteochondrosis: 29 cases (1986–1996). J Am Vet Med Assoc 1997;211(12):1566–70.
7. Hill BD, Sutton RH, Thompson H. Investigation of osteochondrosis in grazing beef cattle. Aust Vet J 1998;76(3):171–5.
8. Davies IH, Munro R. Osteochondrosis in bull beef cattle following lack of dietary mineral and vitamin supplementation. Vet Rec 1999;145:232–3.
9. Scott PR, Rhind S, Brownstein D. Severe osteochondrosis in two 10 month old beef calves. Vet Rec 2000;147:608–9.
10. Ytrehus B, Carlson CS, Ekman S. Etiology and pathogenesis of osteochondrosis. Vet Pathol 2007;44:429–48.
11. Jorgensen B, Andersen S. Genetic parameters for osteochondrosis in Danish Landrace and Yorkshire boars and correlations with leg weakness and production traits. Anim Sci 2000;71:427–34.
12. Van Grevenhof EM, Schurink A, Ducro BJ, et al. Genetic variables of various manifestations of osteochondrosis and their correlations between and within joints in Dutch warmblood horses. J Anim Sci 2009;87:1906–12.
13. Ytrehus B, Ekman S, Carlson CS, et al. Focal changes in blood supply during normal epiphyseal growth are central in the pathogenesis of osteochondrosis in pigs. Bone 2004;35:1294–306.
14. Grondalen T. Osteochondrosis and arthrosis in Norwegian slaughter pigs in 1980 compared to 1970. Nord Vet Med 1981;33:417–22.
15. Bridges CH, Womack JE, Harris ED, et al. Considerations of copper metabolism in osteochondrosis in suckling foals. J Am Vet Med Assoc 1984;185:173–8.
16. Bridges CH, Harris ED. Experimentally induced cartilaginous fractures (osteochondritis dissecans) in foals fed low copper diets. J Am Vet Med Assoc 1988;193:215–21.
17. Bridges CH, Moffitt PG. Influence of variable content of dietary zinc on copper metabolism of weanling foals. Am J Vet Res 1990;51:275–80.
18. Gunson DE, Kowalczyk DF, Shoop CR, et al. Environmental zinc and cadmium pollution associated with generalized osteochondrosis osteoporosis, and nephrocalcinosis in horses. J Am Vet Med Assoc 1982;180:295–9.
19. Rohde C, Anderson DE, Desrochers A, et al. Synovial fluid analysis in cattle: a review of 130 cases. Vet Surg 2000;29:341–6.
20. Van Weeren PR. Osteochondrosis. In: Auer JA, Stick JA, editors. Equine surgery. 4th edition. St Louis (MO): Saunders Elsevier; 2012. p. 1239–55.
21. Beccati F, Chalmers HJ, Dante S, et al. Diagnostic sensitivity and interobserver agreement of radiography and ultrasonography for detecting trochlear ridge osteochondrosis lesions in the equine stifle. Vet Radiol Ultrasound 2013;54(2):176–84.

22. Relave F, Meulyzer M, Alexander K, et al. Comparison of radiography and ultrasonography to detect osteochondrosis lesions in the tarsocrural joint: a prospective study. Equine Vet J 2009;41(1):34–40.
23. Bourzac C, Alexander K, Rossier Y, et al. Comparison of radiography and ultrasonography for the diagnosis of osteochondritis dissecans in the equine femoropatellar joint. Equine Vet J 2009;41(7):686–92.
24. Olstad K, Cnudde V, Masschaele B, et al. Micro-computed tomography of early lesions of osteochondrosis in the tarsus of foals. Bone 2008;43:574–83.
25. Fontaine P, Blond L, Alexander K, et al. Computed tomography and magnetic resonance imaging in the study of joint development in the equine pelvic limb. Vet J 2013;197(1):103–11.
26. Bohndorf K. Osteochondritis (osteochondrosis) dissecans: a review and new MRI classification. Eur Radiol 1998;8:103–12.
27. Hurting MB. Recent developments in the use of arthroscopy in cattle. Vet Clin North Am Food Anim Pract 1985;1(1):175–93.
28. Munroe GA, Gauvin ER. The use of arthroscopy in the treatment of septic arthritis in two Highland calves. Br Vet J 1994;150:439–48.
29. Gaughan EM. Arthroscopy in food animal practice. Vet Clin North Am Food Anim Pract 1996;12(1):233–47.
30. Blaser M, Bertagnoli A, Räber M, et al. Arthroscopic approaches to the fetlock joint of adult cattle: a cadaver study. Vet J 2012;193:701–6.
31. Nixon AJ, Fortier LA, Goodrich LR, et al. Arthroscopic reattachment of osteochondritis dissecans lesions using resorbable polydioxanone pins. Equine Vet J 2004; 36(5):376–83.
32. Sparks HD, Nixon AJ, Fortier LA, et al. Arthroscopic reattachment of osteochondritis dissecans cartilage flaps of the femoropatellar joint: long term results. Equine Vet J 2011;43(6):650–9.
33. Getman LM, Southwood LL, Richardson DW. Palmar carpal osteochondral fragments in racehorses: 31 cases (1994–2004). J Am Vet Med Assoc 2006; 228(10):1551–8.
34. Lacourt M, Gao C, Li A, et al. Relationship between cartilage and subchondral bone lesions in repetitive impact trauma induced equine osteoarthritis. Osteoarthritis Cartilage 2012;20:572–83.
35. Tulleners EP, Nunamaker DM, Richardson DW. Coxofemoral luxations in cattle: 22 cases (1980–1985). J Am Vet Med Assoc 1987;191:569–74.
36. Watts AE, Fortier LA, Nixon AJ, et al. A technique for internal fixation of scapulohumeral luxation using scapulohumeral tension sutures in three alpacas and one miniature steer. Vet Surg 2008;37:161–5.
37. Arighi M, Ducharme NG, Horney FD, et al. Proximal intertarsal subluxation in three Holstein Friesian heifers. Can Vet J 1987;28:710–2.
38. Riley CB, Farrow CS. Partial carpal arthrodesis in a calf with chronic infectious arthritis of the carpus and osteomyelitis of the carpal and metacarpal bones. Can Vet J 1998;39:438–41.
39. Taura Y, Sasaki N, Nishimura R, et al. Histopathological findings on ulcerative lesions of carpal and tarsal joints in Japanese black cattle. J Vet Med Sci 1996;58(2):135–9.
40. Mulon PY, Babkine M, D'Anjou MA, et al. Degenerative disease of the distal interphalangeal joint and sesamoid bone in calves: 9 cases (1995–2004). J Am Vet Med Assoc 2009;234(6):794–9.
41. Desrochers A, St-Jean G, Anderson DE. Use of facilitated ankylosis in the treatment of septic arthritis of the distal interphalangeal joint in cattle: 12 cases (1987–1992). J Am Vet Med Assoc 1995;206(12):1923–7.

42. Starke A, Heppelmann M, Beyerbach M, et al. Septic arthritis of the distal inter-phalangeal joint in cattle: comparison of digital amputation and joint resection by solar approach. Vet Surg 2007;26:350–9.

43. Bicalho RC, Cheong SH, Guard CL. Field technique for the resection of the distal interphalangeal joint and proximal resection of the deep digital flexor tendon in cows. Vet Rec 2007;160:435–9.

44. Desrochers A, Anderson DE, St-Jean G. Surgical diseases and techniques of the digit. Vet Clin North Am Food Anim Pract 2008;24:535–50.

45. Lewis AJ, Sod GA, Gill MS, et al. Distal interphalangeal joint arthrodesis in seven cattle using Acutrak Plus screw. Vet Surg 2009;38:659–63.

46. Bargai U, Cohen R. Tarsal lameness of dairy bulls housed at two artificial insem-ination centers: 24 cases (1975–1987). J Am Vet Med Assoc 1992;201:1068–9.

47. Van Pelt RW, Langham RF. Degenerative joint disease of the carpus and fetlock in cattle. J Am Vet Med Assoc 1970;157:953–61.

48. Huhn JC, Kneller SK, Nelson DR. Radiographic assessment of cranial cruciate ligament rupture in the dairy cow. Vet Rad 1986;27:184–8.

Arthroscopy in Cattle
Technique and Normal Anatomy

Hélène Lardé, Dr Med Vet, DES[a],*, Sylvain Nichols, DMV, MS[b]

KEYWORDS

- Cattle • Arthroscopy • Surgery • Anatomy

KEY POINTS

- Arthroscopy has all the advantages of minimally invasive surgery in cattle.
- Specialized equipment and knowledge of normal joint anatomy of cattle are mandatory for successful arthroscopy.
- The surgical technique is different in cattle compared with the horse. Thick skin and joint capsules complicate movement of the arthroscope within the joints.
- In cattle, septic arthritis and osteochondrosis are the most frequent disorders suitable for arthroscopic treatment.

INTRODUCTION

Arthroscopy in cattle was first described many years ago.[1–3] However, it remains unpopular among food animal surgeons because of the prohibitive cost of the equipment needed and the necessity to do the procedure under general anesthesia. The arthroscopic approach to the bovine joints is described to be similar to that in the horse.[4] Studies have recently highlighted the differences between the two species and have shown that cattle articulations need to be approached differently those of the horse.[5]

This article serves as a guide to bovine arthroscopy. Emphasis is placed on equipment, technique, and normal anatomy. Different disorders that can benefit from arthroscopy are discussed elsewhere in this issue.

ARTHROSCOPY VERSUS ARTHROTOMY

Arthroscopy has all the advantages of minimally invasive surgery. It improves evaluation of the articular cartilage, it allows evaluation of intra-articular structures (meniscus, ligaments, and bones) and pouches, it decreases hospitalization time, and it speeds up recovery.[6] It is a complement to other diagnostic imaging techniques (radiography and ultrasonography) and helps determine the prognosis of joint disease.

[a] Centre Hospitalier Universitaire Vétérinaire (Veterinary Medicine Teaching Hospital), Université de Montréal, 3200 Rue Sicotte, St-Hyacinthe, Quebec J2S 2M2, Canada; [b] Department of Clinical Sciences, Faculty of Veterinary Medicine, Université de Montréal, 3200 Rue Sicotte, St-Hyacinthe, Quebec J2S 2M2, Canada
* Corresponding author.
E-mail address: helene.larde@umontreal.ca

Vet Clin Food Anim 30 (2014) 225–245
http://dx.doi.org/10.1016/j.cvfa.2013.11.004
0749-0720/14/$ – see front matter © 2014 Elsevier Inc. All rights reserved.

Despite these advantages, arthroscopy is not routinely performed on cattle for reasons related to the species and to the practice. First, specialized and expensive equipment is needed to perform arthroscopy and there is a steep learning curve to become familiar with the procedure. In adult cattle, thick joint capsules and thick skin make it difficult to manipulate the scope. Artiodactyl species have smaller distal joints (interphalangeal joints) and range of movement is limited in the metacarpophalangeal joint.[5] Adding to this, abnormal findings like proliferative synovium and fibrin formation make observation of joint structures even more difficult. General anesthesia is another drawback to performing arthroscopy in cattle. It is essential for a thorough and safe arthroscopic examination, which increases the cost of the procedure. All these factors have contributed to make arthroscopy in cattle a procedure exclusive to valuable cows in referral hospitals. However, with the value of purebred cattle continuing to increase, arthroscopic procedures for both septic and nonseptic joint disease should become more popular because the advantages compared with arthrotomy are substantial.

EQUIPMENT AND SURGERY SUITE

The equipment needed for bovine arthroscopy is similar to the equipment used in horses.

Arthroscope

A 4-mm diameter arthroscope, 160 to 180 mm in length, with a 30° viewing angle creating a field of view of 115° is usually used (**Fig. 1**). In narrow joints, a scope with a 70° viewing angle can be used to increase the field of view.

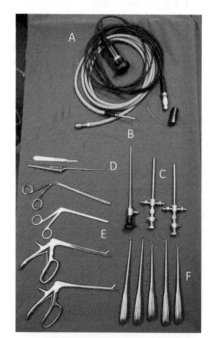

Fig. 1. Instruments needed to perform an arthroscopy. A, light cable and camera; B, 4-mm arthroscope; C, arthroscopic sleeves; D, graduate probe; E, various size and type of Ferris-Smith rongeurs; F, various types and sizes of bone curettes.

Cannula with Adapted Sharp and Blunt Trocars

Blunt or sharp trocars are placed inside the arthroscopic stainless steel sleeve (outer diameter, 5.5 mm; see **Fig. 1**). The skin is sharply incised (1 cm) with a number 10 scalpel blade. The subcutaneous tissue and the joint capsule are incised with a number 11 scalpel blade. The trocar/sleeve unit is inserted through the joint capsule and synovial membrane with a twisting motion until its tip moves freely in the joint. In mature cattle, if the joint capsule is not incised before penetration of the joint, the sharp trocar must be used.

The trocar is then replaced by the arthroscope. The arthroscopic sleeve is essential to protect the scope from bending. Because of the thick joint capsule, stress is often placed on the scope/sleeve unit to see particular areas of the joints. The sleeve also protects the lens from scratches and allows continuous flow of fluids during the procedure.

Light Source

A cold light source is required. It is directly connected to the arthroscope by a fiber light cable. Several light sources are available (xenon, halogen, tungsten, mercury, and so forth), with xenon considered to be the best.

Video Camera

Direct visualization through the eyepiece of the scope is possible, but pictures and videos cannot be recorded and saved this way. The proximity of the surgeon's head also increases the risk of contaminating the surgical field. A video camera is ideally connected directly to the arthroscope and to a processor that projects the images on a monitor. The monitor is on the arthroscopic tower, which can be positioned according to the surgeon's preference.

Video Capture Unit

The procedure can be recorded at low cost on a DVD recorder. The disadvantage of this technology is that the videos are not readily available for computer editing, but it is adequate to keep in the medical record. More expensive medical recording units are available. With this technology, the surgeon can take pictures and control the video recording. The videos are available in many formats that are readily available for computer editing.

Fluid Pump

There are several fluid pump systems available. The most popular is a continuous wave arthroscopy infusion pump. It allows a continuous flow of fluid to maintain pressure within the joint. Lactated Ringer solution is the fluid of choice[7] and, depending on the procedure and the number of joints to be explored, 5 to 20 L are necessary.

Hand Instruments

A blunt graduated probe is useful for evaluating articular cartilage. Variable-size Ferris-Smith rongeurs and bone curettes are used to debride osteochondrosis dissecans lesions or to remove fibrin tags (see **Fig. 1**). Angled or straight curettes are also useful. A flushing cannula is used to remove articular debris, blood clots, and fibrin tags at the end of the procedure. A motorized synovial resector is useful for improving visualization of certain areas of the joint, for removing fibrin tags, or for debriding partial-thickness cartilaginous lesions (fibrillation). Small osteotomes or arthroscopic knives are optional and rarely used in bovine arthroscopy.

Surgery Suite

Arthroscopy, especially on a nonseptic joint, must be performed in a controlled, clean environment with limited access. The animal is placed in dorsal (most commonly) or in lateral recumbency on an adjustable hydraulic surgery table padded with a thick mat. Small calves can be placed in a V-shaped table. The limb is held suspended during aseptic preparation.

Surgical Draping

Waterproof drapes are essential to avoid contamination of the surgical field (**Fig. 2**). An incise drape should ideally be placed over and around the joint. The joint may need to be manipulated to improve visualization of certain areas within it, so the drapes need to be properly secured to the animal.

ANESTHESIA

General anesthesia is recommended for bovine arthroscopy. It increases the likelihood of having a successful outcome. The risk of breaking expensive equipment is reduced with an animal under general anesthesia. Animal movements increase the risk of damaging the cartilage with the instruments. Cost of volatile anesthesia is the main disadvantage.

The authors have performed arthroscopic surgery on calves immobilized with a combination of regional anesthesia and intravenous anesthesia. Epidural and brachial plexus anesthesia are safe and easy to perform on calves and have been described elsewhere.[8,9] Combined with a good sedation (diazepam or xylazine) and injectable general anesthesia (double drip: 5% Glyceryl Guaiacolate or Guaifenesin (GGE) and 2 mg/mL ketamine), the arthroscopies were performed without voluntary movement. This less-expensive approach can only be performed on calves and ideally by a surgeon with some arthroscopic experience to decrease surgical time.

STIFLE (FEMOROPATELLAR, MEDIAL, AND LATERAL FEMOROTIBIAL JOINTS)
Indications

The stifle is frequently affected by disorders suitable for arthroscopy. Osteochondrosis lesions are often located in the stifle.[10] Cruciate ligament rupture and meniscal tears

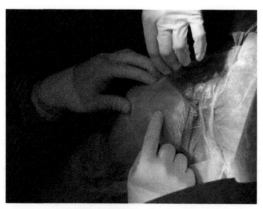

Fig. 2. Impermeable drapes are used to cover the animal during arthroscopy. An incise drape has been placed over the surgical field.

are also reported.[11] In addition, septic arthritis with a hematogenous origin frequently involves the stifle.[12]

Anatomy Review

Three joints form the stifle: the femoropatellar and the lateral and medial femorotibial joints. All these joints communicate in 60% of cases, but the femoropatellar and the medial femorotibial joints always communicate.[13] The lateral femorotibial joint has a large pouch that includes the peroneus tertius and the long digital extensor tendon located proximally on the lateral aspect of the tibia (**Fig. 3**).

In cattle, 3 patellar ligaments attach the patella to the tuberosity of the tibia. These ligaments, along with the medial and lateral collateral ligaments, are important landmarks for arthroscopic portal location. The cranial approach is the safest way to enter the joints because there are no neurovascular structures in that area. The caudal approach is not discussed in this article because its use is only anecdotal.

Surgical Procedure (Dorsal Recumbency with Joint Distension)

Femoropatellar joint

Portal location The limb is in extension. A 1-cm skin incision is made between the median and the lateral patellar ligament halfway between the distal end of the patella and the tibial tuberosity. The subcutaneous fascia is incised using a number 11 blade. A blunt trocar is used to insert the arthroscopic cannula under the patella from a lateral approach. When synovial fluid flows from the open stopcock of the cannula, the blunt

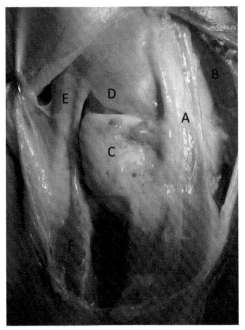

Fig. 3. Lateral view of the lateral femorotibial joint on a cadaver specimen. The skin, the subcutaneous tissue, and the joint capsule have been removed. A, lateral collateral ligament; B, popliteal muscle (origin is intracapsular); C, lateral meniscus; D, lateral femoral condyle; E, tendon of the long digital extensor (origin is intracapsular); F, long digital extensor muscle within the extensor pouch of the lateral femorotibial joint.

trocar is removed and replaced with the arthroscope. The joint is distended and arthroscopic evaluation begins.

Arthroscopic anatomy From this approach the suprapatellar pouch can be viewed. The lateral and medial trochlear ridge, the trochlear groove, and the cartilaginous surface of the patella are seen (**Fig. 4**). The scope can be directed in the lateral pouch next to the lateral trochlear ridge. To enter the medial pouch, the scope must be placed between the median and medial patellar ligament through another portal. The distal aspect of the patella is viewed but is frequently covered by synovium. The distal aspect of the trochlear groove is difficult to evaluate because of the abundant synovium and the difficulty of turning the scope back on itself. Therefore, the communication between the femoropatellar joint and the medial femorotibial joint is rarely seen.

Medial femorotibial joint

Lateral portal location We use the same skin incision already described between the lateral and median patellar ligaments. The joint is then flexed to 60° and the deep fascia is incised with a number 11 blade. A blunt trocar is used to insert the arthroscopic cannula within the abaxial portion of the cranial pouch. When synovial fluid flows from the open stopcock of the cannula, the blunt trocar is removed and replaced with the arthroscope. The joint is distended and arthroscopic evaluation begins.

Arthroscopic anatomy From this approach, the femoral condyle and the dorsal aspect of the medial meniscus are seen (**Fig. 5**).

Medial portal location With the limb extended, a 1-cm skin incision is made between the median and medial patellar ligament, halfway between the distal end of the patella and the tibial tuberosity. The joint is then flexed to 60° and the deep fascia is incised with a number 11 blade. A blunt trocar is used to insert the arthroscopic cannula within the axial portion of the cranial pouch. When synovial fluid flows from the open stopcock of the cannula, the blunt trocar is removed and replaced with the arthroscope. The joint is distended and arthroscopic evaluation begins.

Arthroscopic anatomy From this approach, the scope can easily go in the axial portion of the cranial pouch of the medial femorotibial joint. The tibial intercondylar eminence, the axial portion of the medial femoral condyle, and the medial meniscus are seen.

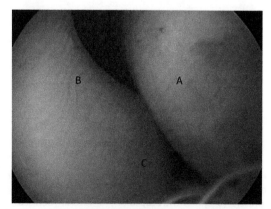

Fig. 4. Arthroscopic view of the patella (A), the trochlear groove (B) and the medial trochlear ridge (C) from the lateral approach of the femoropatellar joint.

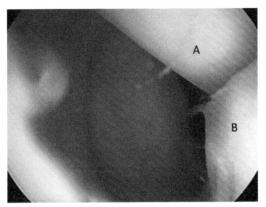

Fig. 5. Arthroscopic view of the medial femoral condyle (A) and the medial meniscus (B) from the lateral approach of the cranial pouch of the medial femorotibial joint.

When looking proximally, the caudal cruciate ligament can be seen in its extrasynovial space (**Fig. 6**).

Lateral femorotibial joint

Medial portal location We use the same skin incision as described previously for the medial portal of the medial femorotibial or femoropatellar joint. The joint is then flexed to 60° and the deep fascia is incised with a number 11 blade. A blunt trocar is used to insert the arthroscopic cannula within the abaxial portion of the cranial pouch. When synovial fluid flows from the open stopcock of the cannula, the blunt trocar is removed and replaced with the arthroscope. The joint is distended and arthroscopic evaluation begins.

Arthroscopic anatomy From this approach, it is possible to slide the scope beneath the long extensor tendon in the abaxial portion of the cranial pouch. Then, the popliteal muscle tendon, the lateral femoral condyle, and the lateral meniscus are seen (**Fig. 7**). A larger portion of the lateral meniscus is seen compared with its medial counterpart.

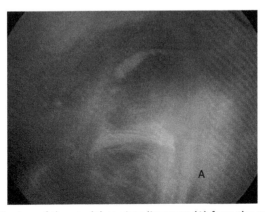

Fig. 6. Arthroscopic view of the caudal cruciate ligament (A) from the medial approach of the cranial pouch of the medial femorotibial joint. The ligament is intracapsular but extrasynovial.

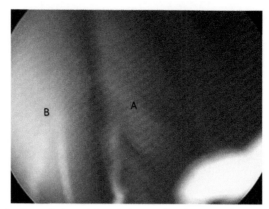

Fig. 7. Arthroscopic view of the origin of the popliteal muscle (A) on the lateral femoral condyle (B) from the medial approach of the cranial pouch of the lateral femorotibial joint.

Lateral portal location The skin incision is located at the same level as the lateral portal for the medial femorotibial and femoropatellar joints. The joint is then flexed to 60° and the deep fascia is incised with a number 11 blade. A blunt trocar is used to insert the arthroscopic cannula within the axial portion of the cranial pouch. When synovial fluid flows from the open stopcock of the cannula, the blunt trocar is removed and replaced with the arthroscope. The joint is distended and arthroscopic evaluation begins.

Arthroscopic anatomy From this approach, the origin of the long digital extensor tendon on the femoral condyle is seen (**Fig. 8**). The axial portion of the lateral femoral condyle and lateral meniscus is seen. The lateral meniscotibial ligament is visualized.

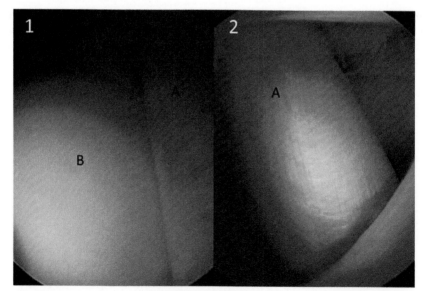

Fig. 8. (1) Arthroscopic view of the origin of the long digital extensor (A) on the lateral femoral condyle (B) from a lateral approach of the cranial pouch of the lateral femorotibial joint. (2) The long digital extensor tendon (A) going distally within the extensor pouch.

The cranial cruciate ligament can be seen in its extrasynovial space in the septum separating the femorotibial joints. This space is filled with fat and the cranial cruciate ligament does not appear clearly except when ruptured (**Fig. 9**).

Extensor pouch evaluation The medial portal is used to slide the scope in the large extensor pouch. Directing the blunt trocar distally offers a better viewing window for evaluation of this pouch.

Technical notes On older cattle, the authors have used sharp trocars to penetrate the fibrotic joint capsule and thickened synovial membrane. Evaluating all 3 joints during the same anesthetic episode is challenging in adult cattle because of fluid extravasation.

HOCK (TARSOCRURAL JOINT)
Indications

As for the stifle, the bovine hock is predisposed to septic arthritis. It is a common site of osteochondrosis and degenerative joint disease.

Anatomy Review

The hock is composed of 4 joints: tarsocrural, proximal intertarsal (PIJ), distal intertarsal (DIJ), and tarsometatarsal joints. The tarsocrural and the PIJ communicate in all cases.[14] Most of the disorders found within the hock involve these articulations. The DIJ and the tarsometatarsal joints communicate in 30% of cases. They rarely communicate with the other joints.

On the dorsal aspect of the joint, the extensor tendons and the peroneus tertius cover the articulation creating a medial and a large lateral dorsal pouch. On the lateral pouch, the cranial branch of the lateral saphenous has to be located before incision of the superficial fascia.

On the plantar aspect of the joint, a medial pouch and a large lateral pouch are present. The medial pouch is smaller because of the deep digital flexor tendon sheath (tarsal sheath). On the medial pouch, the medial saphenous vein and, on the lateral pouch, the caudal branch of the lateral saphenous vein have to be located before incising the superficial fascia.

In cattle, the lateral malleolus is prominent and covers most of the lateral aspect of the large lateral trochlear ridge. The talus has 2 trochleae (**Fig. 10**). The proximal

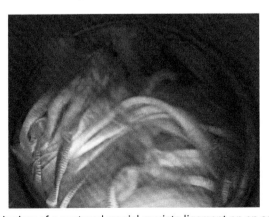

Fig. 9. Arthroscopic view of a ruptured cranial cruciate ligament on an adult bull from the lateral approach of the cranial pouch of the lateral femorotibial joint.

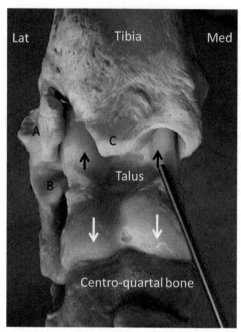

Fig. 10. Tarsocrural and proximal intertarsal joint. The talus has a proximal and a distal trochlea. The black arrow shows the proximal trochlea articulating with the distal tibia. The white arrows show the distal trochlea articulating with the centroquartal bone. A, lateral malleolus; B, calcaneus; C, distal intermediate ridge of the tibia.

trochlea articulates with the distal tibia and the distal trochlea with the centroquartal bone. In cattle, the centroquartal bone results from the fusion of the central and fourth tarsal bones. The second and the third tarsal bones are fused and the first tarsal bone stands alone in a medial and plantar location. The calcaneus articulates with the centroquartal bone, the talus, and the distal tibia (lateral malleolus).

Surgical Procedure (Dorsal Recumbency with Joint Distension)

Dorsal approach

Lateral portal With the joint in extension, the skin is incised 1 cm in the middle of the large lateral pouch. Careful evaluation of the subcutaneous tissue is performed before incising the superficial fascia and the joint capsule with a number 11 blade. A blunt trocar is used to insert the arthroscopic cannula in the lateral pouch. When synovial fluid flows from the open stopcock of the cannula, the blunt trocar is removed and replaced with the arthroscope. The joint is flexed and the arthroscope is directed in the medial pouch. The joint is distended and arthroscopic evaluation begins.

Arthroscopic anatomy The medial malleolus is first visualized (**Fig. 11**). The distal intermediate ridge of the tibia and the lateral malleolus (partially covered with synovium) are then seen. Going back in the medial pouch, the medial trochlear ridge, the trochlear groove, and the lateral trochlear ridge of the talus are seen. The scope is then directed distally to evaluate the calcaneus, the distal end of the lateral malleolus, and the talus (**Fig. 12**).

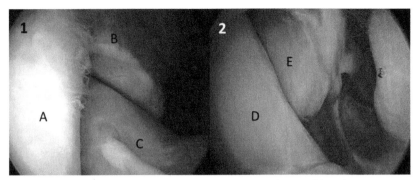

Fig. 11. Lateral approach of dorsal pouch of the tarsocrural joint. (*1*) Arthroscopic view of the lateral malleolus (A), the distal intermediate ridge of the tibia (B), the lateral trochlear ridge of the talus (C). (*2*) With the arthroscope advanced further medially, the medial trochlear ridge of the talus (D), and the medial malleolus (E) are shown.

Medial portal The technique is similar to the lateral portal but the incision is located at the medial aspect of the extensors. It is usually created under arthroscopic guidance with the scope already in the dorsolateral pouch.

Arthroscopic anatomy From this approach the visualization of the lateral malleolus and the lateral trochlear ridge of the talus are improved. The medial structures are difficult to see because the manipulation of the scope is more difficult from the medial approach.

Plantar approach
Lateral portal With the joint in a 45° flexion, a 1-cm skin incision is made in the middle of the lateral pouch. Careful evaluation of the subcutaneous tissue is performed before incising the superficial fascia and the joint capsule with a number 11 blade. A blunt trocar is used to insert the arthroscopic cannula in the lateral pouch. When synovial fluid flows from the open stopcock of the cannula, the blunt trocar is removed and replaced with the arthroscope. The joint is distended and arthroscopic evaluation begins.

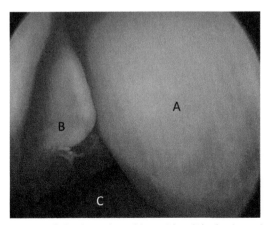

Fig. 12. Arthroscopic view of the lateral trochlear ridge (A), the lateral malleolus (B), and the calcaneus (C) from a lateral approach of the dorsal pouch of the tarsocrural joint.

Arthroscopic anatomy The plantar surface of the talus is first seen. The talocalcaneal joint is then seen distally (**Fig. 13**). Following the calcaneus laterally, the tibiocalcaneal joint can be viewed (**Fig. 14**) (articulation between calcaneus and lateral malleolus). Coming back medially and looking proximally, the medial trochlear ridge and the trochlear groove can be seen by a centrally located opening confined between 2 synovial folds (**Fig. 15**). Because of these folds, the lateral trochlear ridge is difficult to see from this approach. The distal tibia is seen sliding on the trochlear groove of the talus.

Medial portal The technique is similar to that used for the lateral portal. From this approach, the medial saphenous vein has to be localized and care should be taken not to enter the tarsal sheath. This portal is usually created under arthroscopic guidance.

Arthroscopic anatomy From this approach, the lateral trochlear ridge and the trochlear groove can be seen by sliding the scope under the synovial folds previously described. The dorsal aspect of the talus and the calcaneus can be viewed, but the calcaneus cannot be followed laterally as was done from the lateral portal. As for the lateral portal, the medial trochlear ridge is difficult to see from this approach because of the synovial folds.

Technical notes It is easier to start with the lateral approach, either from a dorsal or a plantar approach. Always locate the saphenous veins and the tarsal sheath before entering through the plantaromedial portal. The plantar portals are difficult to create without joint distension. Fluid extravasation should be anticipated if all 4 approaches are performed during the same anesthetic episode.

CARPUS (ANTEBRACHIOCARPAL AND MIDDLE CARPAL JOINTS)
Indications

Septic arthritis of the carpus can be treated by arthroscopic lavage and debridement, similarly to the other joints. Less frequently, osteochondrosis lesions may also be

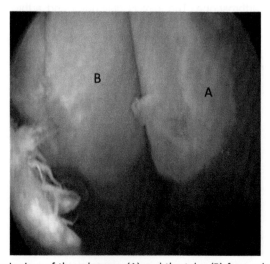

Fig. 13. Arthroscopic view of the calcaneus (A) and the talus (B) from a lateral approach of the plantar pouch of the tarsocrural joint.

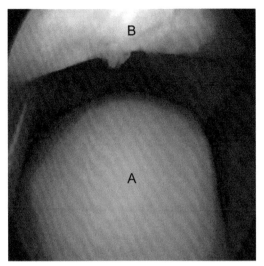

Fig. 14. Arthroscopic view of the calcaneus (A) and the lateral malleolus (B) from a lateral approach of the plantar pouch of the tarsocrural joint.

found in the carpus. They seem to be located in the radiocarpal joint and more frequently involve the distal radius. The lesions are often diffuse and have the appearance of degenerative joint disease rather than osteochondrosis lesions.

Anatomy Review

The carpus is composed of 3 joints: the antebrachiocarpal, middle carpal, and carpometacarpal joints. The middle carpal and carpometacarpal joints communicate in all cases. A communication with the antebrachiocarpal joint is present in 13% of cases.[15]

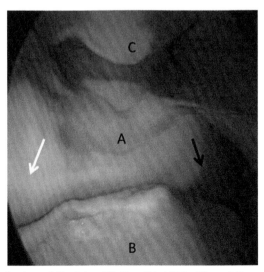

Fig. 15. Arthroscopic view of the talus (A), the distal tibia (B), and the calcaneus (C) from a lateral approach of the plantar pouch of the tarsocrural joint. The black arrow is the medial trochlear ridge and the white arrow is the lateral trochlear ridge of the talus.

The extensor carpi radialis tendon and its sheath separate the dorsal pouch of all three joints creating a medial and a lateral dorsal pouch for arthroscopic evaluation.

The articular surface of the antebrachiocarpal joint is irregular, making it difficult to move the arthroscope from medial to lateral and vice versa. The lateral styloid process of the distal radius extends beyond the joint surface and articulates with the ulnar bone. The cuboidal bones in the first row are, from medial to lateral, the radial, intermediate, and ulnar bones. The distal row includes the fused second and third carpal bones, and the fourth carpal bone (**Fig. 16**). The accessory carpal bone at the palmar aspect of the joint articulates with the ulnar bone.

Surgical Procedure (Dorsal or Lateral Recumbency with Joint Distension)

Antebrachiocarpal joint

Lateral portal The lateral pouch is larger and should be entered first to evaluate the joint cavity. With the joint flexed (135°), a skin incision is made about 1 cm lateral to the extensor carpi radialis tendon, slightly distal to the distal aspect of the radius. The joint is then distended with an 18-G needle attached to a syringe and sterile saline until bulging out. The superficial fascia, the extensor retinaculum, and the joint capsule are incised using a number 11 blade. A blunt trocar is used to insert the arthroscopic cannula in the lateral pouch. When synovial fluid flows from the open stopcock of the cannula, the blunt trocar is removed and replaced by the arthroscope. The scope is passed beneath the extensor tendon into the medial pouch. The joint is distended and arthroscopic evaluation begins.

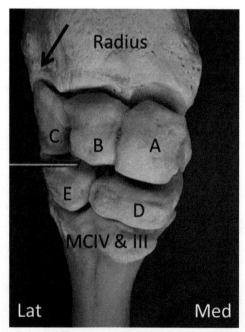

Fig. 16. Antebrachiocarpal, middle carpal, and carpometacarpal joints. A, radial carpal bone; B, intermediate carpal bone; C, ulnar carpal bone (close contact with the large styloid process of the distal radius [*black arrow*]); D, fused second and third carpal bones; E, fourth carpal bone; MCIV & III, Metacarpal bone IV and III.

Arthroscopic anatomy From medial to lateral, the radial bone and the medial joint capsule are first seen. Then the junction between the radial bone and the intermediate bone (**Fig. 17**) is recognized before seeing the junction between the intermediate and the ulnar bone. By increasing flexion of the joint, a small interosseous ligament can be seen between the intermediate and the ulnar bones. Looking proximally at the radius, a normal cleft is seen from each side of the sagittal ridge of the distal radius (**Fig. 18**).

Medial portal The incision is located 0.5 cm medial to the extensor carpi radialis tendon, proximal to the radial bone to be able to slide the arthroscope beyond the sagittal crest of the distal radius. This portal is usually created under arthroscopic guidance with the scope already located in the lateral portal.

Arthroscopic anatomy From this approach, it is difficult to view the radial carpal bone. The intermediate and the ulnar bones are seen. The distal radius can also be evaluated.

Middle carpal joint

Lateral portal The lateral pouch is larger and should be used first to evaluate the joint cavity. With the joint in flexion (135°) and before distension, a skin incision is created about 1 cm lateral to the extensor carpi radialis tendon. The joint is then distended as previously described, and the superficial fascia, the extensor retinaculum, and the joint capsule are incised using a number 11 blade. A blunt trocar is used to insert the arthroscopic cannula in the lateral pouch. When synovial fluid flows from the open stopcock of the cannula, the blunt trocar is removed and replaced by the arthroscope. The scope is passed beneath the extensor tendon into the medial pouch. The joint is distended and arthroscopic evaluation begins.

Arthroscopic anatomy From medial to lateral, the radial carpal bone is first observed. Its junction with the intermediate bone is then viewed before localizing the ulnar bone. The large fused second and third carpal bone is seen distally. Its junction with the fourth carpal bone is viewed by directing the arthroscope laterally (**Fig. 19**).

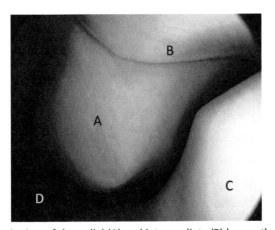

Fig. 17. Arthroscopic view of the radial (A) and intermediate (B) bones, the distal radius (C), and the joint capsule (D) from a lateral approach of the antebrachiocarpal joint.

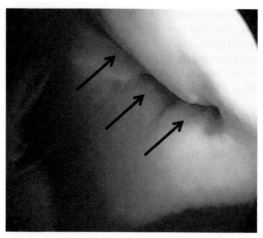

Fig. 18. Arthroscopic view of the distal radius from a lateral approach of the antebrachio-carpal joint. The black arrows show the normal cleft located on each side of the distal sagittal ridge of the radius.

Medial portal This pouch is small and this portal should be created under arthroscopic guidance. The incision is located 0.5 cm medial to the extensor carpi radialis tendon, slightly more distal compared with the lateral portal.

Arthroscopic anatomy In addition to the structures seen from the lateral approach, a small interosseus ligament can be seen between the fused second and third carpal bones and the fourth carpal bone (**Fig. 20**). If the portal is located too proximally within this pouch, it is difficult to slide the arthroscope in the lateral pouch because of the prominent radial bone.

Technical notes The carpal examination should be started from the lateral approach. The correct portal location in the medial pouch is crucial to being able to slide the arthroscope in the lateral pouch. Flexion and extension expose different areas of the joints.

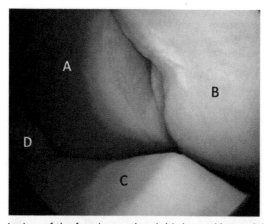

Fig. 19. Arthroscopic view of the fused second and third carpal bones (A), the fourth carpal bone (B), the intermediate carpal bone (C), and the radial carpal bone (D) from a lateral approach of the middle carpal joint.

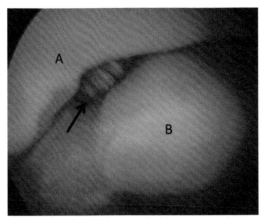

Fig. 20. Arthroscopic view of the middle carpal joint from the medial approach with the joint in complete flexion. Small interosseous ligament (*black arrow*) between the fuse second and third carpal bones (A) and the fourth carpal bone (B).

FETLOCK (METACARPOPHALANGEAL AND METATARSOPHALANGEAL JOINTS)
Indications

Septic arthritis and osteochondral injury are the main indications for fetlock arthroscopy.

Anatomy Review

The fetlock of cattle is divided into a lateral and a medial compartment. These compartments always communicate.[16] However, on the dorsal aspect and sometimes on the palmar/plantar aspect, a fold of synovial membrane separates the joint. This membrane is easily ruptured on the palmar/plantar aspect. On the dorsal aspect, this membrane is thicker and more difficult to rupture without the use of a sharp trocar.

The palmar/plantar pouches are big and spacious on the abaxial aspect of each flexor tendon (lateral and medial). The dorsal pouch is small on the abaxial aspect of the common (forelimb) and long digital extensor tendons (hind limb) and on the abaxial aspect of the lateral digital extensor tendon (forelimb and hind limb). When creating the palmar/plantar portal, care must be taken not to damage the palmar and plantar common digital arteries, veins, and nerves.

Four proximal sesamoid bones and their ligaments, a double condyle metacarpal and metatarsal bone, and 2 proximal phalanges create this articulation (**Fig. 21**).

Surgical Procedure (Dorsal or Lateral Recumbency with Joint Distension)
Dorsal approach
Lateral or medial pouch With the joint extended, a 1-cm skin incision is created about 1 cm abaxial to the extensor tendon in the proximal aspect of the outpouching created following joint distension.[5] The superficial fascia and the joint capsule are incised with a number 11 blade. A blunt trocar is used to insert the arthroscopic cannula in the pouch. When synovial fluid flows from the open stopcock of the cannula, the blunt trocar is removed and replaced by the arthroscope. The joint is distended and arthroscopic evaluation begins. To evaluate the contralateral part of the joint, the arthroscope is removed and a blunt trocar is inserted in the cannula. This unit is then

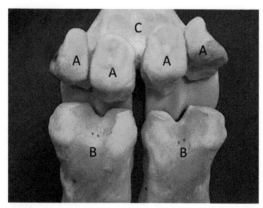

Fig. 21. Palmar/plantar aspect of the fetlock joint in cattle. A, proximal sesamoid bones; B, first phalanges; C, fused third and fourth metacarpal bones.

pushed in the contralateral compartment. The trocar is removed and the arthroscope is replaced. The joint is distended and the evaluation continues.

Arthroscopic anatomy The metacarpal/metatarsal condyle and its prominent sagittal ridge are viewed. The proximal attachment of the joint capsule on the metacarpal/metatarsal bone is seen. Little of the proximal phalanx is seen. The best evaluation is obtained when each compartment is evaluated from its ipsilateral side.

Palmar/plantar approach
Lateral or medial pouch With the joint flexed, a 1-cm skin incision is created in the middle and in the proximal third of the outpouching created following joint distension. The superficial fascia and the joint capsule are incised with a number 11 blade. A blunt trocar is used to insert the arthroscopic cannula in the pouch. When synovial fluid flows from the open stopcock of the cannula, the blunt trocar is removed and replaced by the arthroscope. The joint is distended and arthroscopic evaluation begins.

Arthroscopic anatomy All the palmar structures are visible from the medial or the lateral compartment of the palmar pouch. The 4 proximal sesamoid bones and their suspensory attachments are seen. The palmar aspect of the metacarpal condyle and its sagittal ridge are visualized. The palmar aspect of the proximal phalanges and the cruciate sesamoid ligaments are seen (**Fig. 22**).

Technical notes Make sure that the portal is located in the proximal aspect of the dorsal and palmar/plantar pouch to help with manipulation of the scope. From the dorsal pouch, the contralateral evaluation through the medial septum does not allow complete evaluation of the joint.

OTHER JOINTS
Elbow (Cubital Joint)

The elbow joint has 3 pouches: caudoproximal (olecranon), lateral, and medial.[17] The lateral and medial pouches are separated by the lateral and medial collateral ligaments respectively, which further divide the pouches into cranial and caudal compartments. The large caudoproximal pouch allows an easy arthroscopic evaluation.

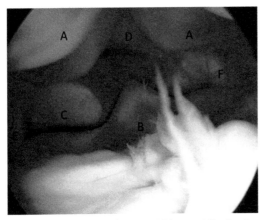

Fig. 22. Arthroscopic view of the proximal sesamoid bones (A), distal metacarpal bone (B), first phalange (C), sesamoid cruciate ligament (D), abaxial (E), and axial (F) collateral ligaments from a proximal approach of the palmar pouch of the metacarpophalangeal joint.

The medial pouch is difficult to reach in cattle because of its proximity to the body wall. Therefore, only the caudoproximal and the craniolateral approaches are discussed here.

The animal is placed in lateral recumbency with the affected limb uppermost, and the joint is distended.

- Craniolateral approach: the arthroscopic portal is created cranially to the lateral collateral ligament. The humeral condyles can be seen, separated by a synovial fossa. Only a small portion of the proximal radius can be evaluated. If needed, a more cranially located portal can be created between the extensor carpi radialis and common digital extensor muscles. From this approach, it is difficult to slide the arthroscope beneath the collateral ligament to evaluate the caudal aspect of the joint.
- Caudoproximal approach: the arthroscopic portal is located between the lateral epicondyle of the humerus and the proximal aspect of the olecranon. The scope is directed cranially and distally toward the anconeal process. The medial and lateral humeral condyles can be seen. The anconeal process is readily located. Flexion and extension of the joint help visualize a larger portion of the condyle.

Shoulder (Scapulohumeral Joint)

The shoulder joint is composed of the humeral head and the glenoid cavity.[18,19] It is a small joint that is only accessible arthroscopically through a craniolateral or caudolateral approach.

With the animal in lateral recumbency and the leg slightly adducted, a spinal needle is inserted in the joint and 60 mL of lactated Ringer solution is infused to achieve maximum distention of the joint. Then, a skin incision is made either cranially or caudally to the tendon of the infraspinatus muscle. From this incision, the arthroscopic sleeve and trocar are directed slightly distally and caudally (craniolateral approach) or slightly distally and cranially (caudolateral approach). The trocar is removed and the arthroscope is inserted to evaluate the joint. Except for the caudal and medial parts of the joint, most of the articular cartilage can be seen with these approaches.

Hip (Coxofemoral Joint)

The hip is formed by the acetabulum and the femoral head.[20,21] It is a deep joint that is difficult to access in adult cattle. A spinal needle is used to distend the joint under ultrasonographic guidance. Longer instruments and arthroscopes may be useful on adult cattle. An arthroscope with a viewing angle of 70° is not mandatory but may improve the examination of the joint.

With the animal in lateral recumbency and with the leg supported, a skin incision is created about 2 cm dorsal to the greater trochanter halfway between its cranial and caudal ends. The arthroscopic sleeve and blunt trocar are introduced in the joint in a cranial and ventral direction. The instrument portal is located 5 cm cranial to the arthroscopic portal. Flexion and extension of the joint improve its evaluation. Traction with the limb in adduction can improve evaluation of the medial aspect of the joint.

ACKNOWLEDGMENTS

The authors thank Dr Marketa Kopal for her support and her help in the preparation of this article.

REFERENCES

1. Hurtig MB. Recent developments in the use of arthroscopy in cattle. Vet Clin North Am Food Anim Pract 1985;1:175–93.
2. Gaughan EM. Arthroscopy in food animal practice. Vet Clin North Am Food Anim Pract 1996;12:233–47.
3. Munroe GA, Cauvin ER. The use of arthroscopy in the treatment of septic arthritis in two Highland calves. Br Vet J 1994;150:439–49.
4. McIlwraith CW, Nixon AJ, Wright IM, et al. Diagnostic and surgical arthroscopy in the horse. 3rd edition. Philadelphia: Mosby Elsevier; 2006.
5. Blaser M, Bertagnoli A, Räber M, et al. Arthroscopic approaches to the fetlock joint of adult cattle: a cadaver study. Vet J 2012;193(3):701–6.
6. Vatistas NJ, Wright IM, Dyson SJ. Comparison of arthroscopy and arthrotomy for the treatment of osteochondritic lesions in the femoropatellar joint of horses. Vet Rec 1995;137(25):629–32.
7. Reagan BF, McInerny VK, Treadwell BV, et al. Irrigating solutions for arthroscopy. A metabolic study. J Bone Joint Surg Am 1983;65(5):629–31.
8. Edmondson MA. Local and regional anesthesia in cattle. Vet Clin North Am Food Anim Pract 2008;24(2):211–26.
9. Iwamoto J, Yamagishi N, Sasaki K, et al. A novel technique of ultrasound-guided brachial plexus block in calves. Res Vet Sci 2012;93(3):1467–71.
10. Trostle SS, Nicoll RG, Forrest LJ, et al. Clinical and radiographic findings, treatment, and outcome in cattle with osteochondrosis: 29 cases (1986-1996). J Am Vet Med Assoc 1997;211(12):1566–70.
11. Ducharme NG. Stifle injuries in cattle. Vet Clin North Am Food Anim Pract 1996; 12(1):59–84.
12. Rohde C, Anderson DE, Desrochers A, et al. Synovial fluid analysis in cattle: a review of 130 cases. Vet Surg 2000;29(4):341–6.
13. Desrochers A, St-Jean G, Cash WC, et al. Characterization of anatomic communications between the femoropatellar joint and lateral and medial femorotibial joints in cattle, using intra-articular latex, positive contrast arthrography, and fluoroscopy. Am J Vet Res 1996;57(6):798–802.

14. Desrochers A. Characterization of anatomic communications of the carpus, fetlock, stifle, and tarsus in cattle using intra-articular latex and positive contrast arthrography [Thesis (MS)]. Manhattan: Kansas State University; 1995. p. 94.
15. Desrochers A, St-Jean G, Cash WC, et al. Characterization of anatomic communications among the antebrachiocarpal, middle carpal, and carpometacarpal joints in cattle, using intra-articular latex, positive-contrast arthrography, and fluoroscopy. Am J Vet Res 1997;58(1):7–10.
16. Desrochers A, St-Jean G, Cash WC, et al. Characterization of anatomic communications of the fetlock in cattle, using intra-articular latex injection and positive-contrast arthrography. Am J Vet Res 1997;58(7):710–2.
17. Nixon AJ. Arthroscopic approaches and intraarticular anatomy of the equine elbow. Vet Surg 1990;19(2):93–101.
18. Nixon AJ. Diagnostic and surgical arthroscopy of the equine shoulder joint. Vet Surg 1987;16(1):44–52.
19. Bertone AL, McIlwraith CW. Arthroscopic surgical approaches and intraarticular anatomy of the equine shoulder joint. Vet Surg 1987;16(4):312–7.
20. Honnas CM, Zamos DT, Ford TS. Arthroscopy of the coxofemoral joint of foals. Vet Surg 1993;22(2):115–21.
21. Nixon AJ. Diagnostic and operative arthroscopy of the coxofemoral joint in horses. Vet Surg 1994;23(5):377–85.

Traumatic Conditions of the Coxofemoral Joint
Luxation, Femoral Head-Neck Fracture, Acetabular Fracture

Emma Marchionatti, DMV*, Gilles Fecteau, DMV,
André Desrochers, DMV, MS

KEYWORDS

- Cattle • Hip • Coxofemoral joint • Coxofemoral luxation • Capital physeal fracture
- Femoral neck fracture • Acetabular fracture

KEY POINTS

- Coxofemoral luxations and fractures are the most common orthopedic problems of the hip in cattle.
- Femoral capital physeal fracture or slipped capital femoral epiphysis is the most common hip injury in young animals.
- Fractures of the femoral neck, the acetabulum, or the greater trochanter may be associated with coxofemoral luxations in adult cows.
- Diagnosis and treatment of hip fractures and luxations remain a challenge for the veterinarian.

INTRODUCTION

Coxofemoral luxations and fractures are the most common orthopedic problem of the hip in cattle.[1,2] Septic arthritis in calves and adult cattle and hip dysplasia in various predisposed breeds have also been reported.[3]

The diagnosis and treatment of hip abnormalities remain a challenge for the veterinarian. The coxofemoral joint is well covered and protected by the gluteal muscles, making palpation and examination difficult. Any joint anomaly without anatomic disruption cannot be noticed easily. Joint distension from septic arthritis or subluxation is subtle and most likely missed during physical examination. However, a fractured greater trochanter or a coxofemoral luxation can be diagnosed with basic knowledge of the normal anatomy.

The authors have nothing to disclose.
Department of Clinical Sciences, Faculty of Veterinary Medicine, Université de Montréal, 3200 rue Sicotte, Saint-Hyacinthe, Québec J2S 2M2, Canada
* Corresponding author.
E-mail address: emma.marchionatti@umontreal.ca

The hip joint is a spheroid-type joint that unites the femur to the coxal bone (**Fig. 1**). The coxal bone receives the femoral head in a cuplike structure formed at the union of the 3 pelvic bones—ilium, ischium, and pubis— the acetabulum. The semilunar articular surface of the acetabulum presents a cranioventral notch and is deepened by a fibrocartilaginous rim, the labrum acetabulare, which is in continuity with the bony margin. The transverse acetabular ligament is a part of the labrum and it crosses the acetabular notch. The joint capsule is attached to the margin of the acetabulum.[4] In cattle, the acetabulum is shallower than in horses, but the labrum is wider.[4,5]

The cylindroid femoral head, supported by the femoral neck, points in an axial direction (**Fig. 2**). The hemispherical articular surface presents a medioventral shallow notch, the fovea capitis, which provides attachment for the femoral head ligament; it is cylindroid and runs from the femoral head to the acetabular fossa. Lateral to the head is the greater trochanter, which provides attachment for the gluteal muscles. The trochanteric fossa separates the greater trochanter and the neck of the femur and provides a site of insertion for the deep hip muscles.[6]

The hip joint stability depends on 3 distinctive structures: the joint capsule, which is reinforced cranially, the cylindroid femoral head ligament and the massive muscle mass formed by the gluteal muscles and the deep hip muscles. The hip joint is naturally flexed when the animal is standing. The significant movements of the hips are the flexion and extension. The gluteal muscles (gluteus superficialis, gluteus medius, gluteus accessorius, gluteus profondus) originate at the coxal bone and end at the greater trochanter and allow the movement of extension, and limited movement of abduction and rotation of the limb. The cranial and caudal gluteal nerves, branches of the sciatic nerve, innervate them. The deep hip muscles (obturatoris externus, gemelli, quadratus femoris) allow very limited adduction and rotation of the limb and are innervated by the sciatic and obturator nerves.[7]

Physical Examination and Diagnostic Procedures Specific to the Hip

The onset of clinical signs is sudden and varies from severe lameness to recumbency. An animal with a chronic hip problem will usually have gluteal atrophy with a prominent greater trochanter. The gluteal muscles of the normal leg can be hypertrophied and

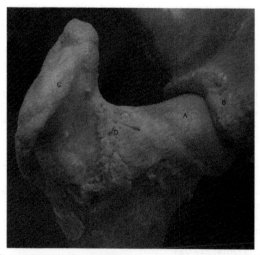

Fig. 1. Right coxofemoral joint of an adult cow, cranial view. A, femoral head; B, acetabulum; C, greater trochanter; D, femoral neck.

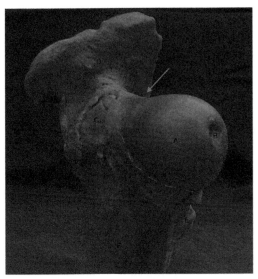

Fig. 2. Right proximal femur, cranial view. A, femoral head; B, fovea capitis; C, femoral neck; D, greater trochanter; E, minor trochanter; F, femoral shaft; dashed line, joint capsule attachment; arrow, trochanteric fossa.

somehow look abnormal. If the animal is young, a varus of the contralateral normal leg is often observed.[8]

Unless there is visible asymmetry between the 2 hips, the diagnosis or location of the painful area is often by ruling out the more common musculoskeletal diseases. The examination of the affected leg starts from the digit up to the hip joint. Unless there is an obvious cause of lameness, the foot should always be pared away to exclude sole abscesses or other painful digital diseases.[8]

Location of the greater trochanter in relation to the ischium and tuber coxae will help to diagnose luxation or femoral head fracture. The examination can be done with the animal standing or in lateral recumbency. If the animal is standing, the limb is abducted gently by an assistant while the clinician puts his hands over and medial to the greater trochanter. Depending on the size and the character of the animal, this manipulation can be done by one person or it may be impossible to do. If crepitation is felt, luxation or fracture of the hip is suspected. Reaction of pain at flexion or extension is more compatible with septic arthritis. In young animals, it is possible to put enough pressure on the hip joint through the muscle by pressing on the greater trochanter to stimulate a painful reaction. It is always better to compare with the normal side, but not always possible because the animal is reluctant to bear weight on the affected leg.[8]

The same examination and manipulation can be done on the recumbent cattle. The animal must be in lateral recumbency position to freely move the coxofemoral joint. As discussed earlier, the size and character of the animal will influence the quality of the examination. A complete musculoskeletal examination, with special attention to both hips, is routinely performed on downer dairy cattle in the authors' clinics: abduction, adduction, flexion, and extension of the leg are done.

Finally, rectal palpation is used to diagnose hip luxation whereby the femoral head can be palpated in the obturator foramen if ventrally luxated.

Ancillary tests of hip conditions are limited because of the depth of the joint; they are difficult to do and special equipment is needed.

Synovial fluid analysis may reveal characteristic changes that may assist diagnosis. However, arthrocentesis of the coxofemoral joint can be a challenge, especially in adults. The joint entry site is cranially to the greater trochanter and to the insertion of the middle gluteus with a caudomedial direction, just dorsal to the femoral neck.[9] An 18-G, 90-mm or longer needle is used. The synovial fluid is usually free flowing; otherwise, a gentle constant aspiration should be performed (**Fig. 3**A). The arthrocentesis can also be performed under ultrasound guidance, thus increasing the precision and decreasing trauma to the joint (see **Fig. 3**B).

Radiographic images are still the most useful ancillary test to evaluate the hip joint. However, a powerful radiography machine is necessary when evaluating adult cattle. The equipment and the technical staff are often available in referral centers only. Practical limitations in the field are considerable and radiographic examination is limited to calves.

Ultrasound is a simple, effective, and noninvasive method that can be used in the proximal hindlimb regions; both soft tissue and bone lesions may be investigated. An experienced ultrasonographer can diagnose joint effusion and coxofemoral luxation in young animals.[10]

Radiography and ultrasound of the hip joint are discussed in more detail in the article on Medical Imaging by Kofler and colleagues in this issue.

COXOFEMORAL LUXATION

Luxation of the coxofemoral joint has been frequently reported in the literature but its frequency in relation to other musculoskeletal problem is unknown.[1,3,10–19] When compared with the horse, the bovine hip has distinctive anatomic particularities predisposing it to luxation: the relatively small femoral head, the shallowness of the acetabulum, the presence of the notches at the acetabular ring margin, and the minimal ligamentous attachments.[1,20] The femoral head ligament is cylindroid and less resistant than in horses and the accessory ligament is absent, which explains the possibility of lateral movements.[4] Therefore, the bovine relies mainly on muscle tone to maintain the intact hip joint.[1]

Coxofemoral luxation may occur in adult animals and in calves. In adults, traumatic injury related to peripartum events, such as milk fever or obstetric paresis, or estrus behavior, are the most frequent causes of hip luxation.[1,3,11–16,21] Bilateral obturator paresis, after dystocia, is a predisposing factor. A cow that develops bilateral

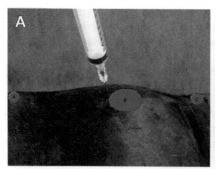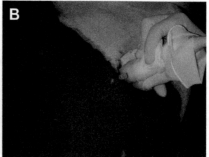

Fig. 3. (*A*) Landmark of the coxofemoral arthrocentesis on a cadaver: the needle is inserted cranially to the greater trochanter and to the insertion of the middle gluteus with a caudomedial direction, just dorsal to the femoral neck. A, tuber coxae; B, greater trochanter; C, tuber ischii. (*B*) Left coxofemoral arthrocentesis under ultrasound guidance on a standing animal.

obturator paresis may go down with both hind legs abducted; hip luxation may develop after the initial trauma or as a result of struggling to stand.[1] In calves, luxations often are subsequent to dystocia and excessive traction during birth. However capital physeal fracture seems to be more frequent as a calving injury.[1,2,17,18]

Four directions of luxation have been described according to the position of the head of the femur in relation to the acetabulum (**Fig. 4**): craniodorsal, caudoventral, caudodorsal, and cranioventral, in order of relative frequency.[1,3,10,14–19,21]

Diagnosis

The diagnosis of coxofemoral luxation in cattle is based on physical examination, but palpation of the femur and pelvic bones can be difficult because of the associated swelling and the surrounding muscle mass.[8,14,22,23] Muscle spasms or damage will prevent any deep palpation. Some animals with a coxofemoral luxation may be recumbent and unable to get up, whereas others may be standing and capable of walking with some easiness. However, minimal weight-bearing is the rule.[3,10–19,21–23] An animal with a craniodorsal coxofemoral luxation is usually unable to bear weight on his leg. The stifle and digits are rotated outward while the hock is rotated inward (**Fig. 5A**). The severe swelling in the gluteal area is another indicator of dorsal hip luxation (see **Fig. 5B**). However, an animal with caudoventral luxation is often incapable of getting up and standing because of the pain engendered by the femoral head position (ventral to the pelvis or in the obturator foramen), the extensive muscle damage, and the potential nerve damage (**Fig. 6**).

The relative position of the greater trochanter to that of the tuber coxae and the tuber ischii should be determined with the animal standing or in lateral recumbency. The normal position of the greater trochanter is ventral to both of these bony prominences and imaginary lines drawn between them will create a "triangle"

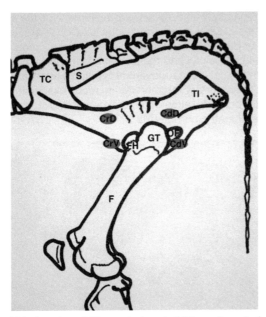

Fig. 4. Directions of hip luxation. CdD, caudodorsal; CdV, caudoventral; CrD, craniodorsal; CrV, cranioventral; F, femur; FH, femoral head; GT, greater trochanter; OF, obturator foramen; S, sacrum; TC, tuber coxae; TI, tuber ischii.

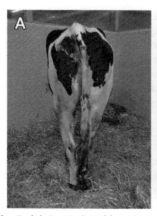
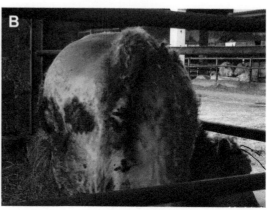

Fig. 5. (*A*) Craniodorsal luxation of the right hip on an adult Holstein cow: there is swelling over the gluteal region. The stifle and digits rotated outward while the hock is rotated inward. (*B*) Male Charolais with a dorsal luxation of the left hip. Notice the severe swelling in the gluteal area. (*Courtesy of* Dr Michele Ballotin, DMV, Miega, Italy.)

(**Fig. 7**).[8,14,22,23] Positioning of the greater trochanter in-line with the tuber coxae and tuber ischii suggests dorsal luxation of the coxofemoral joint.[8,24]

Although the manipulation of the rear limb can be performed standing, a more thorough and complete examination can be achieved when the animal is in lateral recumbency with the affected leg uppermost. Depending on the behavior of the animal, sedation with xylazine might be necessary. In the authors' experience, those manipulations can be performed on dairy cattle without sedation. The entire limb is rotated while performing repeated abduction and adduction, placing one hand on the greater trochanter (**Fig. 8**). Failure to palpate the greater trochanter suggests a ventral luxation. Crepitations and excessive movement of the greater trochanter could be elicited in the case of coxofemoral joint luxation; a greater range of motion of the proximal femur during abduction suggests ventral luxation. The manipulation of a luxated hip could be painful and the animal might not cooperate, rendering the diagnosis difficult. In the case of caudoventral luxation it may be possible to palpate the femoral head in the obturator foramen during rectal examination. In animals with craniodorsal or caudodorsal luxation of the coxofemoral joint, the affected limb may appear to be shorter than the normal side.[8,14,22,23]

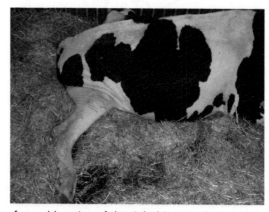

Fig. 6. Ventral coxofemoral luxation of the right hip on a downer cow.

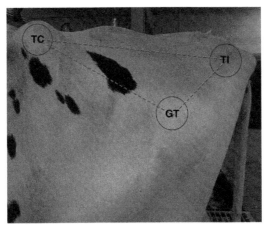

Fig. 7. The triangle formed by the tuber coxae, the tuber ischii, and the greater trochanter. The normal position of the greater trochanter is ventral to both of the bony prominences. GT, greater trochanter; TC, tuber coxae; TI, tuber ischii.

Radiographic views of the hip are useful to confirm coxofemoral luxation, identify associated fractures, and establish a potential treatment and prognosis.[1,22,23,25] Fractures are especially common in caudoventral luxations.[22] Ideally, the animal should be placed in dorsal recumbency with the hind limbs extended caudally and a ventrodorsal

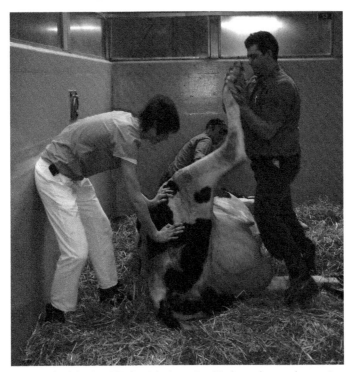

Fig. 8. Manipulation of the hind limb with the animal in lateral recumbency. By performing abduction, adduction, flexion, and extension of the limb, crepitation or excessive movement of the greater trochanter may be felt by placing the hand over it.

view of the pelvis can be obtained (**Figs. 9** and **10**). Depending on the animal's temper, sedation or general anesthesia might be necessary to avoid movements because of the long exposure time. The parameters needed, 100 kV and 200 mA at least, can only be achieved with a powerful fixed radiography machine.[26] A large udder presents additional soft tissue interference, which can be minimized with oblique views (**Fig. 11**).[26] Radiography of the pelvis in the calf can be more readily performed with a portable radiography machine.

A technique for obtaining standing bovine pelvic radiographs has been described.[27] Laterodorsal-lateroventral views were made with the radiographic beam at a 25° to 30° angle to the horizontal plane (**Fig. 12**); the technique required less radiation (70–80 kV and 40–80 mA) than a ventrodorsal view in dorsal recumbency.[25]

Transrectal and transvaginal radiographic examination of the hip joint has also been described in animals standing or in lateral recumbency.[28] The technique requires a flexible, distendable by air pressure, intracavital fixable film holder and the radiographic beam at a 30° to 45° angle. This procedure has been used with good success to identify acetabular fractures, coxarthrosis, and hip luxations,[28] but it is technically demanding, requiring appropriate equipment to avoid unnecessary radiation. Radiographs are less useful in cases of subluxation because of the difficulties in obtaining details in this region.

Ultrasonography has recently been reported as a simple, effective, and noninvasive method for examination of the hip joint in cattle. Normal coxofemoral joint and coxofemoral luxation in different directions have been described in recumbent cows, as well as in standing cows.[10,21,29] Transcutaneous dorsolateral ultrasonographic examination with 5.0-MHz and 3.5-MHz convex transducers allows the identification of the coxofemoral joint in standing and recumbent cows (lateral recumbency) (**Fig. 13**). In the case of luxation the image demonstrates either the ball-shaped femoral head

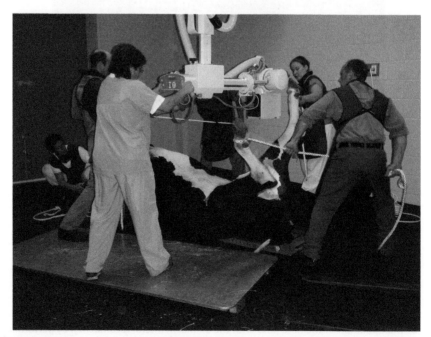

Fig. 9. Positioning of the animal on dorsal recumbency with the hind limbs extended for a radiographic ventrodorsal view of the pelvis.

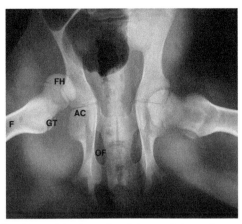

Fig. 10. Ventrodorsal radiographic view of a right cranial coxofemoral luxation on a calf. AC, acetabulum; F, femur; FH, femoral head out of the acetabular cavity; GT, greater trochanter; OF, obturator foramen.

outside the acetabulum or the heterogenic empty joint cavity of the acetabulum, due to fibrin clot/blood and tissue fragments.[21,29]

Transrectal ultrasonography using a 7.5-MHz linear transducer is helpful to diagnose caudoventral luxations by imaging the femoral head in or ventral to the obturator foramen.[21,29]

Treatment

Coxofemoral luxation may be treated by stall rest, closed reduction,[3,12–17] open reduction,[10,11,18,19] or femoral head ostectomy.[30,31]

Although no studies of conservative treatment by stall rest have been published, this approach may lead to the development of pseudoarthrosis in the case of dorsal

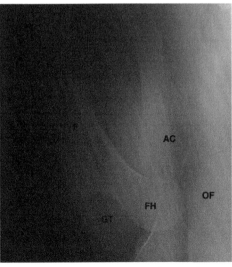

Fig. 11. Ventrodorsal radiographic view of a right caudal coxofemoral luxation on an adult cow. AC, acetabulum; F, femur; FH, femoral head; GT, greater trochanter; OF, obturator foramen.

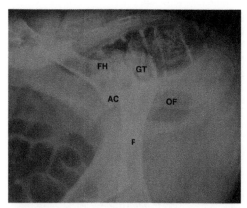

Fig. 12. Lateral oblique radiographic view of a calf with a right dorsocranial coxofemoral luxation. AC, acetabulum; F, femur; FH, femoral head; GT, greater trochanter; OF, obturator foramen.

luxations, as new bone formation occurs on the ilium around the pressure point of the femoral head. However, the animal will remain severely lame and generally not a productive herd member.[1]

Closed reduction of coxofemoral luxations using various techniques has been reported, but recurrence is common.[1] Closed reduction can produce good results if performed within 12 to 24 hours of the injury occurring.[14,15] The prognosis for cases that have been luxated for more than 24 hours is considered to be increasingly poor.[1,14,15] The high likelihood of recurrence following closed reduction can be explained by the inability to accurately achieve adequate reduction. The presence of joint capsule strands, blood, or soft tissue debris into the acetabular cavity may prevent the femoral head from seating properly in the acetabulum[22]; in addition the surrounding damaged muscles and the ruptured joint capsule fail to maintain the femoral head in the acetabular cavity.

If attempting closed reduction, the animal should be sedated and positioned in lateral recumbency with the affected leg uppermost. The cow's pelvis is fixed by a rope placed around the affected leg in the inguinal region to a solid object, as

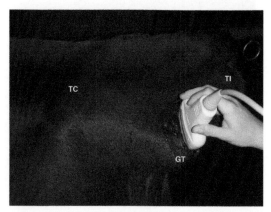

Fig. 13. Ultrasound of the hip joint in standing cattle. The probe is positioned in a transversal plane, parallel to the axis of the femoral neck, or in a oblique plane with craniomedial direction. GT, greater trochanter; TC, tuber coxae; TI, tuber ischii.

a counterforce. A second rope is tied to the distal metatarsal area; while traction is applied, the femur is rotated by pushing down on the craniolateral aspect of stifle and by lifting up the hock.[12–14,16] When the reduction occurs, it is usually accompanied by an audible "clunk." Closed reduction is reported to be successful in 43% to 75% of cases when attempted after or within 12 hours, respectively.[14,15]

Open surgical methods have been described to reduce luxation and stabilize the hip in cattle.[10,11,18,19] Open reduction with removal of soft tissue debris in the acetabulum achieves good results when reconstructive surgical repair is performed rapidly. With time the compromised integrity of bone, joint, and muscles precludes a successful outcome of any surgical technique.

The animal is positioned in lateral recumbency with the affected limb facing up. A standard craniolateral approach to the hip is made by centering the incision over and just cranial to the great trochanter (**Fig. 14**); the incision is prolonged through the fascia lata along the cranial border of the biceps femoris muscle and extended proximally through the gluteal fascia along the cranial border of the superficial gluteal muscle. Retracting the fascia lata cranially, the biceps femoris caudally, and the middle gluteal muscle dorsally allows visualization or palpation of the joint. Partial tenotomy of the tendons of the middle and the deep gluteal muscles or of the origin of the vastus lateralis muscle can be necessary to reach the joint. Once the acetabulum has been cleaned out, traction and rotation of the leg are applied to achieve reduction of the coxofemoral joint.[19,22] In adults the joint capsule usually cannot be sutured because of extended damage; after the muscle, fascia, and skin have been sutured, a stent bandage is placed over the incision. An active suction drain is often used to prevent seroma and decrease infection risk (**Fig. 15**).[22]

A dorsal approach with osteotomy of the greater trochanter, which allows maximal surgical exposure of the joint, has been described.[18] Translocation of the greater

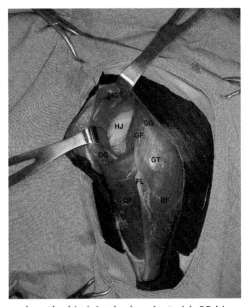

Fig. 14. Surgical approach to the hip joint (cadaveric study). BF, biceps femoris muscle; DG, deep gluteal muscle; FL, fascia lata; GF, gluteal fascia; GT, greater trochanter; HJ, hip joint (capsule); MG, middle gluteal muscle; QF, quadriceps femoral muscle; SG, superficial gluteal muscle.

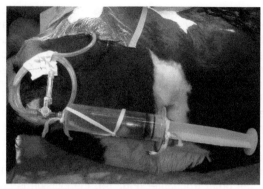

Fig. 15. Active suction drain was placed to prevent seroma after an open reduction of a luxated hip. (*Courtesy of* Dr Hélène Lardé DMV, DES.)

trochanter in a caudal and distal position on the femur temporarily increases tension on the gluteal muscle group, thus resulting in conditions that aid in maintaining reduction of the hip until fibroplasia increases the strength of the surrounding scar.[18]

A modified shuttle pin method, similar to the Knowles operation for dogs, for fixation of the femoral head in the acetabulum, has also been reported.[11,27]

Open reduction is reported to be successful in 75% of calves and 50% of adults with a long-term success rate of 75% for the animals with craniodorsal luxations and 33% for the animals with ventral luxations. The reluxation rate ranges from 17% in calves to 40% in adults.[19]

No matter which technique is used, the recovering animal should be kept in a small stall with deep bedding on a nonslippery floor for 1 week to 2 months after reduction.[22] It is advisable to apply hobbles to the rear legs to prevent their spreading apart. The use of an Ehmer sling, that causes internal rotation of the femur and prevents weight-bearing in the immediate postoperative period, is useful in calves and should be applied for 2 to 4 weeks to allow healing of the joint capsule (**Fig. 16**).

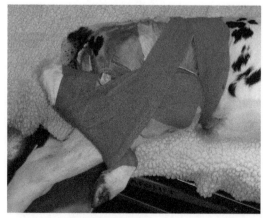

Fig. 16. Ehmer sling on the right hip of a Holstein calf. The Ehmer sling causes internal rotation of the femur and prevents weight-bearing in the postoperative period. (*Courtesy of* Dr Hélène Lardé DMV, DES.)

FRACTURE OF THE FEMORAL HEAD

Femoral capital physeal fracture or slipped capital femoral epiphysis (SCFE) is the most common hip injury in newborn calves and young animals.[2] This condition has been primarily reported after forced extraction during dystocia, particularly in heavily muscled beef calves (Maine Anjou, Charolais, and Simmental).[30,32–34] Traumatic fracture of the proximal femoral physis can also occur in older animals as a result of trauma such as a fall on a hard surface[22]; the condition has been described in young bulls and heifers housed in group pens.[25,35–37] Ossification of the femoral capital epiphysis has been reported to be complete at 42 months of age and SCFE can be expected at any time before complete ossification if forces are great enough.[2] Epiphysiolysis resulting in separation of the proximal femoral epiphysis has rarely been documented in cattle (**Fig. 17**).[34]

Fracture of the femoral capital physis is essentially a Salter-Harris type 1 fracture, but Salter-Harris type 2 fractures are also reported.[34,35]

Diagnosis

The condition is usually diagnosed from the history and clinical signs. Differential diagnosis includes coxofemoral luxation, proximal femoral fracture, and pelvic fracture.

Animals with SCFE may demonstrate a lameness of variable severity; the animal usually is able to stand and ambulate, but will avoid it by laying down most of the time. The limb is typically medially rotated, with the hock and the stifle flexed and only the toe touching the ground.[2,22,23] The conformation of the hip area may appear normal; in chronic cases muscle atrophy is noticeable. Pain and crepitation over the greater trochanter can be elicited when the animal is forced to move or in a recumbent animal with manipulations of the limb involving flexion, extension, and rotation of the hip.[22,23]

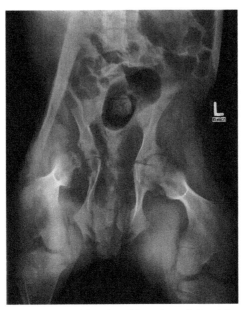

Fig. 17. A 3-week-old calf presented for dorsal luxation of the right coxofemoral joint. A ventrodorsal radiographic view of the pelvis shows a severe septic physitis of the proximal right femur.

Radiographic images of the hip provide a definitive diagnosis, allowing distinguishing SCFE from coxofemoral luxation or, less commonly, femoral neck or acetabular fractures. The radiological examination should be performed with the animal in dorsal recumbency in a frog-leg position and with the limb extended as previously described for coxofemoral luxations.[2,34] Sedation or anesthesia may be required. Because SCFE is a minimally displaced fracture, careful evaluation of the radiographs is essential (**Fig. 18**).

Treatment

The value of the animal will dictate the treatment and success rate differs greatly with the method of treatment. Conservative treatment by stall rest may provide acceptable results to allow growth, but is not recommended for any potential breeding animal.[2] In beef cattle usually the slaughter weight is hardly reached and animals have to be sold sooner. Femoral head excision with formation of pseudoarthrosis might be an alternative solution on young animals or smaller breeds not intended for breeding, unless a heifer is used for ovum pickup or embryo collection. The animal can become comfortable with a small amount of weight-bearing.[2,30,31,34]

The recommended surgical treatment is open reduction and fixation of the fragments. Different implants have been successfully used with or without interfragmentary compression: Knowles pins,[34] Steinmann pins,[36,37] and cannulated screws.[35,36,38] Cannulated screws placed in lag fashion cause compression of the fracture and provide a better stabilization of femoral head compared with divergent pins; in addition they are more resistant to migration.[35] The surgical reduction restores normal limb function if early diagnosis of SCFE is achieved and is considered to have good long-term prognosis.[35,36]

A craniolateral approach through a curvilinear skin incision is made just cranial to the greater trochanter and extended distally to the proximal femur. The fascia lata is incised along the cranial border of the biceps femoris and the superficial gluteal muscles. The superficial gluteal muscle is retracted dorsally and the rectus femoris is retracted caudoventrally; partial tenotomy of the origin of the vastus lateralis to expose joint capsule can be necessary. The capital epiphysis is manipulated digitally to obtain anatomic reduction.

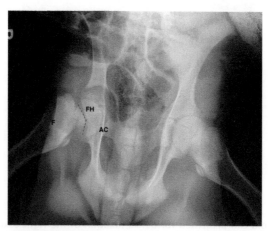

Fig. 18. A vendrodorsal radiographic view of a right SCFE. AC, acetabulum; F, femur; FH, femoral head; dashed line, physis.

Avascular necrosis of the femoral head is a common complication of capital physeal fractures. The blood supply to the femoral capital epiphysis has not been studied in cattle, but the disruption of the blood supply at the time of fracture or surgery is thought to be the cause of avascular necrosis of the femoral head in dogs.[35] Fixation in situ is recommended when displacement is less than one-third of the diameter of the femoral neck; thus, no exposure of the fracture is performed. The correct placement of the screws or the pins in lag fashion should be confirmed by intraoperative radiographs (**Fig. 19**) and manipulation of joint, to detect any crepitus that may indicate penetration of the joint.[35,36,38]

The long-term outcome is reported to be successful in 57% to 90% of animals treated.[35–38] Hobbles to prevent hip abduction and stall rest on nonslipping bedding material are indicated for at least 8 to 10 weeks postoperatively.[22]

FRACTURE OF THE FEMORAL NECK, THE ACETABULUM, AND THE GREATER TROCHANTER

Fractures of the femoral neck, other than SCFE, are very rare in cattle (**Fig. 20**) because the femoral neck is very short and hardly distinct. Clinical signs are similar and the two may only be differentiated by radiographs.[3,22,23] Fractures may be treated successfully by placing Steinmann pins or orthopedic screws across the fracture site.[39]

Fractures involving the acetabulum or the greater trochanter may occur as an isolated entity or in conjunction with hip luxations (**Fig. 21**). The most common cause is a severe trauma, such as a fall on a hard surface. These fractures are most common in adult animals.[22] The diagnosis can be confirmed with radiographs or ultrasound examination.

Greater trochanter fractures normally cause a slight lameness, swelling, and minimal or no crepitus. Healing without treatment is generally very slow and internal fixation is recommended.[22]

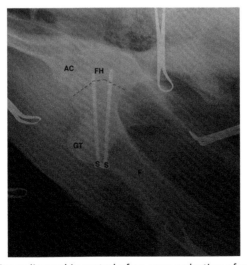

Fig. 19. Intraoperative radiographic control of an open reduction of a right SCFE. AC, acetabulum; CS, cannulated screws; F, femur; FH, femoral head; GT, greater trochanter; dashed line, physis.

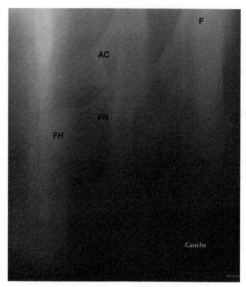

Fig. 20. Oblique ventrodorsal radiographic view of a left femoral neck fracture associated with a caudal hip luxation. AC, acetabulum; F, femur; FH, femoral head; FN, femoral neck; GT, greater trochanter; OF, obturator foramen.

Animals presenting with fractures involving the acetabulum have a mild to severe lameness or are even in decubitus; the prognosis is very guarded because osteoarthritis with a persistent lameness is unavoidable and slaughter is strongly recommended.[1]

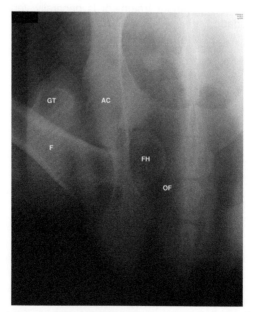

Fig. 21. Oblique ventrodorsal radiographic view of a right greater trochanter fracture associated with a caudal hip luxation. AC, acetabulum; F, femur; FH, femoral head; GT, greater trochanter; OF, obturator foramen.

SUMMARY

Diagnosis and treatment of traumatic conditions of the hip joint in cattle remain a challenge for the veterinarian. This article is intended to give an overview of the most common orthopedic problems of the bovine coxofemoral joint, diagnostic procedures, and treatment options.

REFERENCES

1. Weaver AD. Joint conditions. In: Greenough PR, Weaver AD, editors. Lameness in cattle. 3rd edition. Philadelphia: WB Saunders; 1997. p. 162–80.
2. Ferguson JG. Surgical conditions of the proximal limb. In: Greenough PR, Weaver AD, editors. Lameness in cattle. 3rd edition. Philadelphia: WB Saunders; 1997. p. 262–76.
3. Weaver AD. Hip lameness in cattle. Vet Rec 1969;85:504–12.
4. Barone R. Articulations de la ceinture et du membre pelviens. In: Anatomie comparée des mammifères domestiques. Arthrologie et myologie. Paris: Éditions Vigot; 2000. p. 232–368.
5. Sisson S. Ruminant syndesmology. In: Getty R, editor. Sisson & Grossman's the anatomy of domestic animals. Philadelphia: WB Saunders; 1975. p. 787–90.
6. Barone R. Ceinture et membre pelviens. In: Anatomie comparée des mammifères domestiques. Ostéologie. Paris: Éditions Vigot; 2000. p. 589–737.
7. Barone R. Muscles de la ceinture et du membre pelviens. In: Anatomie comparée des mammifères domestiques. Arthrologie et myologie. Paris: Éditions Vigot; 2000. p. 843–991.
8. Desrochers A, Anderson DE, St-Jean G. Lameness examination in cattle. Vet Clin North Am Food Anim Pract 2001;17:39–51.
9. Greenough PR. Applied anatomy. In: Greenough PR, Weaver AD, editors. Lameness in cattle. 3rd edition. Philadelphia: WB Saunders; 1997. p. 219–32.
10. Starke A, Herzog K, Short J, et al. Diagnostic procedures and surgical treatment of craniodorsal coxofemoral luxation in calves. Vet Surg 2007;36:99–106.
11. Adams OR. Preliminary report on repair of coxofemoral luxation and coxofemoral subluxation in cattle. J Am Vet Med Assoc 1957;130:515–9.
12. Greenough PR. Dislocation of the hip in the cow. Vet Rec 1960;72:180–1.
13. Hart CB. Dislocated hip in the cow. Vet Rec 1950;62:227.
14. Larcombe MT, Malmo J. Dislocation of the coxo-femoral joint in dairy cows. Aust Vet J 1989;66:351–4.
15. Jubb TF, Malmo J, Brightling P, et al. Prognostic factors for recovery from coxofemoral dislocation in cattle. Aust Vet J 1989;66:354–8.
16. Rees HG. Coxo-femoral dislocation in dairy cattle. Vet Rec 1964;76:362–4.
17. Baird AN, Baird DK. What is your diagnosis? Craniodorsal luxation of the left coxofemoral joint. J Am Vet Med Assoc 1995;207:39–40.
18. Madison JB, Johnston JK. Treatement of recurrent coxofemoral luxation in a calf by use of open reduction and translocation of the greater trochanter. J Am Vet Med Assoc 1992;200:83–5.
19. Tulleners EP, Nunamaker DM, Richardson DW. Coxofemoal luxations in cattle: 22 cases (1980-1985). J Am Vet Med Assoc 1987;191:569–74.
20. Sisson S. Equine syndesmology. In: Getty R, editor. Sisson & Grossman's the anatomy of domestic animals. Philadelphia: WB Saunders; 1975. p. 349–75.
21. Taguchi K, Kudo K, Suzuki T, et al. Ultrasonographic appearance of bovine coxofemoral luxation in different directions. J Veterinar Sci Technol 2011;S3:3. http://dx.doi.org/10.4172/2157-7579.S3-003.

22. Hull BL. Fractures and luxations of the pelvis and proximal femur. Vet Clin North Am Food Anim Pract 1996;12:47–58.

23. Nelson DR, Kneller SK. Treatment of proximal hind-limb lameness in cattle. Vet Clin North Am Food Anim Pract 1985;1:153–73.

24. Desrochers A. Coxofemoral luxation. In: Anderson DE, Rings DM, editors. Current veterinary therapy food animal practice. 5th edition. St Louis (MO): Saunders; 2009. p. 268–70.

25. Wenzinger B, Hagen R, Schmid T, et al. Coxofemoral joint radiography in standing cattle. Vet Radiol Ultrasound 2012;53:424–9.

26. Bargai U, Pharr JW, Morgan JP. Radiological diagnosis of the pelvis. In: Bovine radiology. Ames (IA): Iowa State University Press; 1989. p. 145–50.

27. Knowles AT, Knowles JO, Knowles RP. An operation to preserve the continuity of the hip joint. J Am Vet Med Assoc 1953;123:508–15.

28. Nagel E. Transrectal and vaginal routes for radiography of the hip joint in horses and cattle – Transrektale bzw. Vaginale Röntgenuntersuchung des Hüftgelenkes bei Pferd und Rind. In: Internationale Tagung ueber Orthopaedie bei Huf-und Klauentieren. Vienna, 5–7 October, 1983. p. 343–6.

29. Grubelnik M, Kofler J, Martinek B, et al. Ultrasonographic examination of the hip joint region and bony pelvis in cattle – Die sonographische Darstellung der Hü ftgelenksregion und des knöchernen Beckens beim Rind. Berl Munch Tierarztl Wochenschr 2002;115:209–20.

30. Fretz PB, Dingwall J, Horney FD. Excision arthroplasty in calves. Mod Vet Pract 1973;54:67–9.

31. Squire KR, Fessler JF, Toombs JP, et al. Femoral head ostectomy in horses and cattle. Vet Surg 1991;20:453–8.

32. Ferguson JG, Dehghani S, Petrali EH. Fractures of the femur in newborn calves. Can Vet J 1990;31:289–91.

33. Ferguson JG. Femoral fracture in the newborn calf: biomechanics and etiological considerations for practitioners. Can Vet J 1994;35:626–30.

34. Hamilton GF, Turner AS, Ferguson JG, et al. Slipped capital femoral epiphysis in calves. J Am Vet Med Assoc 1978;172:1318–22.

35. Bentley VA, Edwards RB III, Santschi EM, et al. Repair of femoral capital physeal fractures with 7.0-mm cannulated screws in cattle: 20 cases (1988-2002). J Am Vet Med Assoc 2005;227:964–9.

36. Ewoldt JM, Hull BL, Ayars WH. Repair of femoral capital physeal fractures in 12 cattle. Vet Surg 2003;32:30–6.

37. Hull BL, Koenig GJ, Monke DR. Treatment of slipped capital femoral epiphysis in cattle: 11 cases (1974-1988). J Am Vet Med Assoc 1990;197:1509–12.

38. Wilson DG, Crawford WH, Stone WC, et al. Fixation of femoral capital physeal fractures with 7.0 mm cannulated screws in five bulls. Vet Surg 1991;20:240–4.

39. Smyth GB, Hatch P, Mason TA. Surgical repair of femoral neck fractures in two dogs and a calf. Vet Rec 1979;105:248–51.

Stifle Disorders
Cranial Cruciate Ligament, Meniscus, Upward Fixation of the Patella

Rebecca Pentecost, DVM, MS, Andrew Niehaus, DVM, MS*

KEYWORDS

- Cattle • Stifle • Lameness • Cranial cruciate ligament • Meniscus
- Upward fixation of the patella

KEY POINTS

- Stifle injury is a major source of lameness and can be associated with significant production losses in cattle.
- Cranial cruciate ligament injury is a common cause of stifle lameness, and treatment options range from conservative management to ligament replacement techniques.
- Meniscal injury can occur in cattle and is most frequently associated with ligament damage (mainly medial collateral ligament injury).
- Intermittent upward fixation of the patella is a rare condition affecting cattle in North America but is associated with a good prognosis with accurate diagnosis and surgical intervention.

INTRODUCTION

Stifle injury or disease remains a major source of proximal hind limb lameness in cattle. Structures that are commonly affected include the cranial cruciate ligament (CrCL), the medial meniscus, and the collateral ligaments. Osteoarthritis is a common sequela of a primary traumatic injury or degenerative breakdown of one of these structures. Economic losses associated with stifle disease are related to increased recumbency, decreased feed intake, decreased milk production, loss of muscle mass in the affected limb, conception failure in cows, and reluctance to mount in bulls.[1]

RELEVANT ANATOMY

The bovine stifle is composed of the femoropatellar, medial femorotibial, and lateral femorotibial joints. Communication exists between the femoropatellar and medial

Department of Veterinary Clinical Sciences, College of Veterinary Medicine, The Ohio State University, 601 Vernon Tharp Street, Columbus, OH 43210, USA
* Corresponding author.
E-mail address: niehaus.25@osu.edu

Vet Clin Food Anim 30 (2014) 265–281
http://dx.doi.org/10.1016/j.cvfa.2013.11.008
0749-0720/14/$ – see front matter © 2014 Elsevier Inc. All rights reserved.

femorotibial joints in 100% of stifles and between the medial and lateral femorotibial joints in 65% of stifles.[2] Similar to the horse, the bovine patella has a tendinous attachment to the quadriceps apparatus proximally and connects distally to the tibial crest via 3 separate ligaments: the medial, middle, and lateral patellar ligaments. The lateral patellar ligament is continuous with the tendon of the biceps femoris muscle.

The cruciate ligaments are intra-articular and extrasynovial and provide rotational and craniocaudal support to the stifle.[3] The CrCL originates from the intercondylar fossa of the femur and courses craniolaterally to insert on the craniolateral aspect of the tibial eminence (**Fig. 1**). The caudal cruciate ligament (CdCL) lies medial to the CrCL, originates from the intercondylar fossa of the femur, and inserts at the popliteal notch of the caudal tibia.[3,4]

Each femoral condyle is separated from the corresponding tibial plateau by a cartilaginous meniscus that provides cushioning for the joint surfaces (see **Fig. 1**).[5] The lateral meniscus attaches cranially to the tibial eminence and caudally near the attachment of the CdCL with an additional attachment to the intercondylar fossa of the femur via the muscular femoral ligament. The lateral meniscus has no attachment to the lateral collateral ligament. The medial meniscus is attached cranially and caudally to the tibial eminence similarly to the lateral meniscus. In contrast, the medial meniscus is firmly attached to the medial collateral ligament, predisposing the meniscus to concurrent injury in the presence of medial collateral ligament damage.[5,6] Each meniscus is further supported by the intermeniscal ligament. The synovial lining is prolific compared with the equine and can become even more extensive and proliferative in inflammatory conditions associated with joint instability and chronic arthritis.

CRCL RUPTURE

CrCL rupture is a common cause of lameness referable to the stifle. Traumatic rupture of the CrCL is the primary means of injury in cows, whereas bulls are more likely to develop CrCL rupture secondary to accumulative degenerative joint disease.[7,8] It has been suggested that the straightness of the tarsocrural joint in some bulls predisposes to straightness of the stifle, leading to meniscal damage, joint instability, degenerative joint disease, and fraying of the CrCL until rupture.[7] Older cattle may also be at higher risk for degenerative changes to the CrCL predisposing to rupture, as is described in dogs.[9] Falls are common causes of injury, usually secondary to poor

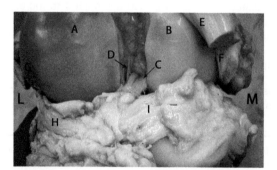

Fig. 1. The right stifle of a bull with normal intra-articular anatomy (cranial view): A, lateral femoral condyle; B, medial femoral condyle; C, cranial cruciate ligament; D, caudal cruciate ligament; E, cut section of the middle patellar ligament; F, cut section of the medial patellar ligament; G, cut section of the lateral patellar ligament; H, lateral meniscus; I, medial meniscus; L, lateral side; M, medial side.

footing, metabolic disturbances around the time of calving, or associated with mounting injuries attributable to normal estrus behavior. Cattle with higher body condition scores are at higher risk, as are older individuals (mean age, 4–5 years).[1,8]

Diagnostic Procedures

Physical examination allows diagnosis in most cases. Stifle injury, particularly CrCL rupture, typically results in evidence of nonspecific lameness. A thorough distal limb and hoof evaluation is necessary to rule out lower limb disorders. Lameness in acute cases can be marked, although some individuals may present with milder lameness or have periodic episodes of lameness interspersed with periods of apparently normal gait. The degree of lameness generally decreases substantially with chronic injuries. In some individuals, a clicking sound may be heard when standing, shifting weight, or walking.[4]

Evaluation of the proximal limb in affected cattle reveals moderate to severe joint effusion. Pain, crepitus, cranial drawer, and increased internal rotation may be found on manipulation of the stifle joint. To elicit cranial drawer, examiners stand behind, place their hands on either side of the limb, and firmly grasp the proximal tibial crest (**Fig. 2**). By quickly pulling caudally on the tibial crest, the examiner may feel movement and hear a clicking noise in the CrCL-deficient stifle. As an alternative, the examiner can attempt to elicit laxity and crepitus through internal rotation of the tibia by placing one hand on the tibial crest and the other on the point of the hock.

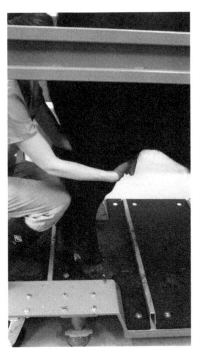

Fig. 2. Cranial drawer in cattle can be elicited to confirm a diagnosis of CrCL rupture. Examiners stand behind the patient and use their knees to brace the hock. The hands are passed along either side of the stifle to grasp the tibial crest firmly. By jerking caudally on the proximal tibia, crepitus associated with a loud clicking noise may be appreciated in the CrCL-deficient stifle.

Radiographic evaluation of the stifle can support a presumptive diagnosis of cranial cruciate rupture in cases in which physical examination findings are suggestive but inconclusive. In normal cattle, the femoral condyles completely overlap the tibial eminences seen on the lateral view (**Fig. 3**A). In CrCL-deficient cattle, the lateral radiograph shows the femoral condyles caudal to the tibial intercondylar eminences (see **Fig. 3**B).[7] In acute, traumatic injuries, avulsion of the CrCL can result in osseous fragments within the joint. In chronic cases, evidence of degenerative joint disease (DJD) may be seen radiographically.[5,7] Craniocaudal views confirm the presence of DJD, avulsion fragments, and can confirm collateral ligament ruptures caused by joint space incongruity.

Arthrocentesis of the bovine joint is best obtained from the area of maximal joint distension. Samples should be acquired from both the femoropatellar and femorotibial joints because the lateral femorotibial joint does not communicate with the other joints in many animals. Analysis of the fluid should indicate sterile inflammation. An 18-gauge needle is sufficient in most cases, although larger needles may be required if the joint fluid is particularly viscous or if proliferative synovium prevents aspiration. Normal joint fluid is transparent with a light yellow color. Normal nucleated cell counts are less than 1000 cells/μL with a total protein of less than 2.5 g/dL. Higher values suggest inflammatory damage or infection.

The gold standard for stifle evaluation in the horse is diagnostic arthroscopy. Arthroscopic evaluation has been reported in the bovine but is uncommonly performed because of economic considerations, lack of necessary equipment, and unfamiliarity with arthroscopic landmarks and techniques.[10] Arthroscopic evaluation allows definitive diagnosis of cruciate rupture and meniscal damage, but can be difficult in heavy cattle with significant periarticular fat or in chronic cases because of extensive proliferative synovitis (**Fig. 4**).

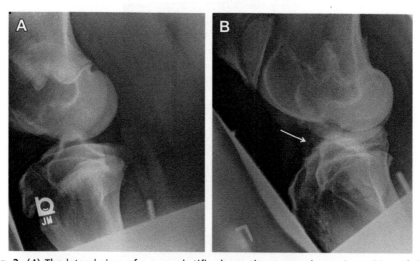

Fig. 3. (*A*) The lateral view of a normal stifle shows the expected superimposition of the femoral condyles over the tibial eminences. (*B*) The lateral view of a CrCL-deficient stifle shows the cranial movement of the proximal tibia with the femoral condyles caudal to the tibial eminences. A small curvilinear osseous body (*arrow*) is seen just cranial to the tibial eminence along with increased opacity in the cranial aspect of the joint. These findings are presumed to be degenerative changes and ossification of the CrCL.

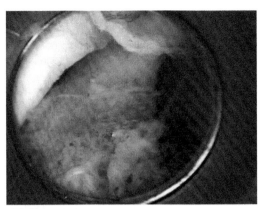

Fig. 4. Arthroscopic imaging of the ruptured CrCL reveals fraying of the ligament fibers. Proliferative synovial villi can impede visibility within the joint in cattle with chronic injuries or preexisting DJD. (*Courtesy of* David Anderson, DVM, MS.)

Treatment

Treatment options vary depending on the perceived economic value of the animal, severity of disease, progression of secondary degenerative joint changes, and availability of the equipment, facilities, and expertise to perform surgical repair. The various options are discussed later.

Salvage may be the best option for affected animals if treatment costs cannot be justified. Without treatment, many animals remain painful and develop progressive DJD leading to increased recumbency, decreased feed intake, generalized weight loss, breakdown of soft tissue support structures in the contralateral limb, and disuse atrophy of the gluteal and quadriceps muscle groups.[4] Stall rest may be effective for cases of partial CrCL rupture, small cattle (<450 kg), or when economic considerations preclude surgery.[4] Limiting activity minimizes cartilage damage secondary to joint instability. Strict stall rest with good footing (dirt floors or manure packs) is important. In addition, it is important to prevent interactions with other cattle. Many affected individuals are overconditioned and benefit from losing weight.

Nonsteroidal antiinflammatory drugs are most commonly used for pain control during long-term management of lameness associated with CrCL rupture (**Table 1**).[11] Of

Table 1 Nonsteroidal antiinflammatory drugs used for medical and surgical management of CrCL rupture			
Drug	**Dose (mg/kg)**	**Route**	**Frequency (h)**
Aspirin	50–100	Oral	Every 12
Phenylbutazone	5	Oral	Every 24–48
	10	Oral	Every 48–72
Meloxicam	0.5–1.0	Oral	Every 24–72
Flunixin meglumine	1–2	IV	Every 12–24
Ketoprofen	1.5	IV or IM	Every 24–48
Carprofen	1.4	IV or SC	—

Abbreviations: IM, intramuscular; IV, intravenous; SC, subcutaneous.

the drugs in **Table 1**, only flunixin meglumine is approved for use in cattle in the United States; therefore, use caution when estimating milk and meat withholding times.[11,12] Also, the use of phenylbutazone is prohibited in lactating dairy cows. One author recommends the use of steroids intra-articularly to decrease inflammation and mitigate pain in nonpregnant animals.[13]

The prognosis for partial ruptures treated conservatively can be good with full return to normal gait and activity. Progressive DJD is likely, which may decrease the productive life of the affected individual despite initial healing. In cattle with complete rupture of the CrCL, long-term prognosis following conservative therapy is poor. Prognosis decreases with increased body weight or greater joint laxity. Cattle that are not accustomed to being handled, aggressive individuals, and those that have a tendency to lie on the affected side are more likely to exacerbate the initial injury, prolonging or impairing healing.[4]

Surgical repair of CrCL injury is the preferred treatment of CrCL rupture. In the author's experience, the best results are seen in cattle that do not have evidence of extensive DJD at the time of surgical intervention. Methods of surgical intervention include extracapsular imbrication of periarticular tissues and ligament replacement.

Joint imbrication accelerates fibrous tissue formation around the stifle. The goal is to delay the onset and progression of DJD by reducing joint laxity. The following are important points to remember when considering the imbrication technique:

1. The extracapsular approach minimizes the potential for iatrogenic intra-articular infection or cartilage damage
2. The procedure is faster compared with implant or graft placement and requires shorter anesthetic times
3. The procedure is technically easy to perform, without the need for special equipment or implants
4. Catastrophic failure is unlikely
5. The imbrication procedure is best reserved for small cattle (<730 kg)

Preoperative antiinflammatory and broad-spectrum antibiotics should be administered before anesthetic induction. The patient is placed in dorsal to dorsolateral recumbency with the affected limb upward. The affected limb is raised to facilitate placement of sutures both medially and laterally (**Fig. 5**). Aseptic preparation and draping are performed.

An S-shaped incision is created over the cranial aspect of the stifle starting 5 to 6 cm proximal to the stifle and ending on the opposite side of the limb approximately 5 to 6 cm distal to the stifle (**Fig. 6**). The incisions are continued deep through the superficial connective tissue until fibrous tissue is encountered. The resulting flaps are undermined bluntly to provide access to the medial and lateral aspects of the joint. Arthrocentesis is performed to remove as much synovial fluid from the joint as possible to maximize the effect of the imbrication procedure; the fluid may be saved and submitted for cytology and culture, if needed (**Fig. 7**).

The limb is placed in full extension, and lateral imbrication sutures are placed. Eight to 10 large, nonabsorbable sutures (the authors routinely use #5 polyester) are placed in a Lembert-style pattern running from the lateral patellar ligament at the level of the distal edge of the patella to the lateral aspect of the tibial crest (**Fig. 8**). The sutures should be placed in 2 rows to maximize the effect of the imbrication; additional rows can be added in large animals. Placing subsequent rows in opposite directions may increase the amount of periarticular fibrosis. The procedure is repeated on the medial aspect of the limb with the Lembert sutures running from the medial patellar ligament at the level of the distal patella to the medial aspect of the tibial crest. Multiple

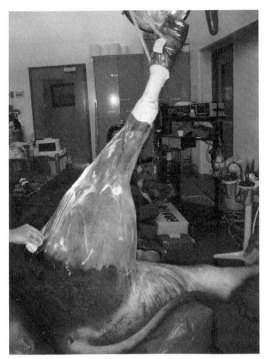

Fig. 5. The patient is placed in dorsal or dorsolateral recumbency with the affected limb up. Hoisting the limb so that the stifle is extended improves access to both the medial and lateral aspects of the limb during imbrication suture placement.

smaller interrupted Lembert sutures can be placed perpendicular to the collateral ligaments to further imbricate the periarticular tissues on either side of the limb. Some descriptions of the imbrication technique suggest the use of an antirotating suture placed from the lateral gastrocnemius attachment on the femoral condyle to the fascia on the tibial crest; however, the risk of peroneal nerve encroachment is high.[4,14] The

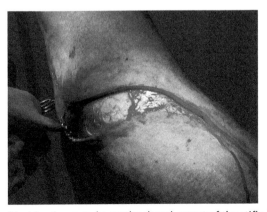

Fig. 6. The S-shaped incision is created over the dorsal aspect of the stifle beginning several centimeters proximal to the stifle on one side of the limb and ending several centimeters distal to the stifle on the opposite side of the limb.

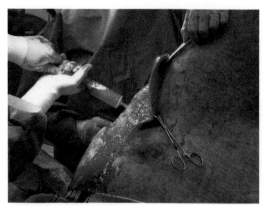

Fig. 7. Synovial fluid is aspirated from the joint to maximize the effect of the imbrication sutures.

subcutaneous and skin closures are routine. A tie-over bandage can be placed to protect the incision after surgery (**Fig. 9**).

Postoperative recovery requires excellent footing. Antibiotics are administered for approximately 7 days, and analgesics up to 2 to 3 months after surgery. After the first 7 to 14 days, an early return to partial weight bearing is desirable to reduce the risk of contralateral limb breakdown. Strict stall rest is continued for a minimum of 4 to 6 months, after which a gradual return to use is recommended. For optimal postoperative performance, lifelong reduction in activity is recommended. Progressive decrease in lameness is expected during the first 6 months with minimal to no ongoing improvement expected thereafter.

Surgical replacement techniques allow for a substitute tissue or implant to replace the function of the damaged CrCL, increasing the stability of the affected stifle. Both autologous grafts and synthetic implants have been described. Important points to remember when considering a replacement technique include:

1. Better stability compared with the imbrication technique
2. The procedure is associated with a faster and more complete return to normal function

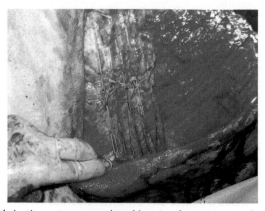

Fig. 8. Multiple imbrication sutures are placed in a Lembert pattern using large nonabsorbable suture (#5 polyester) in 2 or more rows.

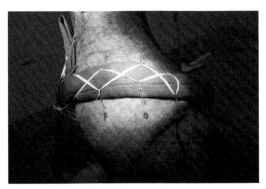

Fig. 9. A tie-over bandage protects the incision during recovery and during the immediate postoperative period. The bandage should be removed and the incision monitored daily for evidence of infection or dehiscence.

3. This technique has reportedly more success in large animals (>730 kg)
4. The technique is a more technically demanding procedure (passing the graft through the joint atraumatically)
5. The technique is more invasive with a higher risk for iatrogenic articular cartilage damage
6. There is an increased risk of postoperative surgical complications including incisional infection, septic arthritis, or graft failure
7. This technique is associated with increased surgical times, increasing the risk for anesthetic complications including myopathies and neuropathies

Comparison of several types of autologous and synthetic implants including skin, fascia, fluorocarbon resin, and polyester fiber was reported in cattle.[15,16] Results suggested that the skin grafts maintained their integrity and size better than fascial grafts.[15] The autologous grafts healed well, were covered with synovial tissue, were less likely to fail, and caused less reactivity than the repairs that incorporated polyester fibers or fluorocarbon resin.[15] All implant types had persistent lameness at 3 weeks and were sound at 6 weeks, suggesting good initial recovery regardless of the implant chosen.

The basic procedure describing placement of an autologous graft was first described by Hofmeyr[17] in 1968. The graft was attached to the tibial crest, passed between the femoral condyles, and was secured to the lateral condyle, effectively replacing the function of the CrCL. Later work by Hamilton and Adams[15] and Hamilton and Nelson[16] compared fascia, skin, polyester suture material, and fluorocarbon resin to determine suitability as potential CrCL replacements. In that study, skin and fascia emerged as the most viable autograft sources.[15,16] Moss and Ferguson[18] evaluated the tensile strength of the CrCL compared with the lateral patellar ligament and the fascia of the gluetobiceps muscle. They later reported the use of the gluteobiceps fascia as a replacement material for cranial cruciate repair in 1988 and the technique was further popularized by Crawford.[1,19] The main advantage is that the fascia of the gluteobiceps is continuous with the lateral patellar tendon and already has a firm attachment to the cranial tibia.

The preoperative anesthetic preparation, patient positioning, and surgical site preparation are as described for the imbrication procedure. The skin incision starts at the greater trochanter extending linearly along the lateral femur to the lateral aspect of the patella. At this level, the incision is redirected to the tibial crest extending sharply through the loose areolar fascia. The incision is extended deeply at the junction of the vastus lateralis and the gluteobiceps, separating the respective muscles throughout the length of the incision. The gluteobiceps are retracted caudally, exposing the cranial edge of the gluteobiceps tendon. Starting at the proximal edge of the incision, a 1.5-cm-wide section of the gluteobiceps tendon is separated, continuing distally to the level of the lateral patellar ligament where it attaches to the tibia. The 1.5-cm-wide section forms the autologous graft to be used as a CrCL replacement. The graft tissue should be kept as long as possible because some tissue will be sacrificed due to unavoidable damage during graft placement through the joint. Graft harvest can result in either craniocaudal or mediolateral splitting of the tendon.[4]

Once the graft has been harvested, it is wrapped in saline-soaked gauze. The graft site along the cranial edge of the gluteobiceps muscle is sutured in a simple continuous pattern. A small arthrotomy is made between the middle and lateral patellar ligaments to allow placement of the graft through the joint. The small size of the arthrotomy incision precludes debridement of the cruciate ligament but maintains joint stability. Older studies report luxation of the patella as a means to facilitate graft passage[1]; however, less aggressive handling of the lateral support tissues is recommended to reduce the risk of postoperative seroma formation and graft failure.[4,5]

A graft passer designed by Crawford[1] and modified from an early description by van Oosterom[20] is used for graft placement (**Fig. 10**). The graft passer is passed into the intercondylar area, emerging as close to the bone over the lateral condyle as possible. Three strands of umbilical tape (6 mm) are placed through the eye of the graft passer and the graft passer is retracted. Two of the strands of umbilical tape are then sutured through the leading end of the autograft with the third strand allowing the passage of additional strands of umbilical tape if needed. The umbilical tape is used to pull the graft through the joint via the intratrochlear space to exit proximal and caudal to the lateral condyle. The damaged end of the graft is resected and secured to the lateral femoral condyle with a plate or orthopedic staples. The gluteobiceps and vastus lateralis are closed as well as the arthrotomy, followed by the subcutaneous tissue and the skin.

Synthetic implants have been proposed as an alternative way to replace the function of the damaged CrCL in cattle. Good synthetic replacements are minimally bioreactive, have similar tensile strength to the CrCL, are resistant to cyclic failure, and must be able to be secured without weakening the implant. A recent in vitro study reported that 3-stranded cords of 200-kg (450-lb) test monofilament nylon fishing line most closely approximated the strength of the CrCL compared with other materials tested.[21] This study also found that the optimal configuration was strands arranged parallel to each other.[21] Successful use of synthetic replacements in clinical patients has occurred but is not widely reported (Anderson, personal communication, 2010).

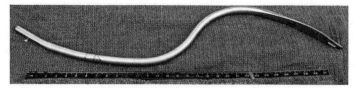

Fig. 10. A graft passer is designed to traverse the bovine intercondylar area and guide umbilical tape and eventually the fascia lata autograft to replace the CrCL. (*Courtesy of Messer Innovative Products, Cottage Grove, Wisconsin.*)

Prognosis

Without treatment, CrCL rupture caries a poor prognosis. Conservative therapy consisting of strict stall rest may allow individuals with partial CrCL tears or low body weights to develop sufficient fibrous tissue to stabilize the joint and allow ongoing productivity. Cattle with complete tears that are not treated surgically generally have progressive deterioration of the joint, lose condition, and must be culled or humanely destroyed.[4] Surgical techniques have better long-term success, with failure occurring more often in heavy individuals or advanced DJD.[1,4,5]

One study reported on 9 cases of CrCL injury diagnosed at 2 referral hospitals.[22] Of these cases, 2 were euthanized without treatment, 2 were treated with strict stall rest, and 5 were treated with extracapsular imbrication. One of the two treated with stall rest and 3 of the 5 (60%) treated surgically regained acceptable use of the joint.[22]

Another study evaluated outcome following extracapsular imbrication in 23 CrCL-deficient stifles in 22 dairy cattle.[14] In these patients, Lembert sutures were placed medially and laterally in the retinaculum in all stifles, and 5 had additional imbrication sutures placed from the femorotibial ligaments to either the lateral or middle patellar ligaments to counteract rotational forces. Thirteen cattle improved markedly (4 of these were considered to have recovered completely), 3 improved moderately with shorter productive periods, and 7 were considered unsuccessful.[14] Unsuccessful cases were commonly associated with moderate to severe DJD.[14]

Fascia lata grafts were evaluated by Crawford[1] in 1990, including 9 experimental animals and 13 clinical cases. Of the 9 experimental animals, all were heifers with no previous evidence of orthopedic disease. The stifle was approached, the CrCL transected, and the fascia lata graft harvested and placed as previously described. One month after surgery, 2 of the 9 heifers retained a noticeable lameness on the operated limb; however, at 2 months after surgery, all heifers were sound.[1] Postmortem examination of all heifers revealed no evidence of iatrogenic articular cartilage damage, no damage to the meniscus, and no osteophyte development indicating DJD.[1] During tensile strength testing, failure of the grafts in all cases was at the attachment point on the caudal femur with pull-out of the graft from the staple.[1] Failure in the normal (unoperated) joints was the middle of the length of the CrCL for most, with 1 failing at the femoral origin of the ligament.[1]

The 13 clinical cases consisted of 9 bulls and 4 cows. Examination findings included cranial subluxation of the tibia (n = 12), pronounced effusion (n = 5), cranial drawer (n = 8), and internal rotation (n = 5).[1] Successful graft placement occurred in 8 of the 13 patients, including 5 bulls and 3 cows.[1] Unsuccessful outcomes in the bulls seemed to be associated with dehiscence of the lateral fascia and joint instability (n = 2) and failure of the graft (n = 2).[1] The cow with an unsuccessful outcome developed severe postoperative radial nerve paralysis and was euthanized. For the clinical patients, mean body weight for the successful cases was 778 kg versus 918 kg for the unsuccessful cases.[1]

A review by Ducharme[4] in 1996 offered outcome data for 6 research animals and 9 clinical cases using the gluteobiceps graft replacement technique.[1,4] Overall success for the experimental animals was 93% (n = 14 of 15).[4] The successful cases had resolved lameness by 2 months after surgery and had grafts present and covered with a vascularized membrane between 3 and 18 months after surgery during postmortem examinations.[4] The mean ultimate tensile strength was found to be 27% to 30% of the original ligament in these individuals.[4]

Success in clinical patients was higher for cows compared with bulls.[4] The overall success rate for cows was 88% (n = 7/8), although 3 of these cows later ruptured their contralateral CrCLs within 6 months to 1 year of surgery. Of these 3 cows, 1 had a partial tear successfully managed with stall rest, 1 was successfully operated, and 1 was euthanized.[4] The success rate in bulls was 43% (n = 6/14).[4] Incisional failure was identified in 6 bulls, with 4 of these bulls developing concurrent septic arthritis.[4] Graft failure led to unsuccessful postoperative outcome in 2 bulls.[4]

MENISCUS

The meniscus performs crucial biomechanical functions by stabilizing the joint, providing a congruent joint surface between the femur and tibial plateau, distributing loads evenly, acting as a shock absorber for the adjacent articular cartilage, and contributing to friction-reduction mechanisms within the joint.[23] Meniscal injury in dogs is often correlated with CrCL rupture, whereas horses are more likely to develop primary meniscal damage.[24–27] However, cattle most commonly acquire medial meniscal damage associated with medial collateral ligament rupture.[6,28] The normal separation of the lateral meniscus from the lateral collateral ligament and the musculature supporting the lateral aspect of the stifle decreases the risk of trauma to the lateral meniscus.[5]

Diagnosis

Diagnosis of medial meniscal damage can generally be made based on physical examination findings. Lameness localized to the stifle, joint effusion, pain on palpation of the medial aspect of the joint, decreased weight bearing, and shortened cranial phase to the stride are common with medial collateral ligament and medial meniscal injury. Most individuals have a tendency to preferentially bear weight on the medial claw. Palpation of the medial stifle reveals a hypermobile meniscus with movement most notable during varus and valgus stress.[6] A distinct separation from the joint capsule is often appreciated. Affected cattle do not have cranial drawer or rotational instability.

Radiographic evaluation of the joint may reveal widening of the medial femorotibial joint that is especially prominent in stressed craniocaudal views. Avulsion fractures at the origin or insertion of the damaged ligament may also be appreciated.

Ultrasonography and arthroscopy are important diagnostic tools for diagnosing meniscal tears in horses[24]; however, use in cattle has remained limited. The limited space between the meniscus and femoral condyles precludes full examination of the meniscus. Ultrasonographic examination of the medial collateral ligament can reveal partial or complete tears that support a presumptive diagnosis of meniscal injury.

Treatment

Prolonged stall confinement for a minimum of 6 to 8 weeks has been suggested for meniscal and medial collateral ligament injury. Conservative therapy is best reserved for cases in which there is no concurrent injury to other joint structures including the CrCL and for mild meniscal injuries.

Diagnostic arthroscopy should ideally be used to confirm the diagnosis and allow debridement of the damaged meniscus.[5] Meniscopexy is performed by creating an approximately 2-cm incision dorsal and parallel to the damaged meniscus. The meniscus is reattached to the medial joint capsule and medial collateral ligament using 3 to 4 nonabsorbable sutures (#0 polypropylene) starting just proximal to the tibia. The knots remain extra-articular to minimize reactivity within the joint. Fixation of the medial collateral ligament can be achieved with cortical bone screws and washers or imbrication of the medial periarticular tissues using large nonabsorbable suture material. The animal should remain confined for 2 to 3 months after surgery, with improvement expected within the first 2 to 4 weeks.[5]

Prognosis

Evaluation of 50 cattle with medial meniscal injury was performed, with arthrotomy in 34 patients.[6,28] Arthrotomy confirmed separation from the medial collateral ligament and joint capsule. Meniscopexy was performed in all 34 individuals undergoing surgery. Follow-up was obtained for 27 operated animals, with improvement in 20 (74% successful).[28] Economics precluded surgery in the remaining 16 cases. Follow-up was available for 11 of these individuals with only 1 showing improvement (9% success rate).[28]

Most of the cattle in this report (76%) were less than 2 years old, suggesting a traumatic injury origin compared with cruciate ruptures, which tend to occur in older animals and may be related to accumulative chronic damage.[6,8] Sequelae of meniscal injury include contralateral limb breakdown injury and varus deformity, which is seen at a higher rate in young, growing animals.

UPWARD FIXATION OF THE PATELLA

Intermittent upward fixation of the patella (IUFP) is a condition that results when the patella becomes engaged by, and fixed on, the proximal aspect of the medial trochlear ridge of the femur. This condition prevents the stifle from flexing and consequently the joint is locked in rigid extension. Because of anatomic differences of the stifle joint, the condition is most commonly seen in the equine species but large ruminants and ruminantlike species can be affected. The condition has been reported in cattle, buffalo, and camels.[29–31]

In India, where ruminants are used for draught purposes, IUFP is seen with a higher prevalence than in North America, where it has mainly featured in small case reports and sporadic retrospective studies.[22,32–34] Brahman cattle and cattle used for draught purposes have an increased predilection of IUFP.[30,35] Females seem to be less affected than males; calves less than 2 years of age are less commonly affected. In India, there is a decrease in incidence in the summer months and animals that are in poor body condition have a higher incidence of IUFP.[30] In nonworking cattle, predisposing factors include late gestation and rapid growth.

Clinical Signs

The predominant clinical sign of IUFP is the failure of the affected animal to flex its stifle; therefore, a rigid extension of the hind leg is noted. When the patella releases, the stifle flexes and the leg is brought forward in a jerky movement (hyperflexion). The disease is frequently seen intermittently but can progress to persistent inability to flex the stifle. In the initial stages, an occasional jerk of the affected limb confined to 1 or 2 steps may be noticed. In chronic cases it may take up to 15 minutes to resolve.[36] Animals can be affected either unilaterally or bilaterally. Increased dorsal toe wear is noted in chronic cases (**Fig. 11**).

Pathophysiology/Causes

Similar to horses, cattle have 3 patellar ligaments originating at the patella and inserting on the tibia. These ligaments are the medial, middle, and lateral patellar ligaments. The loop created by the medial patellar ligament, the patella, and the middle patellar ligament encircle the medial trochlear ridge where it can become caught and prevent

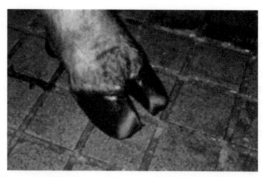

Fig. 11. A cow with upward fixation of the patella has excessive dorsal hoof wear from chronically rolling her toe because of hyperextension of the stifle joint. (*Courtesy of* Nickie Baird, DVM, MS, West Lafayette, IN.)

the stifle joint from flexing. Cattle lack the prominent notch on the medial trochlear ridge of the femur and a medial protuberance on the patella present in horses as part of the equine stay apparatus, making IUFP less common in cattle than in horses. The cause of the upward fixation of the patella is unknown. Ligament laxity has been postulated but the condition has not been able to be experimentally reproduced by ligament elongation.[37] General debility and decrease of the fat between the patellar ligaments has been postulated to predispose to IUFP, and clinical signs in affected animals seem to resolve when the nutritional status of affected animals improved. Heritability as well as working cattle at young ages (<3 years) has also been postulated to lead to IUFP. It has been reported that 97% of affected cattle were working cattle.[36] Hyperextension of the stifle joint, or dragging of the limbs through mud, have been suggested as causes.[36,38]

Treatment

Theories on the pathogenesis include relaxation of the patellar ligaments, which allows the medial and middle patellar ligaments to engage the medial trochlear ridge of the femur. Initial, nonsurgical treatment is intended to reestablish this ligament tone by injection of iodine-based substances into the femoropatellar joint.[35,36] These injections invariably cause lameness, and they are associated with less success than surgical fixation and are not currently recommended for treatment of IUFP. Exercise to increase strength in the quadriceps muscle has been shown to help resolve IUFP in some cases.

Two surgical procedures have been described for treatment of the condition: medial patellar desmotomy and vastus medialis tenotomy. The medial patellar desmotomy is the most common surgical procedure and functions by opening the loop created by the medial patellar ligament, patella, and the lateral patellar ligament, preventing the patella from becoming fixed on the proximomedial trochlear ridge. It can be performed in the standing or recumbent patient. If performed standing, the skin and subcutaneous tissue overlying the medial patellar ligament is infused with local anesthetic. Following a surgical preparation, 5 to 10 mL of lidocaine are infused into the skin and subcutaneous tissues. An incision of 3 to 4 cm is made, oriented vertically over the medial patellar ligament. Blunt dissection exposes the medial patellar ligament, and the ligament is transected close to its insertion on the tibia with a curved bistoury. If transection is performed correctly, the medial patellar ligament becomes nonpalpable. If ligamentous tissue is still palpable in the area of the medial patellar ligament, transection of the ligament should be repeated. The incision is closed routinely. Medial patellar ligament desmotomy should be immediately curative.[39]

A vastus medialis tenotomy is another procedure that has been described for correction of IUFP. It can be performed as a stand-alone procedure or in conjunction with the medial patellar ligament desmotomy. Most surgeons advocate performing this procedure only if the medial patellar ligament desmotomy is not successful. The vastus medialis tenotomy is a more invasive procedure and general anesthesia is recommended.

Postoperative antibiotics are recommended if the procedure was performed in awake, standing animals, in which patient positioning and patient restraint are less controlled. Although controversial, postoperative exercise has been advocated by some to prevent reoccurrence of IUFP. Correction should be immediate and prognosis for complete return to soundness without recurrence is excellent.[39]

REFERENCES

1. Crawford WH. Intra-articular replacement of bovine cranial cruciate ligaments with an autogenous fascial graft. Vet Surg 1990;19(5):380–8.
2. Anderson D, Desrochers A. Musculoskeletal examination in cattle. In: Fubini SL, Ducharme N, editors. Farm animal surgery. St Louis (MO): Saunders; 2004. p. 283–9.
3. Nelson D. Surgery of the stifle joint in cattle. Compendium on Continuing Education for the Practising Veterinarian 1983;5:S300.
4. Ducharme NG. Stifle injuries in cattle. Vet Clin North Am Food Anim Pract 1996; 12(1):59–84.
5. Crawford W, Ducharme N. Ligamentous damage and wounds to the stifle. In: Fubini SL, Ducharme N, editors. Farm animal surgery. St Louis (MO): Saunders; 2004. p. 336–43.
6. Nelson DR, Huhn JC, Kneller SK. Peripheral detachment of the medial meniscus with injury to the medial collateral ligament in 50 cattle. Vet Rec 1990;127(3): 59–60.
7. Bartels J. Femorotibial osteoarthritis in the bull: a correlation of the radiographic findings of the torn meniscus and ruptured cranial cruciate ligament. J American Veterinary Radiology Society 1975;16:159.
8. Huhn J, Kneller S, Nelson D. Radiographic assessment of cranial cruciate ligament rupture in the dairy cow: a retrospective study. Veterinary Radiology 1986;27:184–6.
9. Vasseur PB, Pool RR, Arnoczky SP, et al. Correlative biomechanical and histologic study of the cranial cruciate ligament in dogs. Am J Vet Res 1985;46(9):1842–54.
10. Hurtig MB. Recent developments in the use of arthroscopy in cattle. Vet Clin North Am Food Anim Pract 1985;1(1):175–93.
11. Anderson DE, Edmondson MA. Prevention and management of surgical pain in cattle. Vet Clin North Am Food Anim Pract 2013;29(1):157–84.
12. Anderson DE, Muir WW. Pain management in ruminants. Vet Clin North Am Food Anim Pract 2005;21(1):19–31.
13. Gloobe H. The menisci of the stifle in cattle: an anatomical study. Southwest Vet 1976;29:132.
14. Nelson DR, Koch DB. Surgical stabilisation of the stifle in cranial cruciate ligament injury in cattle. Vet Rec 1982;111(12):259–62.
15. Hamilton GF, Adams OR. Anterior cruciate ligament repair in cattle. J Am Vet Med Assoc 1971;158(2):178–83.

16. Hamilton GF, Nelson AW. The fate of autoplastic and alloplastic implants in the bovine stifle joint. Can Vet J 1970;11(10):209–14.
17. Hofmeyr CF. Reconstruction of the ruptured anterior cruciate ligament in the stifle of a bull. Veterinarian 1968;5(2):89–92.
18. Moss EW, Ferguson TH. Tensile strength of the cranial cruciate ligament in cattle. Am J Vet Res 1980;41(9):1408–11.
19. Moss EW, McCurnin DM, Ferguson TH. Experimental cranial cruciate replacement in cattle using a patellar ligament graft. Can Vet J 1988;29(2): 157–62.
20. van Oosterom R. Intra-articular graftpasser. Vet Surg 1982;11:132–3.
21. Niehaus AJ, Anderson DE, Johnson JK, et al. Comparison of the mechanical characteristics of polymerized caprolactam and monofilament nylon loops constructed in parallel strands or as braided ropes versus cranial cruciate ligaments of cattle. Am J Vet Res 2013;74(3):381–5.
22. Ducharme NG, Stanton ME, Ducharme GR. Stifle lameness in cattle at two veterinary teaching hospitals: a retrospective study of forty-two cases. Can Vet J 1985; 26(7):212–7.
23. Frithian D, Kelly M, Mow V. Material properties and structure-function relationships in the menisci. Clin Orthop 1990;252:19–31.
24. Walmsley JP. Diagnosis and treatment of ligamentous and meniscal injuries in the equine stifle. Vet Clin North Am Equine Pract 2005;21(3):651–72, vii.
25. Kofler J. Ultrasonography as a diagnostic aid in bovine musculoskeletal disorders. Vet Clin North Am Food Anim Pract 2009;25(3):687–731 Table of Contents.
26. Kofler J. Arthrosonography–the use of diagnostic ultrasound in septic and traumatic arthritis in cattle–a retrospective study of 25 patients. Br Vet J 1996; 152(6):683–98.
27. Arnoczky S, Marshall JL. Pathomechanics of cruciate and meniscal injuries. In: Bojrab MJ, editor. Pathophysiology of small animal surgery. Philadelphia: Lea & Febiger; 1981. p. 598–603.
28. Nelson DR, Huhn JC, Kneller SK. Surgical repair of peripheral detachment of the medial meniscus in 34 cattle. Vet Rec 1990;127(23):571–3.
29. Sharma K, Joshi Y, Tanwar R. Report on the incidence of upward fixation of patella (Stringhalt) in bovines of Udaipur area in Rajasthan [India]. Indian Vet J 1984;61.
30. Dass L, Sahay P, Ehsan M, et al. Report on the incidence of upward fixation of patella (Stringhalt) in bovines of Chate Nagpur hilly terrain [India]. Indian Vet J 1983;60.
31. Gahlot T. Lameness in camels. Paper presented at: proceedings of the International Camel Conference “Recent trends in camelids research and future strategies for saving camels”. Rajasthan, India, February 16–17, 2007.
32. Baird AN, Angel KL, Moll HD, et al. Upward fixation of the patella in cattle: 38 cases (1984-1990). J Am Vet Med Assoc 1993;202(3):434–6.
33. Curtis RA. Momentary upward fixation of the patella in a cow, and treatment by patellar desmotomy. Can J Comp Med Vet Sci 1961;25(12):314–6.
34. Johnson R, Ames N. Upward fixation of the patella in a Holstein cow [Orthopedics]. Agri-Practice 1983;4.
35. Tyagi R, Krishnamurthy D, Dhablania D. Upward fixation of patella (stringhalt) in bovines: a survey report. Indian Vet J 1972.
36. Pallai M. A note on chronic luxation of patella among bovines with special reference to its etiology. Indian Vet J 1944;21:48–54.

37. Tyagi R, Krishnamurthy D. Studies on induced upward fixation of patella in bovines and review of mechanism of 'hooking' of patella in animals [India]. Indian Vet J 1978;55.
38. Hanson RR, Peyton LC. Surgical correction of intermittent upward fixation of the patella in a Brahman cow. Can Vet J 1987;28(10):675.
39. Greenough P. Surgical conditions of the proximal limb. In: Greenough P, Weaver A, editors. Lameness in cattle. 3rd edition. Philadelphia: WB Saunders; 1997. p. 269–70.

Index

Note: Page numbers of article titles are in **boldface** type.

A

http://dx.doi.org/10.1016/S0749-0720(14)00009-7
0749-0720/14/$ – see front matter © 2014 Elsevier Inc. All rights reserved.
vetfood.theclinics.com

Moving?

Make sure your subscription moves with you!

To notify us of your new address, find your **Clinics Account Number** (located on your mailing label above your name), and contact customer service at:

Email: journalscustomerservice-usa@elsevier.com

800-654-2452 (subscribers in the U.S. & Canada)
314-447-8871 (subscribers outside of the U.S. & Canada)

Fax number: 314-447-8029

Elsevier Health Sciences Division
Subscription Customer Service
3251 Riverport Lane
Maryland Heights, MO 63043

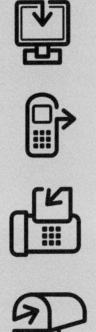

Printed and bound by CPI Group (UK) Ltd, Croydon, CR0 4YY

03/10/2024

01040490-0010